National Key Book Publishing Planning Project of the 13th Five-Year Plan
"十三五" 国家重点图书出版规划项目
International Clinical Medicine Series Based on the Belt and Road Initiative
"一带一路" 背景下国际化临床医学丛书

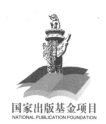

国家出版基金项目
NATIONAL PUBLICATION FOUNDATION

Clinical Oncology

临床肿瘤学

Chief Editor　Ma Wang　Zheng Yanfang　Wang Shusen
主编　马　望　　郑燕芳　　　王树森

U0340110

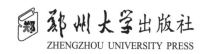
郑州大学出版社
ZHENGZHOU UNIVERSITY PRESS

图书在版编目(CIP)数据

临床肿瘤学 = Clinical Oncology：英文／马望，郑燕芳，王树森主编. — 郑州：郑州大学出版社，2020. 12

（"一带一路"背景下国际化临床医学丛书）

ISBN 978-7-5645-6556-5

Ⅰ. ①临… Ⅱ. ①马…②郑…③王… Ⅲ. ①肿瘤学 – 临床医学 – 英文 Ⅳ. ①R73

中国版本图书馆 CIP 数据核字(2019)第 217869 号

临床肿瘤学 = Clinical Oncology：英文

项 目 负 责 人	孙保营　杨秦予		策 划 编 辑	李龙传
责 任 编 辑	苗瑞敏		装 帧 设 计	苏永生
责 任 校 对	李龙传		责 任 监 制	凌　青　李瑞卿

出 版 发 行	郑州大学出版社有限公司		地　　址	郑州市大学路40号(450052)
出 版 人	孙保营		网　　址	http://www.zzup.cn
经　　销	全国新华书店		发 行 电 话	0371-66966070
印　　刷	河南文华印务有限公司			
开　　本	850 mm×1 168 mm　1／16			
印　　张	17.25		字　　数	670 千字
版　　次	2020 年 12 月第 1 版		印　　次	2020 年 12 月第 1 次印刷

书　　号	ISBN 978-7-5645-6556-5		定　　价	89.00 元

Staff of Expert Steering Committee

Chairmen

Zhong Shizhen   Li Sijin   Lü Chuanzhu

Vice Chairmen

Bai Yuting	Chen Xu	Cui Wen	Huang Gang	Huang Yuanhua
Jiang Zhisheng	Li Yumin	Liu Zhangsuo	Luo Baojun	Lü Yi
Tang Shiying				

Committee Member

An Dongping	Bai Xiaochun	Cao Shanying	Chen Jun	Chen Yijiu
Chen Zhesheng	Chen Zhihong	Chen Zhiqiao	Ding Yueming	Du Hua
Duan Zhongping	Guan Chengnong	Huang Xufeng	Jian Jie	Jiang Yaochuan
Jiao Xiaomin	Li Cairui	Li Guoxin	Li Guoming	Li Jiabin
Li Ling	Li Zhijie	Liu Hongmin	Liu Huifan	Liu Kangdong
Song Weiqun	Tang Chunzhi	Wang Huamin	Wang Huixin	Wang Jiahong
Wang Jiangang	Wang Wenjun	Wang Yuan	Wei Jia	Wen Xiaojun
Wu Jun	Wu Weidong	Wu Xuedong	Xie Xieju	Xue Qing
Yan Wenhai	Yan Xinming	Yang Donghua	Yu Feng	Yu Xiyong
Zhang Lirong	Zhang Mao	Zhang Ming	Zhang Yu'an	Zhang Junjian
Zhao Song	Zhao Yumin	Zheng Weiyang	Zhu Lin	

专家指导委员会

编审委员会

Editorial Staff

作者名单

主　编

马　望　　郑州大学第一附属医院

郑燕芳　　广州医科大学附属肿瘤医院

王树森　　中山大学肿瘤防治中心

副主编

韩苏夏　　西安交通大学第一附属医院

谈东风　　M. D. 安德森癌症中心

闵大六　　上海交通大学附属第六人民医院

李泉旺　　北京中医药大学东方医院

秦健勇　　广州市荔湾中心医院

温居一　　解放军总医院第六医学中心

官成浓　　广东医科大学

编　委（以姓氏汉语拼音为序）

陈美婷　　中山大学肿瘤防治中心

崔久嵬　　吉林大学第一医院肿瘤中心

杜雅冰　　郑州大学第一附属医院

李沂泽　　空军军医大学西京医院

路　平　　新乡医学院第一附属医院

马龙飞　　北京协和医学院

史艳侠　　中山大学肿瘤防治中心

王启鸣　　郑州大学附属肿瘤医院/河南省肿瘤医院

熊　力　　中南大学湘雅二医院

杨　帏　　中山大学肿瘤防治中心

杨忠明　　西南医科大学附属中医医院

昝丽坤　　山西省肿瘤医院

张红梅　　空军军医大学西京医院

张腾飞　　郑州大学第一附属医院

张永高　　郑州大学第一附属医院

Preface

At the Second Belt and Road Summit Forum on International Cooperation in 2019 and the Seventy-third World Health Assembly in 2020, General Secretary Xi Jinping stated the importance for promoting the construction of the "Belt and Road" and jointly build a community for human health. Countries and regions along the "Belt and Road" have a large number of overseas Chinese communities, and shared close geographic proximity, similarities in culture, disease profiles and medical habits. They also shared a profound mass base with ample space for cooperation and exchange in Clinical Medicine. The publication of the International Clinical Medicine series for clinical researchers, medical teachers and students in countries along the "Belt and Road" is a concrete measure to promote the exchange of Chinese and foreign medical science and technology with mutual appreciation and reciprocity.

Zhengzhou University Press coordinated more than 600 medical experts from over 160 renowned medical research institutes, medical schools and clinical hospitals across China. It produced this set of medical tools in English to serve the needs for the construction of the "Belt and Road". It comprehensively coversaspects in the theoretical framework and clinical practicesin Clinical Medicine, including basic science, multiple clinical specialities and social medicine. It reflects the latest academic and technological developments, and the international frontiers of academic advancements in Clinical Medicine. It shared with the world China's latest diagnosis and therapeutic approaches, clinical techniques, and experiences in prescription and medication. It has an important role in disseminating contemporary Chinese medical science and technology innovations, demonstrating the achievements of modern China's economic and social development, and promoting the unique charm of Chinese culture to the world.

The series is the first set of medical tools written in English by Chinese medical experts to serve the needs of the "Belt and Road" construction. It systematically and comprehensively reflects the Chinese characteristics in Clinical Medicine. Also, it presents a landmark achievement in the implementation of the "Belt and Road" initiative in promoting exchanges in medical science and technology. This series is theoretical in nature, with each volume built on the mainlines in traditional disciplines but at the same time introducing contemporary theories that guide clinical practices, diagnosis and treatment methods, echoing the latest research findings in Clinical Medicine.

As the disciplines in Clinical Medicine rapidly advances, different views on knowledge, inclusiveness, and medical ethics may arise. We hope this work will facilitate the exchange of ideas, build common ground while allowing differences, and contribute to the building of a community for human health in a broad spectrum of disciplines and research focuses.

Nick Lemoine

Foreign Academician of the Chinese Academy of Engineering

Dean, Academy of Medical Sciences of Zhengzhou University

Director, Barts Cancer Institute, London, UK

6th August, 2020

Foreword

Malignant tumor becomes one of the major diseases threatening human's health. A considerable amount of effort has been made towards overcoming cancer, although the problem of cancer has not been fundamentally touched, especially the unsatisfactory treatment effect of advanced tumor. However, many new technologies and drugs for the treatment of tumors have emerged, especially coming from the breakthroughs in targeted therapy and immunotherapy, which have greatly extended the survival time of patients with advanced tumors. After more than a century of development, clinical oncology has become one of the most active disciplines in medical field. The focus of clinical oncology is evidence-based medicine, as well as standardized and individualized treatment.

Our purpose in compiling this book is to integrate basic medical sciences and clinical oncology, and establish a complete knowledge system. This book can familiarize the reader with the pathogenesis and characteristics of cancer; master the basic principles of tumor diagnosis and treatment; focus on understanding the concept of comprehensive treatment of tumors, especially the rapid development of targeted therapy and immunotherapy in recent years; get familiar to the basic knowledge and clinical frontiers of cancer research; cultivate readers' clinical thinking ability and lay a solid foundation for their future participate in tumor-related work.

The authors of this textbook come from many well-known medical schools in China, and they are all experts in various oncology fields. Each chapter has been seriously considered to write, so we hope that it will be helpful for reader to study oncology. Due to the rapid development of oncology, there are still deficiencies and shortcomings in the book. We sincerely hope that readers can criticize and correct it so that it can be perfected in the reprint.

Authors

Contents

Chapter 1

Introduction

Cancer is an abnormal growth of tissue, which, if it forms a mass, is commonly referred to as a tumor. This abnormal growth usually (but not always) forms a mass. A cancer can be caused by an abnormal prolifer-ation, which can be caused by genetic mutations. The occurrence of cancer is the result of multiple genes and multistep. Mutations in different genes form different cancers.

Cancer is a gene disease, and its biological basis is gene abnormality. Normal cells have a gene mutation under the action of tumorigenic factors, resulting in normal gene aberration and disorder, thus affecting the biological and genetic characteristics of the cells, forming cancer cells that are different in the shape, metabolism and function of normal ones, and losing the ability to differentiate and mature in different degrees. It grows vigorous and has relative autonomy.

Cancer heterogeneity describes the observation that different tumor cells can show distinct morphological and phenotypic profiles, including cellular morphology, gene expression, metabolism, motility, proliferation, and metastatic potential. This phenomenon occurs both between tumors (inter-tumor heterogeneity) and within tumors (intra-tumor heterogeneity). A minimal level of intra-tumor heterogeneity is a simple consequence of the imperfection of DNA replication: whenever a cell (normal or cancerous) divides, a few mutations are acquired leading to a diverse population of cancer cells. The heterogeneity of cancer cells introduces significant challenges in designing effective treatment strategies. However, research into understanding and characterizing heterogeneity can allow for a better understanding of the causes and progression of disease. In turn, this has the potential to guide the creation of more refined treatment strategies that incorporate knowledge of heterogeneity to yield higher efficacy.

1.1 Development and current situation of oncology

1.1.1 Classification of tumors

According to the biological characteristics of tumors and their hazards to the body, they are generally divided into two categories: benign and malignant. This classification is of great importance in the diagnosis, treatment and prognosis of tumors. A benign tumor is a mass of cells (tumor) that lacks the ability to invade neighboring tissue or metastasize. Benign tumors generally have a slower growth rate than malignant tumors and the tumor cells are usually more differentiated (cells have normal features). They are typically surrounded by an outer surface (fibrous sheath of connective tissue) or remain with the epithelium. Malignant tumors tend to grow rapidly, invasive and metastatic, and are more harmful to humans. If they are not treated in time, they usually lead to death.

Malignant tumors can be divided into two types from histology. Carcinoma is a type of cancer that develops from epithelial cells. Specifically, a carcinoma is a cancer that begins in a tissue that lines the inner or outer surfaces of the body, and that arises from cells originating in the endodermal, mesodermal and ectodermal germ layer during embryogenesis. A sarcoma is a cancer that arises from transformed cells of mesenchymal origin. Thus, malignant tumors made of cancellous bone, cartilage, fat, muscle, vascular, or hematopoietic tissues are, by definition, considered sarcomas. This is in contrast to a malignant tumor originating from epithelial cells, which are termed as carcinoma. Human sarcomas are quite rare. People listened more to cancer than to sarcoma. The incidence of cancer is much more than that of sarcoma. The ratio of cancer to sarcoma is about 9 : 1.

1.1.2　The evolution of pathogenesis and cause of cancers

Human beings have begun the research on cancers to find out how does it occurred and developed since a very long time ago. It has experienced from macro to micro, from its appearance to its nature. It could be classified approximately as the following stages.

1.1.2.1　Visual recognition stage

From the 1500 B. C. to the 1850s, during this 3,000 years period, human beings could only indicate the appearance of the cancers. The Record of "Tumor" in Oracle's Unearthed in Yin Zhou Period 3,500 years ago. However, for the western countries, Hippocrates(400 B. C. −377 B. C.) from the ancient Greeks and Galen from the ancient Rome have described and classified cancers in a certain way. When describing tumors, Hippocrates found that it resembled a crab and grew indefinitely. And the outer circumferential diffusion is difficult to remove and clean, hence the "rab" named such diseases and it has been transformed to the word "cancer" today.

1.1.2.2　Stage of cellular level

In 1850s, along with the invention of microscope, the study of cancers has turned from the appearance into the cellular level, especially during 1858. A German pathologist Virchow whose book, "cytopathology" has brought up some basic arguments about cancers. These view points are the pathological diagnosis for cancer. Those also established the foundations of creation and development for Clinical Oncology. Since from this period, human beings began to discuss pathogenesis of cancers, hence come up with the statement of physical, chemical and virus carcinogenesis. This has led to the inital understanding of pathogenesis and cause of cancers.

1.1.2.3　Subcellular and molecular levels

The appearance of electron microscope makes medicine deep into subcellular level in 1931. The discovery of DNA molecular structure made medicine begin to enter the era of molecular level in 1953. From the 1960s, multiples of inhibition and DNA of the cancers have been found one after another. During 1970s, "cancers is DNA alterative disease" has caused an extension discussion by the scientists. Since the research has made in genetics from 1980s, human beings were able to understand the cancers into another level of Genetic properties. With the deep study of cancer biological behavior at molecular level, humans beings now has much clear and precise understanding of pathogenesis and cause of cancers; from the simple ideas to multiple DNA changes, multiple factors involved and general cause of cancers from multiple evolution etc. The etiology and pathogenesis of tumors will definitely be clearly explained in the near future.

1.1.3　Development and current situation of tumor diagnosis

Throughout the course of development of malignant tumors, it experienced a single pathological diagnosis to the pathological, imaging, and marker comprehensive diagnostic process in breadth, and in depth have gone through the diagnosis from the anatomical site, general morphology diagnosis to the molecular level.

1.1.3.1　Imaging diagnosis

With the development of science and technology, tumor imaging has developed from a variety of original direct imaging, indirect imaging, and contrast media assisted imaging, to today's various checks based on computer processing imaging, including CT, MRI, ultrasound and especially PET, which achieves a unity of biological metabolism of cells and morphology and makes the imaging diagnosis of tumor step to a new level—functional imaging.

1.1.3.2　Histopathological diagnosis

Histopathology is the diagnostic basis of modern clinical oncology. Cell pathology and imunohistochemistry arecomplementary to tumor diagnosis. Electronic endoscopy has brought about breakthroughs in the diagnosis and treatment of tumors. With the development of endoscopic instruments, there are breakthroughs of body examination in both the location and depth. At the same time, because ultrasound technology is applied to endoscopy, the location and depth of tumor can be more precise. Endoscopic therapy has made minimal invasive surgery applicable for tumors and cases, which, instead, need to be solved by conventional surgery before. It also makes it possible for some benign tumors to be minimally invasively treated.

1.1.3.3　Diagnosis of tumor markers

In recent years, molecular diagnosis has been widely applied in clinical practice of tumor diagnosis and treatment. For example, the positive expression of estrogen receptor (ER) and human epidermal growth factor receptor 2 (HER-2) is of guiding significance for the formulation of the treatment scheme; the gene mutation of K-ras and EGFR has a direct relationship with the sensitivity of the tumor to Gefitinib, a protein kinase inhibitor, due to which many hospitals have put these two gene in the list of routine molecular pathological detection. It is worth to noting that, in addition to the changes on the molecular level, immune status also plays an important role in the prognosis of the patients.

1.1.4　The development and current situation of oncotherapy

Treatment of malignant tumors has progressed from the single era of surgical treatment to the era of multidisciplinary synthetic therapy and individualized treatment including surgery, radiation therapy, chemotherapy, biologic therapy, interventional therapy, and palliative care.

1.1.4.1　Surgical therapy of tumors

Ovarian tumor resection operated by Dr. McDowell is the beginning of surgical treatment of tumors. And the radical mastectomy initiated by Dr. Halsted has laid the foundation of the two basic principles of surgical treatment, which including En bloc and lymphadenectomy (surgical removal of lymph nodes). With the update of treatment concept and development of new technology, surgical oncology gradually develops to the high curative and the low incidence of disability direction. In addition to the traditional use of early radical surgery, the scope of modern oncology surgery has changed dramatically in various aspects of oncotherapy, such as cytoreduction, reconstruction, rehabilitation and so on. From wide view of development of surgical oncology, from radical to modified radical, function damage to function preservation, extensive surgery to minimally invasive surgery, the development of surgical oncology goes through the process from single disciplinary to multi-disciplinary participation increasingly.

1.1.4.2   Radiotherapy of tumors

Radiotherapy of biological target based on PET-CT examination; Brachytherapy represented by High-dose-rate post treatment, tissue differential treatment, and particle implantation therapy, etc.; Stereotactic radiotherapy represented by gamma knife, X knife, and radio knife; Intensity-modulated radiotherapy represented by three-dimensional intensity modulation and volume modulation; As well as the clinical application of protons and heavy ion therapy presents a vision of multi-directional development and multi-directional development.

1.1.4.3   Chemotherapy of tumors

Application of nitrogen mustard in the treatment of lymphoma has unveiled the curtain for modern cancer chemotherapy. The concept of combination chemotherapy was proposed and a longer period of disease remission was obtained in childhood (acute lymphoblastic leukemia, ALL), laying the foundation for cancer chemotherapy. The continuous availability of new drugs with different mechanisms of action has enriched the choice of chemotherapy and further improved the efficacy. With the advancement of molecular biology, drug-related genetic information has gradually been acquired, such as genetic polymorphisms of drug transporters, screening of drug sensitivity and drug resistance sites, and differences in drug metabolism enzymology. In order to guide clinical drug selection, predict efficacy, reduce adverse reactions, resulting in the concept of individualized chemotherapy, and become the future direction of cancer chemotherapy.

1.1.4.4   Biotherapy of tumors

The biological treatment of tumors is based on the development of immunotherapy. Dr. Coley prepared streptococcus and serratia lysates into coley toxins for the treatment of cancer patients, opening a new chapter in biotherapy. Dr. Oldman proposed the concept of biological therapy as the fourth model of cancer treatment, further establishing the status of cancer biological therapy. Tumor immunotherapy, molecular targeted therapy and gene therapy have enormous therapeutic potential, especially molecular targeted therapies. They have achieved remarkable curative effect in clinical practice, triggered the revolution in the concept of anti-cancer therapy, and promoted the treatment of cancer to an unprecedented new phase.

1.1.4.5   Interventional treatment of tumors

Interventional treatment for cancer is a new discipline that integrates radiological imaging and clinical therapeutics developed in recent years. It's characterized by less trauma, fewer complications, accurate positioning, and safe treatment. Interventional treatment of tumors originated in 1904, Dr. Dawbam injected embolus made of petrolatum and wax into the external carotid artery to perform preoperative embolization of tumors. And Swedish radiologist Seldinger invented percutaneous puncture and cannulation, which laid the foundation for modern tumor vascular interventional therapy. In recent 20 years, endovascular stent implantation, local tumor ablation, and radioactive seed implantation have opened up a new era of non-vascular interventions.

1.1.4.6   Other treatments for tumors

Including tumor palliative care, psychotherapy, nutritional support therapy and traditional Chinese medi-cine treatment. These treatments focus on improving symptoms, improving the quality of life of patients, and prolonging the survival period. They have become an important component of comprehensive cancer treatment.

1.2　Introduction to cancer epidemiology

Cancer epidemiology is the study of risk factors for certain tumor population and related health problems, the development and the outcome, discussing and developing effective preventive measures of a discipline. Over the years through epidemiological investigations and clinical observations, it has been found that malignant tumors are a chronic and complex disease with multiple factors involved. The surrounding environment and lifestyle have great influence on the occurrence of malignant tumors. Intrinsic factors such as genetic and immune mechanisms also play an important role in tumor development.

1.2.1　Cancer around the world

At present, malignant tumor has become the second cause of human death, after angiocardiopathy. According to the American Cancer Association and the National Program of Cancer Registries, in the United States, from 2005 to 2014, the incidence of cancer in women was relatively stable, for men that was reduced by about 2% annually, and from 2006 to 2015, the cancer mortality rate decreased by about 1.5% annually, and the total cancer death rate decreased by 26% from 1991 to 2015, equivalent to 2,378,600 death cases. In 2018, 1,735,350 new cancer cases and 609,640 cancer deaths were predicted (Figure 1–1).

Estimated New Cases

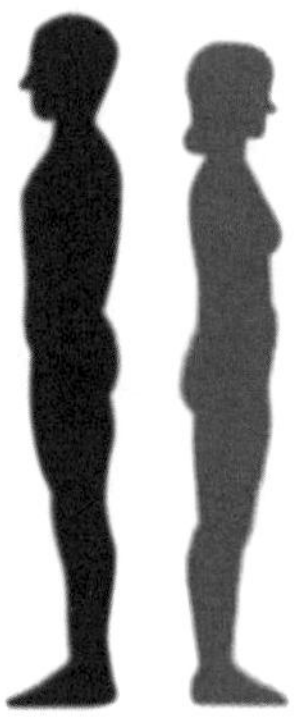

Males

Prostate	164,690	19%
Lung & bronchus	121,680	14%
Colon & rectum	75,610	9%
Urinary bladder	62,380	7%
Melanoma of the skin	55,150	6%
Kidney & renal pelvis	42,680	5%
Non-Hodgkin's lymphoma	41,730	5%
Oral cavity & pharynx	37,160	4%
Leukemia	35,030	4%
Liver intrahepatic bile duct	30,610	4%
All sites	856,370	100%

Females

Breast	266,120	30%
Lung & bronchus	112,350	13%
Colon & rectum	64,640	7%
Uterine corpus	63,230	7%
Thyroid	40,900	5%
Melanoma of the skin	36,120	4%
Non-Hodgkin's lymphoma	32,950	4%
Pancreas	26,240	3%
Leukemia	25,270	3%
Kidney renal pelvis	22,660	3%
All sites	878,980	100%

Estimated New Cases

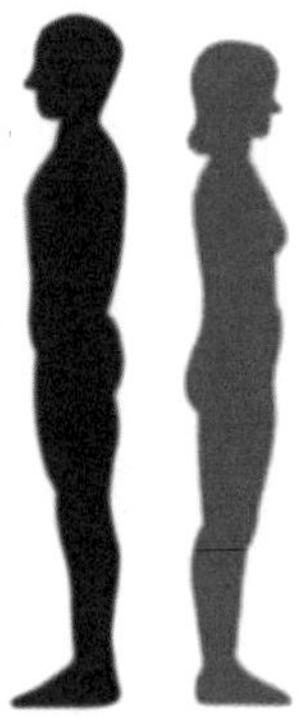

Males

Lung & bronchus	83,550	26%
Prostate	29,430	9%
Colon & rectum	27,390	8%
Pancreas	23,020	7%
Liver & intrahepatic bile duct	20,540	6%
Leukemia	14,270	4%
Esophagus	12,850	4%
Urinary bladder	12,520	4%
Non-Hodgkin's lymphoma	11,510	4%
Kidney & renal pelvis	10,010	3%
All sites	323,630	100%

Females

Lung & bronchus	70,500	25%
Breast	40,920	14%
Colon & rectum	23,240	8%
Pancreas	21,310	7%
Ovary	14,070	5%
Uterine corpus	11,350	4%
Leukemia	10,100	4%
Liver & intrahepatic bile duct	9,660	3%
Non-Hodgkin's lymphoma	8,400	3%
Brain other nervous system	7,340	3%
All sites	286,010	100%

Figure 1–1　Ten leading cancer types for the estimated new cancer cases and deaths by sex (the United States, 2018)

In 2012, the world increased 14. 1 million cancer cases, of which 8. 2 million died. Among them, China has increased 3. 7 million cancer patients, and about 2. 2 million people have died, accounting for 21. 9% and 26. 8% of the global total, respectively. In 2012, nearly half of the world's newly increased cancer cases occur in Asia, most of which are in China. Despite this, China has not entered the ranks of the highest cancer incidence and death rates in 2012, but Chinese huge population base makes new cancer cases and total annual cancer deaths ranked first in the world.

All over the world, the highest incidence of cancer is lung cancer. In 2012, new lung cancer cases were 1. 8 million, and the number of deaths was 1. 5 million, of which more than 1/3 appeared in China. In other cancers, about 50% of the world's newly increased cases of liver cancer and esophageal cancer appear in China. Since the beginning of twenty-first Century, Lung cancer is the first place of morbidity and mortality in China, and it is rising rapidly. As a respiratory disease, the incidence of lung cancer is increasing rapidly, which is closely related to air pollution and smoking. With the implementation of tobacco control policy in recent years, the smoking rate in China has shown a slight downward trend. The WHO has established the outdoor air pollution as a carcinogen in 2013 and is now the most widely spread carcinogen. Therefore, air pollution based on PM 2. 5 is the most important cause of high incidence of lung cancer.

In liver cancer and esophageal death cases, China accounts for about 51% and 49% , respectively. In China, the number of new cases and death cases in gastric cancer accounted for more than 40% of the worldwide. In addition, upper gastrointestinal tumor is still a common killer of rural residents in China, while lung cancer, breast cancer, colorectal cancer and so on are also increasing year by year. The distribution of cancer in urban areas is similar to that in developed countries. Lung cancer, breast cancer, colorectal cancer show an increasing trend. The rising trend of thyroid cancer in women is obvious.

1.2.2   Epidemiology of malignant tumors in china

With high-quality data from an additional number of population-based registries now available through the National Central Cancer Registry of China, the authors ana-lyzed data from 72 local, population-based cancer registries (2009-2011), representing 6. 5% of the population, to estimate the number of new cases and cancer deaths for 2015. Data from 22 registries were used for trend analyses (2000-2011). The results indicated that an estimated 4, 292, 000 new cancer cases and 2, 814, 000 cancer deaths would occur in China in 2015 (Table 1-1 to Table 1-3).

Residents of rural areas had significantly higher age-standardized (Segi population) incidence and mortality rates for all cancers combined than urban residents (213. 6 per 100, 000 *vs* 191. 5 per 100, 000 for incidence; 149. 0 per 100, 000 *vs* 109. 5 per 100, 000 for mortality, respectively). For all cancers combined, the incidence rates were stable during 2000 through 2011 for males (10. 2% per year), whereas they increased significantly (12. 2% per year) among females. In contrast, the mortality rates since 2006 have decreased significantly for both males (21. 4% per year) and females (21. 1% per year).

Therefore, China's cancer prevention and control work needs to formulate effective and feasible strategies according to different regions.

Table 1-1　Estimated new cancer cases and deaths (thousands) by sex:China,2015

Site	ICD-10	Incidence			Mortality		
		Total	Males	Females	Total	Males	Females
Lip,oral cavity,& pharynx (except nasopharynx)	C00-C10,C12-C14	48.1	31.1	16.9	22.1	15.3	6.8
Nasopharynx	C11	60.6	43.3	17.3	34.1	24.9	9.2
Esophagus	C15	477.9	320.8	157.2	375.0	253.8	121.3
Stomach	C16	679.1	477.7	201.4	498.0	339.3	158.7
Colorectum	C18-C21	376.3	215.7	160.6	191.0	111.1	80.0
Liver	C22	466.1	343.7	122.3	422.1	310.6	111.5
Gallbladder	C23-C24	52.8	24.5	28.3	40.7	18.8	21.8
Pancreas	C25	90.1	52.2	37.9	79.4	45.6	33.8
Larynx	C32	26.4	23.7	2.6	14.5	12.6	1.9
Lung	C33-C34	733.3	509.3	224.0	610.2	432.4	177.8
Other thoracic organs	C37-C38	13.2	8.2	5.0	6.5	4.1	2.3
Bone	C40-C41	28.0	16.4	11.6	20.7	12.4	8.3
Melanoma of the skin	C43	8.0	4.3	3.7	3.2	1.8	1.5
Breast	C50	272.4	3.8	268.6	70.7	1.2	69.5
Cervix	C53	98.9	—	98.9	30.5	—	30.5
Uterus	C54-C55	63.4	—	63.4	21.8	—	21.8
Ovary	C56	52.1	—	52.1	22.5	—	22.5
Prostate	C61	60.3	60.3	—	26.6	26.6	—
Testis	C62	4.0	4.0	—	1.0	1.0	—
Kidney	C64-C66,C68	66.8	43.2	23.6	23.4	15.2	8.2
Bladder	C67	80.5	62.1	18.4	32.9	25.1	7.8
Brain,CNS	C70-C72	101.6	52.3	49.3	61.0	35.8	25.2
Thyroid	C73	90.0	22.2	67.9	6.8	2.5	4.3
Lymphoma	C81-C85,C88, C90,C96	88.2	53.0	35.2	52.1	32.7	19.4
Leukemia	C91-C95	75.3	44.4	30.9	53.4	32.0	21.3
All other sites and unspecified	A_O	178.1	95.5	82.6	94.0	55.0	39.0
All sites	All	4,291.6	2,512.1	1,779.5	2,814.2	1,809.9	1,004.4

Table 1-2　Estimated new cancer cases and deaths (thousands) for selected cancers by age groups：China，2015

Cancer		Birth to 49		50 to 59		60 to 69		70		Birth to death	
Breast	Female	1.9	(1 in 52)	2.3	(1 in 43)	3.4	(1 in 29)	6.8	(1 in 15)	12.4	(1 in 8)
Colorectum	Male	0.3	(1 in 287)	0.7	(1 in 145)	1.2	(1 in 85)	3.4	(1 in 29)	4.5	(1 in 22)
	Female	0.3	(1 in 306)	0.5	(1 in 194)	0.8	(1 in 122)	3.1	(1 in 32)	4.2	(1 in 24)
Kidney & renal pelvis	Male	0.2	(1 in 456)	0.4	(1 in 284)	0.6	(1 in 155)	1.3	(1 in 74)	2.1	(1 in 48)
	Female	0.1	(1 in 706)	0.2	(1 in 579)	0.3	(1 in 320)	0.7	(1 in 136)	1.2	(1 in 83)
Leukemia	Male	0.2	(1 in 400)	0.2	(1 in 573)	0.4	(1 in 260)	1.4	(1 in 71)	1.8	(1 in 56)
	Female	0.2	(1 in 515)	0.1	(1 in 887)	0.2	(1 in 446)	0.9	(1 in 111)	1.3	(1 in 80)
Lung & bronchus	Male	0.1	(1 in 682)	0.7	(1 in 154)	1.9	(1 in 54)	6.1	(1 in 16)	6.9	(1 in 15)
	Female	0.2	(1 in 635)	0.6	(1 in 178)	1.4	(1 in 70)	4.8	(1 in 21)	5.9	(1 in 17)
Melanoma of the skin	Male	0.5	(1 in 218)	0.5	(1 in 191)	0.9	(1 in 106)	2.6	(1 in 38)	3.6	(1 in 27)
	Female	0.7	(1 in 152)	0.4	(1 in 254)	0.5	(1 in 202)	1.1	(1 in 91)	2.4	(1 in 42)
Non-Hodgkin lymphoma	Male	0.3	(1 in 382)	0.3	(1 in 349)	0.6	(1 in 174)	1.8	(1 in 54)	2.4	(1 in 42)
	Female	0.2	(1 in 545)	0.2	(1 in 480)	0.4	(1 in 248)	1.3	(1 in 74)	1.9	(1 in 54)
Prostate	Male	0.2	(1 in 403)	1.7	(1 in 58)	4.8	(1 in 21)	8.2	(1 in 12)	11.6	(1 in 9)
Thyroid	Male	0.2	(1 in 517)	0.1	(1 in 791)	0.2	(1 in 606)	0.2	(1 in 425)	0.6	(1 in 160)
	Female	0.8	(1 in 124)	0.4	(1 in 271)	0.3	(1 in 289)	0.4	(1 in 256)	1.8	(1 in 56)
Uterine cervix	Female	0.3	(1 in 368)	0.1	(1 in 845)	0.1	(1 in 942)	0.2	(1 in 605)	0.6	(1 in 162)
Uterine corpus	Female	0.3	(1 in 342)	0.6	(1 in 166)	1.0	(1 in 103)	1.3	(1 in 75)	2.8	(1 in 35)
All sites	Male	3.4	(1 in 30)	6.1	(1 in 16)	13.4	(1 in 7)	32.2	(1 in 3)	39.7	(1 in 3)
	Female	5.5	(1 in 18)	6.1	(1 in 16)	9.9	(1 in 10)	26.0	(1 in 4)	37.6	(1 in 3)

Table 1-3　Expected 5-year survival for all cancers combined by sex and geographic area：China,2015

Areas	Gender	Asr incidence	Ash deaths	1-(M/I)/%
All areas	Male	234.9	165.9	29.3
	Female	168.7	88.8	47.3
	Total	201.1	126.9	36.9
Urban areas	Male	215.9	142.9	33.8
	Female	168.9	77.1	54.4
	Total	191.5	109.5	42.8
Rural areas	Male	259.6	195.1	24.8
	Female	168.5	103.8	38.4
	Total	213.6	149.0	30.3
North China	Male	240.3	171.9	28.5
	Female	187.0	97.5	47.9
	Total	213.2	134.5	36.9

Continue to Table 1-3

Areas	Sex	Asr incidence	Ash deaths	1-(M/I)/%
Northeast	Total	189.2	116.4	38.5
	Male	208.4	146.9	29.5
	Female	169.8	85.5	49.6
East China	Total	193.7	115.6	40.3
	Male	224.1	152.8	31.8
	Female	165.8	80.6	51.4
Central China	Total	185.5	109.4	41.0
	Male	208.3	142.2	31.7
	Female	164.7	77.9	52.7
South China	Total	202.4	122.4	39.5
	Male	242.1	168.7	30.3
	Female	165.2	77.5	53.1
Southwest	Total	226.7	170.2	24.9
	Male	281.4	219.5	22.0
	Female	170.9	119.7	29.9
Northwest	Total	207.9	133.2	36.0
	Male	253.9	171.5	32.5
	Female	158.5	91.9	42.0

1.2.3   The research on tumor epidemiology

Cancer epidemiology research can be summarized as the following:
(1)Distribution of malignant tumors and main factors affecting distribution.
(2)Study and discuss the main factors affecting the development of malignant tumors.
(3)Understanding of the natural history of cancer.
(4)Predicting the probability of developing a tumor.
(5)Monitor malignant tumors and predict tumor progression.
(6)Study and formulate prevention strategies and evaluate implementation effects.

1.3   The expectation of clinical oncology

At present, clinical oncology has become a secondary clinical discipline. In the future development, the characteristics of the individualized diagnosis and treatment of multidisciplinary cooperation should be highlighted, and the principle of prevention, early diagnosis and early treatment should be carried out, and the incidence and mortality of the tumor should be reduced. In this process, it is necessary to use the achievements of translational medicine to intervene in the essence of the occurrence and development of the tumor, block the initiation of the tumor, find the molecular targets to effectively control the tumor, and develop effective drugs and treatment methods for these targets. At the same time, the treatment modalities of all kinds of tumor including surgery, radiotherapy, chemotherapy, biological therapy and minimally invasive treatment should be optimized and combined to achieve overall control of tumors at different levels.

To conquer the tumor, saving the life and maintaining the health are the sacred mission of the time endowed with medicine and the subject of clinical oncology, especially the oncology professionals. The needs of society and the needs of oncology development are calling for the growth of scholars generations to generations, inspiring the research efforts of scholars generations to generations.

Lu Ping

Chapter 2

Tumor Epidemiology

With the extension of human life expectancy and the change of lifestyle, cancer has become a disease that seriously threatens human health. Cancer has become the world's largest public health problem. According to the report of the International Agency for Research on Cancer (IARC), in 2012 worldwide, there were 14.1 million new cancer cases, 8.2 million cancer deaths, and 32.6 million people living with cancer within 5 years of diagnosis. 57% (8 million) of those new cancer cases, 65% (5.3 million) of the cancer deaths, and 48% (15.6 million) of the 5-year prevalent cancer cases occurred in the less developed regions. It is estimated that there will be 20 million new cases in the world by 2020, and the number of deaths will reach 12 million.

The occurrence of cancer is the coefficient consequence of environmental factors and genetic factors. In order to radically reduce the incidence of cancer and improve human health, we should continuously explore etiology and take positive precautions. Cancer epidemiology has made great contributions to the research on etiology and prevention of tumors. Cancer epidemiology lays a foundation for in-depth discussion on the etiology and pathogenesis of tumors by studying the distribution of cancer among different regions and populations, as well as studying the relationship between cancer occurrence and environmental factors including lifestyle. At the same time, cancer molecular epidemiology has developed from cancer epidemiology with the contribution of modern molecular biology, molecular immunology and other advanced technologies. Through studying the relationship of polygenetic changes and tumorigenesis, cancer molecular epidemiology explores the role of gene-environment interaction in tumorigenesis and provides the basis for screening and prevention for individuals at risk.

This chapter will focus on the concept of cancer epidemiology, research content, common research methods, cancer etiology and prevention.

2.1 Overview

2.1.1 Definition of cancer epidemiology

Cancer epidemiology is an important branch of epidemiology, which studies the distribution of cancer in the population and its influencing factors, to formulate corresponding preventive strategies and measures.

The research contents of cancer epidemiology can be summarized as follows:

- The incidence, mortality and distribution of cancer in different population, time and region.

- The influencing factors of cancer prevalence, including environmental factors, genetic factors and the interaction between them, and explore its pathogenesis.

- The corresponding preventive strategies and measures, including elimination and avoidance of exposure to carcinogenic factors, intervention for pathogenic factors, early diagnosis and treatment, and screening, etc.

2.1.2　Principle and application of cancer epidemiology

2.1.2.1　Principle of cancer epidemiology

Malignant neoplasms are not randomly distributed in the population, showing specific characteristics of time, region and population distribution. As a result of the existence of such differences, cancer epidemiology explores the cause of this distribution through comparing the different time, regions and distribution of cancer in the population. The aim of cancer epidemiology is to develop prevention strategies for the cause and take preventive measures to prevent or reduce the harm of cancer to human health. Based on the characteristics of cancer incidence and distribution, the principle of cancer epidemiology can be summarized as:

- The prevalence and pathogenesis of cancer in the population, including the exposure of carcinogenic factors to the development of the tumor, which is pathogenesis.

- The factors affecting the occurrence of cancer, including the interaction of environmental factors with the organism, namely etiology.

- Principles and strategies for cancer prevention, including tertiary prevention of cancer.

It should be emphasized that modern cancer epidemiology is different from traditional epidemiology. Cancer is a complex systemic disease and a multi-stage process with multiple factors, involving the natural and social environment factors and human physiological, mental, and spiritual aspects of the internal environment factors. Therefore, in etiology, the interaction of environmental factors and the host factors should be fully considered. In the prevention and control of cancer, we should take into account all factors and emphasize the joint participation of governments, medical workers and the general public.

2.1.2.2　Application of cancer epidemiology

With the rapid development of modern epidemiology, statistical methods and molecular biology techniques, the application of cancer epidemiology has become wider and wider, penetrating into all aspects of medical care and public health. According to different research methods and properties, cancer epidemiology can be divided into nutritional epidemiology, clinical epidemiology, molecular epidemiology, immigration epidemiology and so on.

The main application scope of cancer epidemiology is summarized as follows:

(1) Prevention and control of cancer

One of the main research contents and tasks of cancer epidemiology is cancer prevention. The ultimate goal of cancer prevention is to reduce the morbidity and mortality of cancer and improve the quality of life of cancer patients, which is also the guiding principle for the tertiary prevention of cancer. Cancer epidemiology plays an important role in the prevention and control of cancer and has made remarkable achievements, such as screening and prevention of cervical cancer.

(2) Cancer surveillance

Cancer surveillance is an important measure to prevent and control cancer. Cancer monitoring refers to the long-term, continuous and systematic information collection of cancer dynamic distribution and influencing factors. The information can be reported and analyzed for feedback, so as to take timely intervention measures and evaluate its effect.

(3) Research on the etiology and risk factors of cancer

The cause of cancer is complex, and it is the result of interaction of many factors. One of the important application of cancer epidemiology is using modern epidemiological methods to identify the etiology and risk factors of cancer, and then control the risk factors.

(4) Evaluation of the effectiveness of cancer prevention

The final assessment of the effectiveness of cancer prevention must be based on cancer epidemiology. For example, whether the reduction of smoking in the whole society can reduce the incidence of lung cancer needs to be carried out by epidemiological analysis. Whether large-scale nutritional interventions in communities can reduce the incidence of malignancy also requires epidemiological approaches to evaluate.

In short, cancer epidemiology has a very wide range of application, involving both cancer etiology exploration and control effect evaluation, both fundamental research and clinical research, touching all aspects of the medical and health fields.

2.1.3 The prevalence and trends of cancer

2.1.3.1 Overall trends in global cancer incidence

With the development of economy and the progress of the society, the average human lifespan is extended, and the disease spectrum has also undergone tremendous changes. Most infectious diseases are effectively controlled. However, chronic diseases such as cardiovascular disease and cancer have become serious threats to human health. It is estimated that there will be 20 million new cases in the world by 2020, and the number of deaths will reach 12 million.

The incidence of cancer in different countries and regions of the world is significantly different. The estimated age-standardized rates in the world (per 100,000) is shown in Figure 2-1. The overall age-standardized cancer incidence rate is almost 25% higher in men than in women, with rates of 205 and 165 cases per 100,000 person-years, respectively. Cancer incidence rates among males vary by a factor of almost 5 across the various regions of the world, with annual rates ranging from 79 cases per 100,000 males in western Africa to 365 cases per 100,000 males in Australia/New Zealand (with high rates of prostate cancer constituting a significant contribution to the latter). There is less variation among females, with annual cancer incidence rates varying by a factor of about 3, ranging from 103 cases per 100,000 females in south-central Asia to 295 cases per 100,000 females in North America.

There is less regional variability in mortality than in incidence; the mortality rates in more developed regions are 15% higher in men and 8% higher in women than the corresponding rates in less developed regions. In men, the rate (per 100 000) is highest in central and eastern Europe (173 deaths per year) and lowest in western Africa (69 deaths per year). In contrast, the highest rates in women are seen in Melanesia (119 deaths per year) and eastern Africa (111 deaths per year), and the lowest rates are in Central America (72 deaths per year) and south-central Asia (65 deaths per year).

According to the analysis of the prevalence trend of cancer, lung cancer is the highest in both incidence and mortality (13% and 19%, respectively). Breast cancer is the second most common cancer in the world (12%), and liver cancer has the second highest mortality (9.1%). The incidence of colorectal cancer is on the rise in the world. The estimated incidence, mortality and 5-year prevalence of cancers in the world is shown in Figure 2-2.

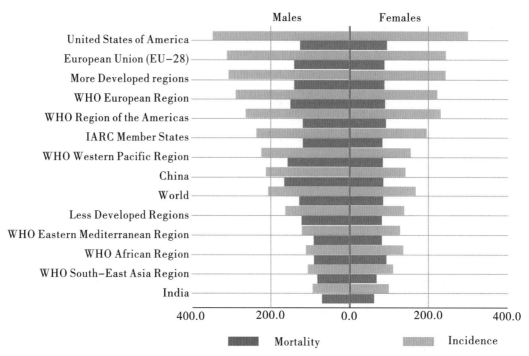

Figure 2-1   The estimated age-standardized rates in the world (IARC)

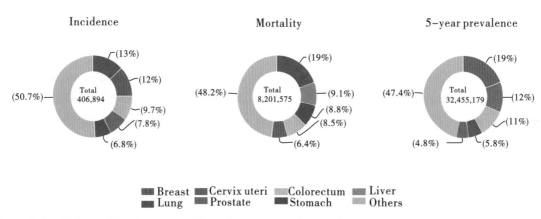

Figure 2-2   Estimated incidence, mortality and 5-year prevalence of cancers in the world:both sexes (IARC)

2.1.3.2   The incidence of cancer in China

Over the past 30 years, cancer death rates have risen significantly in China. Cancer has become the first cause of death among urban and rural residents, with one in every four Chinese people dying of cancer. Among male patients, lung cancer, liver cancer, stomach cancer and esophageal cancer are common. Among women, lung cancer, breast cancer, stomach cancer and colorectal cancer are high-incidence cancers. At the same time, the incidence of lung cancer, colorectal cancer and breast cancer are also rising significantly, which makes the prevention and treatment of cancer in China more difficult.

Over all, the prevalence trend of cancer is not optimistic, and positive efforts should be taken in the whole society. Cancer prevention is the priority, and we should strive to control cancer in the early stage, to reduce cancer incidence and mortality for the purpose of improving human health.

2.2   Risk factors for cancer

The occurrence of cancer is a multi-stage pathological process with multiple factors involved in. Risk factors for cancer include environmental factors and genetic factors. Environmental factors include chemical, physical and biological factors. At present, 85% of the causes of cancer occurrence are due to environmental factors including lifestyle, and the occurrence of most cancer is the result of cumulative exposure to environmental pathogenic factors.

2.2.1   Environmental factors

Environmental factors, such as occupational exposure and lifestyle, have been recognized since the 16th century. As Ramazzini noted in 1700, the incidence of breast cancer in nuns was higher than that of women. In 1775, Pott found that the workers who sweep the smokestacks had high incidence of scrotal carcinoma. In 1894, Unna found that sunlight exposure was associated with skin cancer; in 1895, Rehn discovered that exposure to aromatic amine was associated with the onset of bladder cancer. At the beginning of the 20th century, the chemical carcinogen animal model was established, providing a direct experimental evidence for chemical carcinogens. In 1915, Japanese scholars Yamagiwa and Ichikawa found that smearing a rabbit ear's surface with coal tar might lead to skin cancer. However, the establishment of environmental risk factors for cancer etiology mainly comes from a series of epidemiological studies; for example, a cohort study of smoking and lung cancer from Doll & Hill, provides the epidemiological evidence that cigarette smoking is a risk factor for lung cancer. In addition to occupational exposure and lifestyle factors, nutritional status, and inflammatory processes caused by bacterial and viral infections are also important environmental risk factors. In 1982, Doll &Peto proposed that 85% of the causes of cancer were induced by environmental factors, and the consensus was reached.

Environmental factors include chemical, physical and biological factors. Among them, chemical factors are the most important factor of cancer risk, including chemical carcinogens such as alkanes, polycyclic aromatic hydrocarbons, aromatic amines, azo dyes, nitrite compounds and so on. Physical factors include ionizing radiation, ultraviolet radiation, thermal radiation, strong electromagnetic field, mechanical stimulation, asbestos and so on. Biological factors include bacteria, fungi, viruses and parasites.

2.2.1.1   Chemical carcinogen

(1)Classification of chemical carcinogens

Chemical carcinogen is currently considered as a chemical carcinogen that can cause tumor formation or humans or animals. In recent years, it has been found that there are more than 2,000 kinds of chemicals, some of which are related to the formation of human tumors.

According to the role of chemical carcinogen, it can be divided into direct carcinogen, indirect carcinogen and promoting carcinogen. Direct carcinogen refers to the direct action of chemical substances with the cells in the body, which can induce the carcinogenesis of normal cells without metabolic activation. Indirect carcinogen is the chemical substance that needs to be activated by oxidase in the body to have a carcinogenic effect. Promoting carcinogen is a kind of chemical substance that does not show carcinogenesis alone, but can promote other carcinogens to induce the formation of tumor.

(2)DNA damage caused by chemical carcinogens

Indirect carcinogens can form the final carcinogens with electrophilic group through metabolic activation and be combined with the biological macromolecules of cells, where DNA is the main target of the final carcinogen. Finally, carcinogen combines with DNA to form carcinogen-DNA adduct.

Carcinogen-DNA adduct can cause a variety of DNA damage forms, such as bases insertions and deletions, DNA single or double strands breaks, DNA cross-linking, etc., these lesions can affect DNA replication and transcription, resulting in cell malignant transformation.

Since carcinogen-DNA adduct is both an exposure marker and an effect marker, it has special significance in tumor monitoring. In recent years, with the development of molecular biology technology, different methods can be used to detect the level of adduct in cells or humor, which can be used as a marker for carcinogens exposure to human body. For example, the status of aflatoxin was evaluated for the determination of aflatoxin-guanine admixture in urine.

2.2.1.2　Physical carcinogen

The range of physical factors is very wide, including electromagnetic waves, ultraviolet radiation, thermal radiation, mechanical stimulation, etc. Ionizing radiation is the main physical carcinogen, which mainly includes the radiation of electromagnetic wave with short wave and high frequency and the radiation of electron, proton, neutron and so on.

For miners, because of long-term exposure to radioactive cobalt, radon, uranium or other radioactive dust, the incidence of lung cancer significantly increased; the incidence of leukemia among survivors of the second world war and those receiving X-rays was significantly higher. The mechanism of damage caused by ionizing radiation is mainly forming ionizing and free radicals. The nature of free radicals is very active, which can cause DNA single strand breaks or changes in base structure. In addition, ultraviolet radiation can induce skin cancer in the face, the back of the hand and other sites exposed to sun. The mechanism of DNA damage induced by ultraviolet light at different wavelengths is also different.

2.2.1.3　Biological carcinogen

Biological factors include bacteria, fungi, viruses and parasites. Whether bacteria and fungi themselves are carcinogenic has not been determined. A large number of epidemiological evidence suggests that *Helicobacter pylori*(*h. pylori*) infection is closely related to the occurrence of gastric adenocarcinoma. Compared with non-infected persons, infected individuals showed a significantly higher risk of developing gastric cancer. Therefore, in 1992, WHO identified it as a human carcinogen. The inflammatory process induced by helicobacter pylori plays an important role in the occurrence of gastric cancer. In the process of inflammation, the production of free radicals such as endogenous NO^-, O_2, and OH^- can induce DNA damage and cell malignant transformation. In addition, the infection can change the local environment in the body and thus influence the endogenous synthesis, activation of the carcinogen metabolism process, have the effect of auxiliary carcinogenic.

Although the aetiological relationship between the virus and human cancer has not been fully elucidated, an increasing amount of evidence suggests that some virus is related to human certain cancers, such as Epstein-Barr virus infection related to nasopharyngeal carcinoma, hepatitis B virus (HBV) infection related to liver cancer, especially human papilloma virus (HPV) infection as the cause of cervical cancer. All of these evidences have greatly enriched the awareness of the relationship between viral infections and cancer.

The relationship of parasitic infection with tumor incidence was found as early as 1900. There was evidence showing that the high incidence of schistosomiasis correlates with bladder cancer in Egypt. In addition, in the African continent, the prevalence of malaria has been accompanied by the high incidence of Burgett's lymphoma, which is now believed to be due to EBV infection during the malaria infection.

2.2.2   Genetic factors

It is believed that environmental factors are the initiating factors of cancer, while individual genetic characteristics determine the susceptibility to cancers. Through the study of inherited or familial tumor syndrome, some oncogenes were identified. Since these genes are in cancer pathways, carriers with its germ cell mutation have very high risk of cancer. However, in fact, the inherited tumor is only a very small part, and most human tumors are caused by environmental factors, which are the result of the interaction of gene-environment factors.

2.2.2.1   Hereditary familial tumor syndrome

Inherited tumor syndrome is also known as hereditary tumors, such as: *Rb* gene mutations leading to retinoblastoma, *p*53 gene mutations leading to the Li-Fraumeni syndrome, APC gene mutations leading to familial adenomatous polyposis.

Compared with sporadic tumors, inherited tumors have the following features:

● Obvious familial aggregation. Almost every generation has individuals who suffer from the same tumor or multiple different tumors. At present, most inherited tumor syndromes were found as single-gene autosomal dominant inheritance.

● Early onset. For example, the onset of familial hereditary breast cancer and colorectal cancer patients are 10–30 years earlier than sporadic patients.

● Multiple primary cancer, sometimes bilateral cancer incidence in pair organs.

● Often accompanied by other abnormalities, such as some non-vital organs deformity, low sexual function and immune function.

● Genetic abnormalities can be detected in somatic cells. The gene that causes a genetic tumor is usually a tumor suppressor gene, and the loss of function will cause cells to grow out of control and thus form a tumor.

It needs to be emphasized that hereditary tumors account for only a very small proportion of the overall tumor incidence, and most tumors are the result of the combination of environmental factors and individual genetic susceptibility factors.

2.2.2.2   Cancer genetic susceptibility

Most common cancers are sporadic, not familial, and the genetic predisposition of sporadic tumors is not fully understood. In recent years, domestic and overseas scholars have done a lot of work on cancer susceptibility genes, and found some susceptibility gene polymorphism are closely related to the risk of some sporadic tumors.

Genetic polymorphism is essentially the difference in the sequence of nucleotide in chromosome DNA, and the frequency in the population is not less than 1%. Among them, single nucleotide polymorphisms (SNPs) is the most important polymorphic form, which is an important material basis for determining the genetic difference between individuals, accounting for more than 90% of all known polymorphism. SNP is widely available in the human genome, with an average of one out of every 500–1,000 base pairs, estimated to be up to 3 million or more. It is generally believed that SNP is an important step towards the application of the human genome project. This is mainly because the SNP would provide a powerful tool, used for high individual discovery, identification of disease genes, drug design and basic research in biology, etc. A large number of SNP sites exist, giving researchers the opportunity to discover genetic variants associated with various diseases, including tumors. Some SNPs are not directly responsible for gene expression, but become important markers because they are adjacent to certain disease genes.

Association study based on population is the most commonly used method to study the association of SNPs with tumors. With the development of high-throughput technology, the genome-wide association study (GWAS) was born. GWAS can study and analyze tens of thousands to hundreds of thousands or even millions of genetic variants at the full genome level at the same time. Therefore, GWAS is a groundbreaking method to study tumor associated genes and guide the direction for cancer research, offering a new opportunity for cancer prevention, diagnosis and treatment.

2.3　Research methods of cancer epidemiology

Cancer epidemiology is usually divided into descriptive epidemiology, analytical epidemiology, experimental epidemiology and theoretical epidemiology. Descriptive epidemiology is mainly based on the whole society or community data, such as the distribution of cancer in the population, and it plays a role in revealing the phenomenon and providing clues for making hypotheses. Analytical epidemiology includes case-control studies and cohort studies for testing or verification of hypotheses. Experimental epidemiology includes clinical trials and intervention trials, which are used to confirm or corroborate hypotheses. Theoretical epidemiology is using mathematical formula that reflects the relationship between the etiology, the host and the environment to clarify the epidemiological law. There is no absolute limit among various epidemiological methods, which are interrelated.

The following is the main introduction of descriptive epidemiology, analytical epidemiology and experimental epidemiology.

2.3.1　Descriptive epidemiology

Descriptive epidemiology is the method to describe the frequency distribution of cancer in population, time and space (region). Information is usually derived from tumor monitoring data or data obtained through special investigations. Descriptive epidemiology is not only the starting point of epidemiological studies, but also the basis of other epidemiological study methods.

Common indicators of describing cancer distribution include: cancer incidence, cancer prevalence, cancer mortality and cancer survival rate, etc.

2.3.1.1　Common indicators of describing cancer distribution

(1) Cancer incidence

Cancer incidence refers to the frequency of the occurrence of new cancer cases in a certain population within a certain period of time. Observation time units are usually expressed in terms of years.

Cancer incidence can be calculated according to different characteristics (such as age, sex, race, etc.). Since the incidence is affected by many factors, the composition of age, gender and other factors should be taken into consideration when comparing different data to standardize the incidence. By comparing cancer incidence of different characteristics, it can be used to evaluate the etiology and control measures.

(2) Cancer prevalence

Cancer prevalence refers to the proportion of old and new cases of cancer in a certain population within a certain period of time. Cancer prevalence can be divided into the point prevalence and the period prevalence according to the observation time. The point prevalence is generally not more than one month, and the period prevalence is usually more than one month.

Cancer prevalence is a common indicator of cross-sectional studies, often used to reflect the prevalence of malignancy and the impact on population health. Cancer prevalence can provide scientific basis for the planning of medical facilities, the requirement of health man power, and the input of medical expenses.

(3) Cancer mortality

The cancer mortality rate indicates that in a certain period of time, the frequency of people die from cancer in a certain population.

Cancer mortality can also be calculated according to different characteristics (such as age, sex, race, etc.). When comparing mortality rates in different regions, it is necessary to scale the mortality rate before comparison. For cancer with a high fatality rate, mortality and incidence are very close, and the accuracy of mortality is higher than the incidence rate, so it is commonly used as an indicator of etiology.

(4) Cancer survival rate

Cancer survival rate refers to the proportion of survival patients after several years (usually 1, 3, 5 years) in patients who have received some kind of treatment.

Cancer survival rate reflects the extent to which cancer is harmful to life and can also be used to evaluate the long-term efficacy of a treatment. The 5-year survival rate is an important index for clinical evaluation of tumor prognosis.

2.3.1.2　Prevalence survey

Prevalence survey, also known as cross-sectional study, is the main research type of descriptive research. Prevalence survey describes the distribution of cancer and related factors in the crowd, by systematically collected morbidity and mortality of cancer and demographic data at a specific time and specific scope of the crowd. It provides etiological clues and hypotheses, as the preliminary basis of researching the etiology. Prevalence survey only provides clues for establishing causal links, and no causal inference can be made from it.

The types of prevalence survey include census and sampling survey. Census is a full investigation, referring to in a specific period; all people within a certain range are the research object of investigation. For example, the investigation of the death of the whole population, and the screening of cervical cancer in certain groups. Sampling survey is a more commonly used research methods than census. Sampling survey refers to the survey of a representative sample of a population at a given time and within a certain range by means of random sampling, that is to infer the overall situation by investigating the subjects in the sample.

2.3.2　Analytical epidemiology

Analytical epidemiology is based on the preliminary etiological hypothesis of descriptive epidemiology, using elaborate design, testing or validating the etiological hypothesis presented by descriptive epidemiology. Analytical epidemiology usually includes case-control study and cohort study.

2.3.2.1　Case-control study

Case-control study is one of the most basic and commonly used research types in epidemiological methods. In case-control study, patients diagnosed with certain diseases (such as cancer or precancerous lesions) are selected as a case group, people who are not suffering from the disease but otherwise matched are selected as control group. Through investigation and laboratory examination, the exposure of various risk factors in the case group and the control group is compared, to determine whether the exposure factors are the risk factors for the disease.

Case-control study is a retrospective study method of finding the etiology of the results, therefore, it is also called retrospective study. Due to different case sources, case-control studies are divided into population-based and hospital-based case-control studies, with the former being more representative than the latter.

(1) Major design types of case-control study

The main design types of case-control studies include: matching in case and control; mismatching in case and control.

1) Matching

Matching, which requires the control to be consistent with the case in certain factors or characteristics, is intended to exclude the interference of confounding factors in comparison between the two groups. For example, when comparing two groups of data with age as the matching factor, it can avoid the influence of the differences of age between the two groups on the relationship between the tumor and the etiological factors. Matching is divided into frequency matching and individual matching.

Once a certain factor has been matched in the case-control study, the relationship between the factor and the tumor cannot be analyzed, and the interaction with other factors cannot be analyzed. Therefore, matching of? unnecessary factors should be avoided.

2) Mismatching

In the case and control groups specified in the design, generally, the number of control should be equal to or more than the number of cases. There are no special rules for control selection.

(2) Derivative case-control studies

Derivative case-control studies include nested case-control studies and case-cohort studies, among which nested case-control studies are frequently used in the cancer epidemiology.

Nested case-control study is a research method combining the traditional case-control studies and cohort studies, that is, based on the follow-up observation of a predetermined queue, the design thoughts of case-control study are studied.

Nested case-control studies are performed in a particular cohort, characterized by the advantages of both case-control studies and cohort studies.

(3) Statistical analysis method

Case-control studies cannot calculate relative risk due to the inability to calculate morbidity. In case-control studies, the index of association strength between disease and exposure is the odds ratio (or). $OR>1$ indicates that there is a "positive" association between exposure and disease, $OR<1$ indicates a "negative" relationship between exposure and disease. Case control study data collation and OR calculation methods are shown in Table 2-1.

Table 2-1　Case control study data collation and statistical methods

Project	Cases	Control
Exposed	a	b
Non-exposed	c	d

$$\text{odds ratio}(OR)=\frac{ad}{bc}$$

2.3.2.2　Cohort study

Cohort study, also known as prospective study and follow-up study, is one of the most important methods in analytical epidemiology. It collects data on the factors related to cancer incidence in specific populations; thereafter, follow-up observation and comparison of the outcomes of different populations with different risk factors, such as morbidity and mortality are performed to investigate the relationship between risk factors and the observed outcome, and to verify the etiological hypothesis. Compared with case-control study, the efficacy of cohort study is better than that of case-control study, so cohort study is widely used in the etiology of cancer epidemiology.

(1) Main research types of cohort study

In cohort study, the research objects are chosen in a specific population, and divided into exposed group and non-exposed group according to the risk factors of study, thereafter, followed up for a period of time to compare cancer morbidity or mortality. According to the different time of observation start and termination of research object, cohort study is divided into prospective cohort study, historical cohort study and ambispective cohort study.

1) Prospective cohort study

Prospective cohort study is the basic form of cohort study. The grouping of the research objectsis determined according to the present exposure status of the research objects. At this point, the effects of exposed factors on cancer have not yet occurred and need to be observed for a period of time.

The advantage of prospective cohort study is that it can directly obtain first-hand information about the exposure and outcome, avoiding the retrospective bias and the subjective bias of the researcher, and the results can be trusted. The disadvantage is that the studys need to be carried for a long time and be expensive, thus affecting their feasibility.

2) Historical cohort study

At the beginning of the study the researchers had historical data on the exposed status of research objects at some point in the past. The grouping of the research objects is based on this historical data; therefore the outcome of the study has emerged at the beginning of the study.

Although the method of collecting data in historical cohort study is retrospective, its property still belongs to the prospective observation, therefore, it is a popular fast cohort study method, with time-saving and labor-saving characteristics. The disadvantage is that the data accumulation is not controlled by the researcher, so it may not meet the requirements.

3) Ambispective cohort study

Ambispective cohort study is also known as hybrid cohort study, which is based on the historical cohort study, continues to observe for a period of time. It is a design pattern combining the prospective cohort study with the historical cohort study, so it can compensate for their shortcomings.

(2) Statistical analysis method

The greatest advantage of prospective cohort study is that it can directly calculate the cancer incidence in the study subjects, so it can directly calculate relative risk (RR). The greater the RR, the greater the correlation between exposure and tumor. The prospective cohort study data collation and RR calculation are shown in Table 2-2.

Table 2-2   Data collation and statistical methods of the prospective cohort study

Project	Cases	Control	Research objects
Exposed	a	b	$a+b$
Non-exposed	c	d	$c+d$

$$\text{relative risk}(RR) = \frac{a}{a+b} \Big/ \frac{c}{c+d}$$

2.3.3 Experimental epidemiology

Experimental epidemiology is one of the main methods of epidemiological study, which refers to the randomization of groups in a population. Because of the artificial intervention factors in the study, it is often referred to as the intervention study.

Currently there is no uniform classification standard for the types of experimental epidemiology. According to the characteristics of the cancer epidemiology research, experimental studies are usually divided into clinical trials and site and community intervention trial, the former refers to the patients as the research object of the test, the latter refers to the general population as the research object to carry out the experiment.

2.3.3.1 Clinical trial

Clinical trial is an experimental study of patients. Clinical trial is a commonly used method in the research of cancer epidemiology. It is often used to evaluate anti-tumor therapy and provide scientific basis for cancer treatment and prevention.

Clinical trials must be forward-looking and performed under strict quality control conditions. Clinical trial design should follow the following principles.

(1) Randomization

The randomization principle should be followed in the allocation of research objects, so that the background information affecting treatment effect and measurement result should be as similar as possible between the two experimental groups.

(2) Control

Standard treatment is often used in clinical trials as a control, that is to compare with conventional or current best treatment.

(3) Blind method

Blind method is adopted to avoid the influence of subjective factors of researchers and subjects on the study effect.

(4) Multi-center study

Multi-center clinical trials are clinical trials conducted by multiple researchers using the same method in accordance with the same test plan. Multi-center clinical trials can avoid the limitations of a single research institution.

(5) Ethical morality

Ethical morality is the basic premise of clinical trial.

2.3.3.2 Three stages of clinical trials

(1) Phase I clinical trial

Phase I clinical trial is the starting of small-scale test, mainly to observe the safety of drugs, to ensure the safe and effective dose for clinical use. Therefore, clinical pharmacokinetic studies, including the maximum tolerated dose (MTD) and dose-limiting toxicity (DLT), were mainly carried out. The study subjects were generally 10–30 people.

Because the research emphasis of phase I clinical trials is not antitumor effect, the patients diagnosed with advanced cancer are chosen, conventional treatment is no longer valid to them, but need to be generally in good condition, liver, kidney, heart and other organs have normal function, in order to objectively evaluate the side effects of drugs.

(2) Phase Ⅱ clinical trial

The purpose of phase Ⅱ clinical trial is to find out the drug effective tumor types, and to evaluate the effect of drugs, observe the relationship between curative effect and the dosage regimen, to further evaluate the safety of drugs. The study subjects were generally 100–300 people.

Phase Ⅱ clinical trial should be first tested in patients that are most likely to have efficacy, and these patients usually have no other effective treatment options available. Phase Ⅱ clinical trials are best used in patients who have never received chemotherapy.

(3) Phase Ⅲ clinical trial

Phase Ⅲ clinical trial is commonly referred to as randomized controlled clinical trials (RCT). Its purpose is to further evaluate the effect of new drugs, indications, adverse reactions and drug interactions in a larger scope, to provide a scientific basis for drug administration to approve new drugs from trial production to formal production. The study subjects were generally 1,000 to 3,000 people.

Phase Ⅲ clinical trial should be multi-center, and the inclusion criteria should be universal in order to promote the application.

2.4   Cancer prevention

At present, the cause of cancer is not yet entirely clear, the complex biological behavior of cancer is still not understood, and most cancers are found mostly in the middle and late stages with poor treatment, so cancer has become a major threat to human health. For cancer, prevention is better than treatment. According to the cancer report from world health organization (WHO), up to a third of cancers are preventable. As long as the governments, medical workers and the general public taking positive action through the adjustment of public health resources and strategies, focusing on the study of cancer prevention, more than a third, even nearly half of all cancers can be prevented.

Cancer prevention includes population screening, early diagnosis, health education, behavioral intervention, chemoprophylaxis, rehabilitation and other aspects. Cancer prevention is classified into three levels:

• Primary prevention: prevention of causes and intervention for risk factors. For example, targeted intervention is carried out for a high-risk population to remove certain pathogenic factors to reduce the incidence of cancer.

• Secondary prevention: early detection, early diagnosis and early treatment of cancer, to improve cure rate and survival rate and reduce mortality.

• Tertiary prevention: measures to alleviate suffering, improve the quality of life and extend life through clinical treatment, rehabilitation and palliative care.

2.4.1   Tertiary prevention strategies

2.4.1.1   Primary prevention

The main risk factors of cancer can be effectively controlled and eliminated by taking positive preventive measures against the specific carcinogenic factors.

Controlling risk factors is the focus of cancer prevention. Cancer incidence trend is directly related to human lifestyle, including diet, smoking, drinking, and infection, especially in developing countries; due to the speeding up of urbanization, the tumor incidence increased dramatically. More than 85% of the reasons for the occurrence of human cancer are environmental factors, including lifestyle. Therefore, the purpose of inhibition and reduction of cancer can be achieved by reducing exposure to these risk factors.

Since the 1980s, the United States, China, Finland, Japan all have conducted primary prevention against cancer etiology, using chemical intervention methods such as added vitamin E and C, beta-carotene, trace elements expected to reduce the onset of cancer or precancerous lesions. Unfortunately, the majority of the test results are not encouraging. The biological effects of these chemicals and the nutrients needed for long-term metabolism of natural foods such as fresh vegetables still confuse researchers.

Till now, we have seen the initial results of cancer incidence reduction achieved through primary prevention. With a major breakthrough in the cause of cervical cancer, cervical cancer has become the world's fastest declining cancer. The infection of HPV was reduced by sexual education. Simple pap smear test can be sensitive to detect severe epithelial precancerous lesions and early cervical carcinoma, cervical cancer incidence and mortality decreased by 78% and 79%, respectively. At the same time, with the success of the HPV vaccine, cervical cancer is expected to be the first human tumor to be fully controlled through vaccination. In addition, since the emergence of hepatitis B virus (HBV) vaccine and vaccination, the natural transmission and prevalence of HBV has been effectively curbed. For example, the infection rate of HBV has been significantly reduced in China since the introduction of HBV vaccine in children, indicating a significant decrease in the incidence of liver cancer. In addition, it is expected to reduce the incidence and mortality of gastric cancer by eradicating helicobacter pylori infection. Currently, three intervention trials in China and Colombia show that the precancerous lesion of gastric cancer is obviously reversed after the eradication of helicobacter pylori infection.

Moreover, it is of great significance in preventing cancer and improving human health by changing unhealthy lifestyles, proper diet and strengthening physical exercise. Other important prevention methods including tobacco control, less alcohol consumption, eliminating excessive tension, paying attention to the nutrition balance, reducing the fat and cholesterol intake, eating more food with rich vitamin A, vitamin C, vitamin E and fiber, not eating mildewed, salty or overheated food, etc.

2.4.1.2 Secondary prevention

Secondary prevention is mainly using simple screening and early diagnosis. Preventive screening of high-risk groups, actively treating precancerous lesions and blocking the cancer, will achieve higher rate of early discovery, early diagnosis and early treatment.

Screening is an important means of early detection of tumors, improvement of cure rate and mortality. For example, breast cancer is still a highly lethal cancer in women, but organized breast census, such as breast B ultrasound and molybdenum palladium examination can improve the sensitivity and specificity of detection of breast cancer, significantly improve the patient's survival rate and the quality of life.

The screening methods used for population screening must be simple, effective, economical and acceptable to the recipient. There are not many cancers that have efficient screen methods, which can be screened on a large scale. Now common screening includes detection of HPV infection and cervical exfoliated cells smear screening for cervical cancer; breast self-inspection and X-ray screening for breast cancer; fecal occult blood, anal finger diagnosis, colonoscopy screening of colorectal cancer; serum prostate specific antigen detection of prostate cancer; etc.

Although there is no standard screening program for gastric cancer, the screening of gastric cancer is progressing in some parts of the world, among which Japan is the most significant. Since the 1950s, large-scale gastric cancer screening has been carried out in Japan. Due to the improvement and popularization of endoscopic technology in the past 10 years, the rate of early diagnosis of gastric cancer has exceeded 50%. In China, since the late 1970s, in areas prone to stomach cancer and the high-risk population, different methods have carried gastric cancer screening to about 90,000 people, more than 400 cases of gastric carcinoma were detected, the early gastric cancer accounts for 27.8% –71.0%.

2.4.1.3　Tertiary prevention

Tertiary prevention is mainly using the existing medical technology and means to treat patients rationally, and using rehabilitation and palliative care to alleviate the suffering of patients, improve the quality of life and prolong life.

With the continuous improvement of modern diagnosis and treatment and the deepening of research on the pathogenesis of tumor, comprehensive treatment and individualized treatment should be actively advocated. Rehabilitation and palliative care for cancer patients should be carried out, so as to reduce the suffering of patients and improve the quality of life of cancer patients.

2.4.2　Cancer chemoprevention

Cancer chemoprevention is an important part of cancer prevention. Chemical prevention is also called chemo-intervention, refers to the use of certain natural or synthetic compounds to inhibit, reverse, or prevent the process of tumorigenesis, and to promote the application of specific research results in healthy population, for the purpose of reducing tumor morbidity and mortality.

The ideal chemoprevention agent should havecharacteristics such as non-toxic or slight toxic side effect, highly efficient, convenient for oral administration, and clear anti-cancer mechanism. Currently there are not many drugs used for cancer chemo-intervention with clear intervention mechanism, but such as vitamin C, vitamin E can reduce carcinogen endogenous synthesis or reduce the DNA damage of free radicals and reactive oxygen species produced in carcinogenic process. Non-steroidal anti-inflammatory drugs (NSAIDs) can inhibit cell proliferation and angiogenesis, thereby inhibiting tumor.

Common tumor chemical prevention agents include: NSAIDs, vitamin C, vitamin E, tamoxifen, etc.

2.4.3　Strategies for cancer prevention and control

In recent years, people have gradually realized that although the level of diagnosis and treatment of cancer has been continuously improved, it is still not effective to preventcancer incidence increasing year by year. More and more countries and governments have come to realize the enormous financial burden of malignant tumors. It has become a major public health problem that needs to be solved as soon as possible to curb the rise of cancer morbidity and mortality. Many countries have begun to shift their focus from treatment to prevention of cancer.

Since the 1980s, the United States has strengthened the fundamental and epidemiology research with the purpose of prevention, by the implementation of preventive measures such as tobacco control, advocating a healthy lifestyle and eating habits. In the 1990s, the incidence of cancer in the United States dropped by 0.7% a year, including lung, colon and prostate cancers. Between 1991 and 1995, there was a decline of 2.6%. Among them, men fell by 4.3% and women by 1.1%. The rise in morbidity and mortality of cancer in the United States has finally been effectively curbed.

The public health policy in our country are also undergoing gratifying changes. At the end of 2003, the ministry of health issued the China cancer prevention and control plan for 2004–2010, clearly put forward by giving priority to prevention and controlling the main risk factors, including tobacco control, infection control, proposing reasonable diet and sports. It emphasized strengthening of the early diagnosis and treatment, including cervical screening and early diagnosis and treatment of cervical cancer; screening and early diagnosis of esophageal cancer, stomach cancer, liver cancer and nasopharyngeal carcinoma in high-risk groups; screening and early diagnosis of colorectal cancer and breast cancer in urban communities. China has begun to gradually adjust its health strategy, and has increased the human, material and financial resources of cancer prevention significantly. In short, the prevention of cancer should be highly valued by governments, researchers and public health workers.

However, cancer prevention and control in our country are still in its infancy and is facing enormous challenges. It requires a concerted effort by the whole society to focus on prevention and ultimately achieve the goal of reducing cancer morbidity and mortality and improving human health.

Zheng Yanfang

Chapter 3

Etiology and Pathogenesis of Tumor

3.1 Genetic factors

The occurrence and development of malignant tumors are caused by both external environmental factors and intrinsic genetic factors. The external environmental factors mainly include physical factors, chemical factors, and biological factors, etc. This part has been described in Chapter 1, and the following will describe the Internal factors of tumorigenesis—genetic factors.

Molecular genetics suggests that the occurrence of malignant tumors is an integrated effect of the activation of the proto-oncogene, the inactivation of the tumor suppressor gene, or both of them. The mutation of these genes cause corresponding changes of the transcriptional translation of biologically functional proteins, mainly involved in the regulation of cell proliferation, cell synthesis metabolism, cell senescence and death, resulting in the process of transforming normal cells into malignant cells, which is characterized by rapid proliferation, no aging and death, etc.

(1) Proto-oncogenes

Proto-oncogenes fall into two categories: cellular oncogenes and virus oncogenes. Proto-oncogenes are normal genes found in human and animal cells and play an important role in the regulation of cell growth and differentiation. Normally, these genes are a dormant or low expression, having no carcinogenic activity. When the proto-oncogene is abnormally activated caused by the physical, chemical, biological and other factors, it will become an oncogenic gene, which will transform normal cells into malignant tumor cells. The activation methods mainly include point mutations, chromosomal rearrangements, amplification, and others.

The protein products encoded by oncogenes are classified into the following two categories, according to their biological functions.

1) Protein kinases

● Transmembrane growth factor receptor with tyrosine protein kinase activity, such as neu, erbB, forms, ret, etc.

● Non-receptor tyrosine-protein kinase, such as Src family: Src, Syn, Fyn, Abl, Lck, Ros, Yes, Met, Trk, and others.

● Serine/threonine protein kinases, such as Raf, Raf-1, Mos, Pim-1, and others.

2) Signal transduction

● Small G protein, with GTP binding and GTPase activity, such as ras family: K-ras, N-ras, H-ras, and Mel, Ral, etc.

● Growth factors, such as Sis (PDGF-β), Fgf family (Int-2, Csf-1), etc.

● Transcription factors, such as Myc family, Fos family, Jun family, Ets family, Rel, Erb A.

(2) Tumor suppressor gene

Tumor suppressor gene is a gene that inhibits cell consistent growing and protects a cell from cancelation, which can be grouped into categories including caretaker genes, gatekeeper genes, and landscaper genes. When inactivated, the tumor suppressor gene may assist in oncogene to fully exert its function, resulting in the occurrence of a malignant tumor. The role of several tumor suppressor genes is discussed simply below.

1) Human retinoblastoma gene (Retinoblastoma, Rb)

Rb gene is the earliest tumor suppressor gene, encoding the 105 KD nucleoprotein p105RB with the function of transcriptional regulation. Phosphorylation is its inactive form and dephosphorylation is its active state. Normally, dephosphorylated p105RB can bind to E2F transcription factor to inhibit its transcriptional activity, leading to cell growth stoppage. When there is a point mutation or fragment deletion in the Rb gene, some other products can bind to p105RB. Therefore they lose the ability to bind to E2F, resulting in continuous cell growth and proliferation.

2) $p53$

In normal cells, the expression level of $p53$ is very low. When DNA damage occurs, $p53$ can be activated to stoppage of cell growth, allowing them to repair DNA. On the other hand, $p53$ can induce cell apoptosis if DNA damage cannot be repaired. Inactivation of $p53$ mutations cannot function as a "monitor" for DNA damage, resulting in the accumulation of erroneous DNA and genomic instability, subsequently, causing mutations in other genes and leading to tumorigenesis.

However, single oncogene activation or inactivation of tumor suppressor gene does not result in cell malignancy. Only when both mutations occur, complementing each other, and when there is a certain accumulation of them that could induce malignancy. Therefore, it can be seen that tumorigenesis is a multi-step, multi-factor, multi-gene involved and comprehensive biological process.

3.1.1 Overview of the DNA damage response

3.1.1.1 Introduction to DNA damage

DNA damage is a result of changes in the composition and structure of the DNA sequence. Both intrinsic factors including copying errors, the instability or normal cell metabolites, and exogenous elements including physical, chemical or biological factors can cause alterations resulting in as many as one million individual molecular lesions per cell per day. Different changes can cause various alterations like simple base changes including deletions, fusions and translocations, and complex changes including DNA backbone damages, DNA double-strand break, and cross-links. One kind of change can cause many damages at the same time(Figure 3–1).

(1) Causes of DNA damage

Both intrinsic factors and external factors can cause DNA damage. Intrinsic factors include DNA replication errors, instability of DNA itself, active oxygen in the process of body's metabolism, etc. External factors include physical factors: radiation(IR), ultraviolet light(UV); and chemical factors: free radicals, base analogs, alkylation agent (O-6-E-G) and embedding dye. Biological factors mainly refer to the virus, such as measles, rubella virus and so on.

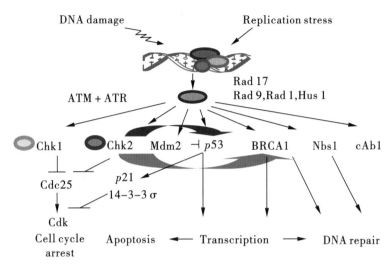

Figure 3-1　DNA-damage response(DDR)

(2)The type of DNA damage

The type of DNA damage included DNA base damages, DNA backbone damages, and cross-links.

1)DNA Base Damages

Base damages include O6-methylguanine, thymine glycols, and other reduced, oxidized, or fragmented bases in DNA that are produced by reactive oxygen species or by ionizing radiation. Ultraviolet (UV) radiation also gives rise to these species indirectly by generating reactive oxygen species, as well as producing specific products such as cyclobutane pyrimidine dimers and (6-4) photoproducts.

2)DNA Backbone

Backbone damages include abasic sites and single-and double-strand DNA breaks.

3)Cross-links

Bifunctional agents such as cisplatin, nitrogen mustard, mitomycin D, and psoralen form interstrand cross-links and DNA-protein cross-links.

(3)Meaning & Consequence

Generally speaking, damage usually has two biological effects. One is to bring a permanent structural change to the DNA molecules, that is, a mutation, and lateral teroreliminate the cells' ability to transcribe the gene. The other is to make the damaged DNA loses its function as a template for replication or transcription. In this way, the affected DNA will influence the survival of its daughter cells after it undergoes mitosis, leading to cell dysfunction and final death to induce potentially harmful mutations in the cell's genome.

As a result, DNA damage is of both positive and negative significance. For individuals, DNA damage is the basis of single cell death or the development of organism disease. However, for the long term development of species, mutation is the molecular basis of evolution and differentiation.

3.1.1.2　DNA damage recognition

There are four main strategies utilized for human identification of DNA damage: direct damage recognition, multistep damage recognition, recognition by proxy and recognition of DNA repair intermediates. The whole processes ask for proteins that bind to a specific sequence or structure in DNA, that is, the sensors. In contrast to enzymes with simple substrates, damage sensors must recognize their target in the vast excess of related structures.

Different DNA damages can be recognized by corresponding sensors, but there is not a one-to-one mapping between damages and recognition mechanisms. Such a non-interactive relationship makes the detection of DNA damage more sensitive and efficient to guarantee the stability of life activities.

Remarkably, DNA damage sensors not only bind to damaged DNA in the process of damage search but also contact undamaged DNA through specific binding. Thus, DNA damage sensors spend far more time associated with undamaged DNA In the presence of their high concentrations to carry out their specific functions. To solve this problem, DNA damage recognition is usually a multistep reaction to ensure a low probability that all of the steps will occur after the initial contact with undamaged DNA. Rather, although all the processes are operative at all times, the magnitudes of the repair or checkpoint reactions are amplified by the presence of DNA damage. However, the discrimination between undamaged and damaged DNA is still not absolute.

(1) Direct damage recognition

In its simplest recognition form, direct damage recognition consists of complementarity between a particular DNA damage and cognate protein, usually an enzyme like photolyase and DNA glycosylases. It is not by a simple binary reaction involving surface complementarity, but is rather by an induced fit mechanism, like Escherichia coli photolyase, which contains two steps: backbone recognition and dinucleotide flipping.

(2) Multistep damage recognition

Two types of recognition are involved: the molecular matchmakers and the combinatorial recognition.

The molecular matchmaker is a protein brings two compatible, but otherwise single macromolecules together promotes their association by a conformational change and then dissociates from the complex.

It utilizes the energy from ATP hydrolysis and can proactively identify the damage. Examples include RFC ineukaryotic DNA replicationand Uvr Aand XPC inbacterial and mammali an nucleotide excision repair.

Combinatorial recognition is common for transcriptional regulation, but relatively rare in DNA repair. It is utilized in a broad sense for several DNA repair functions. For example, in the absence of light, photolyase binds to the dimer to facilitate the binding of UvrA and promote the subsequent nucleotide excision processes.

(3) Recognition by proxy

Proteins that carry out functions not directly related to DNA repair can also become part of the recognition process. Instead of actively recognition, they just arrest targets at the damage sites and recruiting a repair mechanism, as exemplified by bacterial transcription-repair coupling factor(TRCF) that binds to the stalled RNA polymerase and recruits the damage-recognition complex, UvrA2/UvrB1, to the damage site during transcription-coupled repair of *E. coli*.

(4) Recognition of DNA repair intermediates

DNA repair reactions can produce intermediates like single-strand nicks, gaps, flap structures, double-strand breaks, or joint molecules. Such structures might be recognized by other damage-sensing systems, which may initiate an alternative set of reactions of both four main DNA damage response pathways.

3.1.1.3 Introduction to DNA damage response pathways

DNA damage is a common event in a cell's life. It can not only perturb the cellular steady-state quasi-equilibrium but also lead to the death of the single cell and the aging of multicellular organisms. For the sake of removal of damage, eukaryotes have developed a series of DNA damage response (DDR) pathways.

Different DNA damage can be identified by the corresponding mechanism, and later activate or amplify certain biochemical pathways which help to coordinate DNA replication with damage response, or reduce serious harmful effects through cell death or aging.

Currently, there are four kinds of generally acknowledged response pathways: DNA damage checkpoints, DNA damage repair, transcriptional response, and apoptosis. All of them may function independently, but frequently a protein primarily involved in one response may participate in others. One kind of DNA damage can activate multiple response pathways, while one response pathway can also repair a variety of damages.

Defects in any of these pathways may cause genomic instability. Therefore, maintaining a good balance between DNA damage and response is essential for maintaining biological stability and diversity. Due to space limitations in this textbook, we mainly introduce the first two pathways.

3.1.2　DNA damage checkpoints

3.1.2.1　Molecular components

Control mechanisms enforcing dependency in the cell cycle are here called checkpoints. DNA damage checkpoints are biochemical pathways that delay or arrest cell cycle progression in response to DNA damage to provide time for DNA damage repair. Sometimes it can induce DNA repair genes and apoptosis, but both of them can function independently of cell-cycle arrest machinery.

Related proteins can be roughly divided into four kinds of components: sensors, mediators, transducers, and effectors. However, there isn't an absolute demarcation among them. Both proteins can play different roles in more than one step of checkpoint response and even participate in multiple response pathways and damage sites. Thus the division just based on their prominent roles in specific checkpoints. Besides, such proteins serve as well in the normal physiological processes of the cell, which ensures the sensitivity of real-time monitoring.

(1) Sensors

The major DNA damage sensors in eukaryotic cells are the phosphoinositide 3-kinase-like kinases (PIKKs), such as the ATM, ATR, and 9－1－1 complexes. ATM is an oligomeric protein with a size of 350 kDa. It has a protein kinase activity. After exposure to ionizing radiation, ATM can phosphorylate many proteins, such as Chk2, $p53$, Nijmegen break syndrome (NBS1), and breast cancer. Sense 1 (BRCA1) and its serine and threonine sites. Studies have shown that ATM can prevent single-stranded damage DNA replication, promote its repair, and then prevent DNA double-strand damage.

ATR is a protein kinase specific to the serine and threonine sites of the SQ/TQ sequence that phosphorylates all proteins that are phosphorylated by ATM. Unlike ATM, ATR is activated by ultraviolet light instead of ionizing radiation. The Rad17-RFC complex is a structural homolog of replication factor C (RFC). RFCs are pentamers formed from $p140$, $p40$, $p38$, $p37$, and $p36$. The 9－1－1 complex is a cyclic structure homologous to proliferating cell nuclear antigen (PCNA). The roles of Rad17-RFC and 9－1－1 complexes in the injury checkpoint reaction are currently considered to be similar to those of RFC and PCNA in replication. Studies have found that Rad17-RFC recruits and binds the 9－1－1 complex in an ATP-dependent manner to form the Rad17-RFC/9－1－1 supercomplex with the participation of Rad9 and Rad17.

(2) Mediators

There are three kinds of human regulators: 53BP1, TopBP1, MDC1. In addition to these real regulators, other proteins such as H2AX, BRCA1, M/R/N (MRE11-Rad50-NBS1) complexes and structural maintenance of chromatin 1 (SMC1) also respond at the DNA damage checkpoint and play important roles. In response to DNA damage checkpoints, mediators interact with damage sensors, signal transducers, and effectors. The decrease or deletion of these proteins can limit the DNA damage checkpoint activity; weaken the radiosensitivity of the tumor.

(3) Transducers

In humans, there are two kinases, Chk1 and Chk2, which strictly activateorin activate other proteins that indirectly or directly participate in cell cycle regulation and checkpoint responses. Both Chk1 and Chk2 are specific serine/threonine kinases. ATM recognizes double-strand breaks caused by radiation and transmits damage signals to effectors through Chk2. ATR recognizes ultraviolet damage and transmits damage signals through Chk1 to effectors. Studies have found that Chk1 is significantly overexpressed in urothelial tumors, colorectal cancer, non-small cell lung cancer, and gastric cancer.

Chk2 mutations have been found in a variety of tumors, and their mutations may prevent damage recognition, injury repair, or apoptosis by inhibiting DNA damage checkpoint pathways, leading to tumorigenesis.

(4) Effectors

There are three main effectors in human cells, namely Cdc25A, Cdc25B, and Cdc25C, which are phosphatases that regulate cell cycle-dependent kinases. After Cdc25 is phosphorylated, its activity is inhibited in three ways: outside the nucleus, causing its degradation, or both. When normal cells are mitosis, Cdc25 protein is separated from 14-3-3 protein, activated and transported to the nucleus, allowing mitosis to proceed normally. When ionizing radiation or ultraviolet rays cause DNA damage, ATR/ATM recognizes damage and phosphorylates Cdc25 protein through Chk1/Chk2 to bind to 14-3-3 protein. The latter transports Cdc25 into the cytoplasm and disable Cdc25.

3.1.2.2 DNA damage checkpoints

After DNA damage, eukaryotic cells can activate DNA damage response, which can activate DNA damage checkpoint pathway, change transcription level, and activate DNA damage repair pathway and apoptosis. Four checkpoints are involved: G1/S, intra-S, G2/M and S/M checkpoint. This chapter focuses on the mechanism of DNA damage checkpoint pathways and their role.

(1) The G1/S checkpoint

The G1/S injury checkpoint prevents cells from entering the S phase in the event of DNA damage by inhibiting the initiation of replication. At present, the path of G1/S injury checkpoints in human cells has been elucidated. Whether the cell cycle arrest is caused by the ATM-Chk2-Cdc25A pathway or the ATR-Chk1-Cdc25A pathway, a sustained block of G1/S phase is mediated by $p53$.

(2) The intra-S-phase checkpoint

An unrepaired lesion at the G1/S checkpoint or an injury at S phase activates the intra-S-phase checkpoint pathway, leading to cell cycle arrest, activation of the DNA damage repair system, and affect the accuracy and integrity of DNA replication followed by cell injury. Although there is some evidence that the activation of the S-phase injury checkpoint can slow down the replication fork process, the main mechanism of the S-phase block is still to inhibit the opening of the replication origin. Mainly through two routes: ATM/ATR-Chk2-Cdc25A-Cdk2 pathway, ATM-BRCA1-NBS1-SMC1 pathway.

(3) The G2/M checkpoint

The G2/M injury checkpoint prevents cells from entering the M phase in the event of DNA damage and undergoes mitosis. According to the type of DNA damage, different signal pathways are slightly different. The single-strand DNA breaks caused by ultraviolet radiation cause activation of the ATR-Chk1-Cdc25 pathway, blocking G2/M phase progression, and ionizing radiation-mediated double-strand breaks that cause ATM-Chk2-Activation of the Cdc25 pathway blocks progression in the G2/M phase. Cdc25A is a key molecule that regulates the G2/M checkpoint.

(4)The S/M checkpoint

The copy damage checkpoint (also known as the S/M checkpoint) refers to the process of inhibiting mitosis when DNA replication is ongoing or blocked. DNA damage or deletion of nucleotides can cause the process of replication fork formation to block and initiate the replication damage checkpoint pathway. The replication injury checkpoint blocks cell cycle progression through the same ATR-Chk1-Cdc25 signaling pathway as the G2/M injury checkpoint.

3.1.3 DNA damage repair mechanism

The stability of cellular genetic material is affected by its conditions and external conditions. There are many types of DNA damage, such as DNA alkylation, oxidation, mismatch, loop formation, fragmentation, and atypical structures. The human body undergoes natural evolution and establishes a variety of repair mechanisms for DNA damage. By identifying DNA damage sites, a series of biochemical pathways are activated, DNA replication and transcription are coordinated, damaged DNA is repaired, and the body is relatively independent and stable. Among them, base excision repair, nucleotide excision repair, mismatch repair, double-strand break repair, and cross-injury synthesis repair play a key role and is the main route of DNA damage repair. This chapter focuses on the description of DNA damage repair types and molecular mechanisms. It aims to promote readers' understanding of the importance of this field and provide a theoretical basis for exploring the application of DNA damage repair pathways in cancer therapy.

3.1.3.1 Base excision repair

BER was discovered and proposed by Professor Lindahl in 1974 and was awarded the Nobel Prize in Chemistry in 2015 for his outstanding contribution in related fields.

Studies on BER have found that this pathway is initiated by a DNA glycosylase that recognizes base deletions such as deletions, oxidations, alkylations, deaminations, and mismatches. Purine/pyrimidine (AP) endonucleases, purine/pyrimidine (AP) lyase, break the phosphodiester bond at both ends of the damage site near the damage site recognized by DNA glycosylase, and DNA glycosylase. In addition to damaging the base, an abasic site (AP site) is created. According to the number of removed bases, the AP sites to be repaired can be divided into two short sequences (single nucleotides) and long sequences (2–10 nucleotides). The corresponding DNA polymerase is recruited according to the length of the formed AP locus. Usually, DNA polymerase β participates in short sequence repair, and DNA polymerase σ and ε participate in long sequence repair. The AP site was filled with a complex formed by DNA polymerase, poly ADP ribose polymerase 1 and X-ray repair cross-complement factor 1. After the AP site is filled, the two ends are connected to the broken DNA strands with DNA ligase 1, DNA ligase 3, and X-ray repair cross-complement factor 1.

3.1.3.2 Nucleotide excision repair

NER is a major repair pathway for a large number of DNA damages caused by external factors. It is essential for all organisms and has always been a focus and hotspot in the field of DNA damage repair.

ATP was used to hydrolyze about 25bp double-stranded DNA structure in and around the injured area to form stable precursor complex 1; a more stable precursor complex two was formed under the action of XPG; XPF · ERCC1 was recruited to the site of injury, irreversible precursor complex three is formed. XPG was excised from the 3' end of the lesion. XPA cleaved the 5' end upstream of the lesion and released about 20–30 bp oligomers with the help of PCNA; DNA Pol δ/ε/K, PCNA, and RFC will fill the missing nucleotide fragments complete DNA ligase will be stranded connection.

An important feature of nucleic acid excision repair is that it can repair a large number of different

DNA structural damages and does not rely on a damage recognition enzyme to initiate the repair process. He received the 2015 Nobel Prize in chemistry for his outstanding contribution in elucidating the molecular mechanisms of NER.

3.1.3.3 Mismatch repair

MMR mainly corrects base pairing errors caused by various causes and inserts and deletion bases. From low to advanced organisms have a conservative system of mismatch repair. MMR is initiated by binding of the MutS dimer (MSH2/MSH6) or the MutSb dimer (MSH2/MSH3) to the mismatched base and the inserted or deleted base, respectively. MLH1-hMLH3, PMS1/PMS2, and EXO1, RPA, RFC, and DNA polymerase were sequentially recruited and integrated into the DNA damage complex, excising mismatched bases, and reassembling the correct DNA.

MMR dysfunction results in DNA microsatellite instability (MSI), which in turn causes mutations in some proto-oncogenes or tumor suppressor genes (such as BRAF, MRE11A, KRAS).

3.1.3.4 Double-strand break repair

The double-strand break is produced by reactive oxygen species, ionizing radiation and chemicals, acts as a normal result of V(D)J recombination and immunoglobulin class-switching processes or occur as a consequence of replication fork arrest and collapse. It can be repaired either by homologous recombination (HR) or non-homologous end-joining (NHEJ) mechanisms.

(1) Homologous recombination (HR)

HR happens during a late period of S to G2. It is a slow process with high fidelity in low-grade eukaryotes, initiated by a collapsed fork. Three steps are involved: strand invasion by Rad51 depending on homologous duplex, branch migration by DNA Pol, and Holliday junction formation. The Holliday junction is then resolved into two duplexes by the structure-specific endonucleases, MUS81/MMS4 complex, and the gap is ligated by Ligases. Because the lost information is retrieved from a homologous duplex, a not exactly same one can cause a mutation.

(2) Non-homologous end-joining(NHEJ) mechanisms

In contrast to HR, NHEJ can quickly respond to damage caused by ionizing radiation and V(D)J recombination in mammalians' cells of the whole cycle. The non-homologous end-joining (NHEJ) repair pathway mainly involves seven core proteins, namely Ku70, Ku80, DNA-PKcs, Artemis, XRCC4-like factor (XLF), XRCC4 and DNA ligase IV.

This process includes three steps: identifying the site of double-strand breaks; multiple enzymes involved in the processing of the damaged DNA ends; the XRCC4-DNA ligase IV complex with the help of the XLF reconnectsthe processed DSB ends. It is a dynamic process involving multiple protein complexes, which is flexible and changeable.

For instance, the Ku heterodimer binds to the two ends of a double-strand break and recruits DNA-PKcs and the Ligase4-XRCC4 heterodimer, which then ligates the two duplex termini regardless of whether the two ends come from the same chromosome.

3.1.3.5 Translesion synthesis

TLS repair is an important method of DNA damage tolerance in the body. When the double-stranded DNA damage occurs extensively, and the repair system cannot be effectively repaired by the above four approaches, the low-fidelity DNA polymerase will displace the high-fidelity DNA polymerase that is arrested at the DNA damage, allowing the DNA replication complex to cross the damage. To continue replication, this DNA damage compensation mechanism is TLS.

Because the low-fidelity DNA polymerase does not depend on the principle of base pairing when inserting nucleotides in the TLS process, the TLS repair approach also has a high probability of error and a propensity for mutagenesis. Despite these drawbacks, the TLS repair approach can avoid the serious consequences of incomplete DNA replication.

After more than half a century of hard work, many important breakthroughs have been made in the field of DNA damage repair. The value of intervention in DNA damage repair has gradually become evident in clinical research, becoming a hot spot in cancer targeting therapy and tumor radiosensitizaer.

3.1.4   Transcriptional response and apoptosis

Compared with DNA repair and DNA damage checkpoints which play a relatively unique role in DDR, transcriptional response and apoptosis are ubiquitous phenomena during the cells' activities.

Transcriptional response regulates multiple proteins involved in DNA repair, cell cycle checkpoint control, protein trafficking, and degradation to take part in the harmed DNA mending process. The corresponding damage can stimulate modification of transcriptional factors (TF) or enzymes to enable the activation/inactivation of TF. Transcriptional activators can promote transcription by combining cis-acting elements or by interacting with general TF. The transcriptional suppressor can inhibit transcription by interfering with the basic transcriptional device or by inhibiting the transcription activator. Also, a variety of non-coding RNA is also involved in the process.

Apoptosis is a process of programmed cell death that occurs in multicellular organisms. Biochemical events lead to characteristic cell changes: blebbing, cell shrinkage, nuclear fragmentation, chromatin condensation, chromosomal DNA fragmentation, and global mRNA decay. In this process, organisms can clear up these damaged cells and limit the risk of transmitting the wrong genetic information to the offspring.

3.1.5   Summary

The stability of cell genetic material is influenced by a variety of factors, both intrinsic and external, which can cause different types of DNA damage, such as DNA alkylation, oxidation, mismatching, loop structure, atypical DNA structure, single strand break, double-strand breaks, etc. These DNA damages disrupt cellular homeostasis and dynamic equilibrium, which cause gene mutations, chromosomal abnormalities, even degradation, aging and death at different biological levels. There are four main strategies utilized for human identification of DNA damage: direct damage recognition, multistep damage recognition, recognition by proxy and recognition of DNA repair intermediates. By searching and identifying DNA damage sites, cell initiates DNA damage response reactions, activates series of biochemical pathways and coordinates the progress of DNA replication and transcription, then repairs the damages. Among the responses, DNA damage checkpoints, DNA damage repair, transcriptional response, and apoptosis play a key role. In this way, the cell maintains its independence and stability. This section shows recent research results in DNA damage responses and focuses on how the DNA damage checkpoints and DNA damage repair pathways are activated after DNA damage, as well as the functional mechanism of them. This section details the molecular components and different types of DNA damage checkpoints, details different types, and mechanisms of DNA damage repair pathways, briefly introduces the role of transcriptional response and apoptosis in DNA damage response.

This section aims to promote the readers understanding the great significance of this field and provide a theoretical basis for exploring its application in clinical cancer therapy.

3.2 Virus and cancer

Virus infection is one of the important causes of tumorigenesis. The virus which can cause human or animal tumors or malignant transformation of cells in vitro is known as an oncogenic virus. The tumors caused by the virus infection account for about 20% of the overall tumor incidence.

Oncogenic viruses can be divided into DNA virus and RNA virus by nucleic acid type. To determine whether a virus is an oncogenic virus, it must meet the following five conditions. The virus is infected before the tumor formation; viruses, viral nucleic acids, and viral antigens can be found in the tumor; the corresponding virus or viral antigen can be produced by the tumor cells cultured In vitro; the virus can induce malignant transformation of normal cell, and can induce tumors in animals; preventing viral infection with immune intervention can reduce the incidence of tumors.

The detailed molecular mechanism of oncogenic virus-induced tumorigenesis is not fully elucidated. The current studies have shown that the virus gene integrates with the DNA of the host cell after infection, which affects the composition and expression regulation of the host gene, initiates a series of molecular events, and interferes with host cell differentiation, proliferation, and apoptosis, resulting in malignant transformation. With the development of molecular biology, the molecular mechanism of an oncogenic virus will be more clear.

3.2.1 Definition of an oncogenic virus

An oncogenic virus or oncovirus is a virus which can cause human or animal tumors or malignant transformation of cells cultured *in vitro*. Oncogenic viruses can be divided into DNA virus and RNA virus. Although the detailed molecular mechanism of virus-induced tumorigenesis has not yet been fully elucidated, with the development of molecular biology, researchers have conducted a large number of studies on the isolation and identification of oncogenic viruses and related function. The results from a genetic origin, cell cycle, signal transduction, bioinformatics and other aspects of the oncogenic virus confirmed that oncogenes play a key role in the occurrence and the development of cancer.

3.2.2 History of the oncogenic virus

The theory that tumor could be caused by a virus began with the experiments of Vilhelm Ellerman and Oluf Bang in 1908, who first show that avian erythroblastosis could be transmitted by cell-free extracts. This was subsequently confirmed for solid tumors in chickens in 1910 by Peyton Rous. Peyton Rous demonstrated that chickens inoculate by spontaneous sarcoma cell extracts would result in solid tumors. Later, scientists came to realize that certain murine malignancies and mammalian malignancies are caused by viruses. These oncogenic viruses belong to the family of retroviruses and have definite malignant transformation functions without killing the host cells. Retroviruses can be prevalent in many species, such as mice and chickens. For example, most chickens will be infected with the virus a few months after hatching. In most cases, the infected virus appears as a transient form of viremia without causing obvious symptoms.

Animals can also be innately infected and subsequently develop immune tolerance to the virus, which later on exhibits long-term toxemia. Retroviral strains with rapid transformation and high oncogenicity are more likely to induce malignant transformation, such as Rous Sarcoma Virus, a rare and well-studied virus isolated by Rous.

Researchers divided oncogenic retroviruses into two groups based on their rate of malignant transformation: the first group included a rare, rapidly transformable, transducible oncogenic retrovirus. These viruses are highly oncogenic and have a tumorigenic rate of up to 100% in animals infected for days. Subsequent studies have found that they can transform cultured susceptible animal cells; the second group is non-transduced oncogenic retroviruses. Not all animals develop tumors after being infected with these viruses, and the virus can infect the host for several weeks to several months. In the late 1980s, a third oncogenic retrovirus was found that showed long-term latent infection and rarely caused the tumor to occur, months or even years after infection.

Each type of oncogenic retrovirus causes tumor with a special mechanism. Retroviruses cause cancers because their genome contains genes that transduce cells, which can become oncogenic when expressed in host cells. Proteins encoded by these genes can cause transformation or tumorigenesis. The gene carried by this virus that causes malignant transformation of cells is called the v-oncogenes, and its copy in normal cells is called the c-oncogenes or proto-oncogenes. Non-transduced retroviruses do not encode cell-derived oncogenes, and when the virus is integrated into the vicinity of the proto-oncogene of the host cell's genome, transcription of the proto-oncogene is inappropriately activated. The products of viral oncogenes are not effective for the retrovirus's own proliferative infection, however, studying the retrovirus's oncogenes and oncogenesis are of great importance for us to understand the origin of the tumor.

3.2.3   Types of oncogenic virus

3.2.3.1   Oncogenic RNA virus

Oncogenic RNA viruses belong to the family of retroviruses. According to the morphology of the virus, the genome integrity, the life cycle of the virus and the oncogenic mechanism, it can be divided into four types: A, B, C, and D. The type C oncogenic RNA virus has a definite etiological relationship with the tumorigenesis. The type B virus has a less etiological relationship with the tumorigenesis than type C. Type A may be immature B/C type. Type D virus is isolated from Rhesus Macaque and has no direct evidence of tumorigenicity. Due to the differences in the genome structure of the virus, it can be divided into non-defective and defective oncogenic RNA viruses according to whether they need a helper virus to produce a complete virus particle when cultured in vitro. The sarcoma virus with the SRC oncogene contains the complete gag, pol and env genes, so it belongs to the non-defective virus. The defective RNA virus is lacking in the pol and env genes but contains oncogenes. These oncogenes often form gap-fusion genes and produce fusion proteins such as gag-yes, gag-actin-fgr, and gag-rat. The structural genes in this virus are exchanged or lost to the cellular genome when cells are infected so that the virus needs the help of a helper virus to produce the complete virion. Oncogenic RNA viruses are divided into acute and chronic oncogenic RNA viruses based on the tumorigenic ability in animals. Acute oncogenic RNA virus can induce tumors in 3–4 weeks after inoculation of animals. Chronic oncogenic RNA virus causes tumor in animals using a 5–12 months time period. Chronic oncogenic RNA virus does not carry an oncogene. Only when the virus's LTR (Long Terminal Repeat) DNA integrates into the host cell then cause abnormal overexpression of the host cell's gene, it causes a tumor.

Retroviruses infect and exchange genes with host cells. The captured gene are genetically modified to produce an active combinatorial gene called protooncogene, usually denoted v. The same gene of the cell is denoted c. For example, the oncogene in the Rous sarcoma virus genome is called v-Src, and the same gene is called c-Src in the cell. The origin of the oncogene can be discerned from v-matched and c-matched genes. It has been found that there are more than 30 kinds of cellular oncogenes in the retroviral genome, and same oncogenes can be found in different the retroviral strains.

The retrovirus life cycle is the replication of genetic material using RNA and DNA as templates. First, the viral RNA is reverse-transcribed into single-stranded DNA by the host cell's RNA polymerase after the virus infects the cells, and then the double-stranded DNA is synthesized and finally integrated into the host genome. The double-stranded DNA can be transcribed into infectious RNA, involve in the production of retroviral particles.

3.2.3.2 Oncogenic DNA virus

There are double-stranded DNA Viruses and single-stranded DNA viruses.

The double-stranded DNA viral genome is composed of double-stranded or partially double-stranded DNA. Viruses with double-stranded DNA genome can be divided into 22 families. Oncogenic DNA viruses that infect mammals include adenoviridae, herpesviridae, papillomaviruses, polyomavirus and poxviridae. Some of these double-stranded DNA genomes are linear. The others are ring-shaped. The synthesis of viral mRNAs depends on the host's RNA polymerase.

The currently known viruses with single-strand DNA genome have five families, among which the Circoviridae and parvoviridae families contain viruses that can infect mammals. The single-strand genome is produced by the action of cellular DNA polymerases. The mRNA requires double-stranded DNA as a template for synthesis. Therefore, whether the single-stranded DNA is the sense or antisense strand, the synthesis of DNA must be completed before the mRNA synthesis in the viral replication cycle.

After DNA virus infects cells, transcription of genes is initiated immediately. The expression product of these early genes are usually transforming proteins that activate the expression of middle and late genes. The infections of DNA virus can be divided into lytic infection and abortive infection. The former is a virus that infects the host cells and can then enter DNA replication and eventually lead to cell death. These cells are often the natural host of the virus, called permissive cells. An abortive infection is a virus that infects a non-host cell. In that case, viral DNA replication is very inefficient and even viral DNA can't replicate. Permissive infection is a complete virus life cycle process from adsorption, invasion, DNA replication, transcription, capsid generation, assembly, and viral particle release. Then the newly released viruses infect neighboring cells. Non-permissive infection is the integration of the viral genome into the host cell genome, causing the cell to undergo malignant transformation. At present, the DNA oncogenic viruses associated with human tumors include EBV, HPV, HHVB, HBV, etc. They can cause tumors of nasopharyngeal carcinoma, cervical carcinoma, burkitt lymphoma, and liver cancer, respectively.

3.2.4 The pathogenic mechanism of oncogenic virus

Although oncogenic viruses belong to different families, they still share many common features. In theory, any virus that can encode a protein to promote the progression of the cell cycle or inhibit apoptosis has the potential to transform cells and cause tumors. An important characteristic of oncogenic viruses is the ability to infect but not kill host cells. Some viruses can induce the secretion of certain proteins or cytokines to stimulate the growth of uninfected cells, induce tissue proliferation, or down-regulate the killing effect of the immune system on infected cells. Such viruses also have the potential to cause tumorigenesis.

In recent years, researchers have put forward a number of mechanisms that explain howviruses cause cancer. One of the most widely accepted theories is that when an oncogenic virus infects cells, its genetic material tends to integrate into the host chromosomes, causing the cell to become cancerous. This phenomenon is also known as cellular transformation. Transformation can cause uncontrolled cell growth and eventually tumor formation. Existing studies have shown that transformation is an independent process. All or part of the viral genome will be present in the transformed cells, generally accompanied by the expression of specific viral genes. On the other hand, when a particular viral gene is expressed, infectious virus particles are no longer required (except for some retroviruses) anymore. Viral transforming proteins change the proliferation properties of cells through a limited number of molecular mechanisms.

3.2.4.1 Viral oncogenes

Based on the differences in sequence similarity between viral oncogenes and cellular genes, virus oncogenes are divided into two categories. The first type of viral oncogene has very high similarities to cellular genes, such as viral oncogenes of transduced retroviruses and some herpes viruses. It is clear that the sequence of these viral oncogenesis captured by the virus from the infected cell genome. Retroviral particles need to contain some cellular RNA and undergo recombination during reverse transcription to produce transduced retroviruses. The limiting factor for the production of transduced retroviruses may be the frequency with which cellular mRNA molecules are packaged into viral particles.

Cellular proto-oncogenes are highly conserved during evolution, and numerous studies have found that many vertebrate proto-oncogenes share homology with yeast. Therefore, it can, therefore, be concluded that the products of these genes must have indispensable functions for eukaryotic cells. Also, a single copy of the viral oncogene is sufficient to transform the infected cells, indicating that their function must exceed that of the proto-oncogene that they are homologous to. Therefore, the viral oncogene is a dominant transforming gene.

The second type of viral oncogene has no significant correlation with cellular genes. But the short amino acid sequences contained in the encoded products of these genes also exist in cellular proteins. As for the true origin of these oncogenes, it is still unclear.

3.2.4.2 The integration of viral DNA

Viral DNA is usually retained in the nuclei of oncogenic virus-transformed cells. These DNA sequences are part of the sequence of the infected DNA genome. Viral DNA integration refers to the integration of viral DNA into the genome of a host cell's nuclei after certain oncogenic viruses infect cells. And the integrated DNA can be transmitted from the parent to the offspring as part of normal genetic material as the cells proliferate.

Integration of proviral DNA by viral integrase is an important step in the retrovirus's life cycle. This proviral DNA can be randomly integrated at any site in cellular DNA. For transduced retroviruses, where the viral oncogene carried by it causes cancerous cells, it does not matter at which site in the genome, because it is integrated. In contrast, for non-transduced retroviruses, its integration into specific regions of the cell genome is the key to inducing tumorigenesis. For tumors resulting from the transformation of this type of virus, each tumor cell has the same proviral chromosomal location, indicating that the tumor is originated from a single transformed cell, and therefore the tumor is considered to be monoclonal.

The integration of viral DNA sequences is not a prerequisite for successful replication of all oncogenic DNA viruses. However, integration is the rule for adenoviruses or polyomaviruses to transform cells. Because these viruses contain specific genes inserted into the host genome, random recombination between cells and viral DNA sequences can occur. Therefore, integration can occur at many sites in the genome of a cell, and it is not necessary to retain specific viral DNA sequences to link with the cellular DNA.

Most of the cells infected with adenovirus or polyomavirus retain only a portion of the viral genome. In different cell lines transformed by the same virus, the integrated genomic sequences are diverse, but one thing in common is that the smallest unit of viral genes is retained. 1–10 or 20 copies of viral DNA can be integrated into each cell, and there can be multiple integration sites. However, there is little evidence that this difference in the integrated copy number is related to the difference in the phenotype of transformed cells.

The second mechanism for the presence of viral DNA in transformed cells is the presence of a stable exosomal free masses, such as the situation of B-cell EB virus and papillomavirus. Along with the synthesis of cellular DNA, the viral genome also replicates, and the replicated viral DNA is systematically distributed to progeny cells, thereby maintaining tens to hundreds of copies of the viral genome episome in each cell. Therefore, in order to permanently change the cell growth traits, in addition to the viral genes that are required to regulate cell growth and proliferation directly, there is also a need for genes for episomal replication.

3.2.4.3   viral protein's function in transformation

Classical genetics methods have been used to identify transforming genes of the oncogenic virus, to explore viral products and viral genes expressed in transformed cell lines, and to analyze the transformability of viral DNA fragments. For example, it was discovered that murine polyomavirus temperature-sensitive mutants have the ability to transform, indicating that early viral transcription units are sufficient to initiate and maintain transformation. The more valuable discovery was the isolation of mutant retrovirus strains, particularly two mutants of the Rous sarcoma virus discovered in the early 1970s. The first mutant is a strain that spontaneously lost nearly 20% of the viral genome. This mutant no longer transforms the infected cells but still replicates. The second mutant is a temperature-sensitive mutant that can only transform cells at a suitable temperature, but cell replication is not temperature-regulated. The above mechanism indicates that cell transformation and virus replication are two completely different processes.

The presence of a cellular oncogene in the viral genome is a feature of a transduced retrovirus. It has also been discussed that acquisition of a cellular oncogene sequence is a small probability event for a virus. Transduced retroviruses are replication-defective due to the loss of all or part of the virus-encoding gene when capturing the cell gene. However, this type of virus can spread when mixed with a helper virus which provides necessary viral protein for viral replication.

In many viral oncogenes, the viral and cellular protein coding sequences are fused. The presence of a viral sequence can increase the efficiency of oncogene mRNA translation, stabilize the protein, or determine the localization of a protein in the cell. Overexpression of cellular genes caused by the promoters of several viral oncogeneses sufficient to cause transformation, but in most cases viral oncogenes have different mutants and have the potential to promote transformation. These mutations include nucleic acid changes, truncations, rearrangements of one or both ends of the viral gene, and affect the normal function of the gene.

DNA-mediated transformation can assess the effect of different viral oncogenes (or DNA sequences encoding a single viral protein) on cell growth and proliferation. This strategy can also be used to study the viral transforming proteins. Transformation of primary cells by adenoviruses, papillomaviruses, and polyomaviruses requires two or more viral gene products. Most of these viral proteins have the ability to alter cell traits in the absence of other viral proteins. Certain viral genes are only required in specific transformed phenotype or are required only under specific conditions (such as the SV40 small T antigen, bovine polyomavirus type 1 E7). Some genes alone are not active. The adenovirus E1B gene is a typical example of this phenomenon. E1B gene, in synergy with the E1A gene, can transform cultured rodent cells, but itself does not have the ability of phenotypic transformation.

Han Suxia

Chapter 4

Biological Behavior of Tumor

The formation of a tumor is a complex, multi-staged process that can span decades. Uncontrolled cellular proliferation, caused by mutations present within transformed cells, results in the formation of a tumor body. The growth and biological processes of a typical malignant tumor cell can be divided into four stages: a single cell malignant transformation → clonal hyperplasia of transformed cells → local invasion → distant metastasis. The intrinsic characteristics of malignant transformed cells, such as doubling time and the host immune response, affect growth and progression of the tumor. This chapter will focus on the biological behavior of tumors.

4. 1   The growth kinetics and regulatory mechanisms of tumor cells

4.1.1   Kinetics of tumor growth

The growth rate of tumors may vary between tissues and individuals. Generally, benign tumors are usually well-differentiated and grow more slowly, while the malignant tumors are poorly-differentiated, less mature, and grow more rapidly. There are several factors affecting tumor growth rate, such as doubling time, growth score, the ratio of generation and loss.

4.1.1.1   Doubling time

Doubling time is defined as the time that is required for an initial population of cells to double. The doubling time of most malignant tumor cells is not shorter than normal cells; typically the doubling time of malignant tumor cells is similar to or longer than normal cells. Thus, the doubling time does not solely determine the growth rate of malignant tumors.

In clinical practice, the doubling time is defined as the time required for tumor volume to increase by a factor of one. The doubling time of most primary tumors is between 2 to 3 months; however, in the same patient the doubling time of a metastatic tumor is shorter. During the early stage of tumor growth the doubling time is shorter; as the tumor grows, the doubling time gradually increases.

4.1.1.2 The growth fraction of tumor cells

Growth fraction (GF) of tumor cells is defined as the proportion of cells in the proliferating phase (S phase and G2 phase). A larger GF is positively correlated with rapid tumor growth and a smaller GF is negatively correlated with rapid tumor growth. In the early stage of malignant transformation, the vast majority of cells are in the proliferative phase thereby contributing to a higher GF.

4.1.1.3 The generation and loss of tumor cells

Normal cells maintain homeostasis through growth and loss. Many factors such as contact inhibition, apoptosis, necrosis, lack of nutrition, and host anti-tumor immune response affect the growth of the tumor. The balance between the generation and loss directly affects the growth rate of tumor tissue. Tumor cells grow more quickly than they turn over thereby contributing to the tumor growth and invasion.

4.1.2 The regulatory mechanism of tumor cell growth

Tumor growth is affected by many factors, including the following aspects.

4.1.2.1 The cell cycle and tumor cell growth

At its core, cancer is a progressive disease caused by several varieties of genomic mutations ranging from simple base-pair indels to complex chromosomal rearrangements. Most oncogenes and suppressor genes exert their function by regulating cell cycle. Gene mutations affecting transcript initiation/termination and protein functioning of key cell cycle molecules may potentially contribute to hyper-proliferation and decreased apoptosis. Therefore, cancer may be classified as a disease of the cell cycle.

(1) Cell cycle

The cell cycle or cell-division cycle is the series of events that take place in cell leading to the duplication of its DNA (DNA replication) and subsequent division into two daughter cells. The cell cycle consists of four distinct phases: G1 phase, S phase (synthesis), G2 phase (collectively known as interphase) and M phase (mitosis). In normal individuals, the cell cycle of stem cells is accelerated while the cell cycle of more differentiated cells proceeds slower. If the cell cycle becomes misregulated, the cell may initiate a cascade of events that leads to apoptosis; however, certain aberrant events may also promote tumorigenesis.

(2) The regulatory mechanisms of tumor's cell cycle

Every individual has a sophisticated program or "biological clock" which determines whether or when cells begin to grow, divide, or die. This sophisticated program is the cell cycle regulatory mechanism, which is under the control of the cell cycle related genes. Normal execution of the cell cycle program may promote cell growth, division and death depending on which genes are expressed.

1) The key regulation of cell cycle

The key regulatory mechanism of the cell cycle is a group of protein kinases (called cyclin-dependent kinases, CDKs). They are activated at a specific time during cell cycle by phosphorylating substrates that promote completion of the cell cycle. The activation of CDKs relies on that the accumulation and binding of cyclin proteins, which are expressed and degraded in a cell-cycle dependent manner.

2) Restriction Point of cell cycle regulation

The first phase within interphase is called G1 (G1 phase); it is also called the growth phase. The main regulatory point, known as the "restriction point", that determines whether the cell cycle can proceed into S phase occurs during the latter half of the G1 phase.

The progression of the cell cycle through restriction points is due to signaling pathways that are stimulated via the binding of extracellular growth factors with their associated transmembrane receptors. As long as the related growth factor exists, the cell can proceed through the restriction point. Once the restriction point is passed, the cells can finish G1, G2 and M phases without growth factors. However, if the cell lacks the related growth factor at G1, the cell cycle enters a quiescent state, called G0 phase. During this period, cells can survive for a long time without proliferation, and once they are stimulated by growth factors or other extracellular signals, they typically reenter the cell cycle.

3) Regulate checkpoint of cell cycle

Completion of the cell cycle also requires faithful duplication of the cell's genetic material. If the previous cell cycle phase has not yet been completed (such as incomplete DNA synthesis or repair), the start of the next phase of a cell cycle will be delayed. This precise sequence of cell cycle progression is achieved through the use of checkpoints.

There are two types of checkpoints during the cell cycle: one is the DNA damage check point which checks for any form of DNA damage or incomplete DNA synthesis. If any damage is detected, the cell will either attempt to correct it or proceed to apoptosis.

(3) Cell cycle and tumor therapy

Sensitivity to treatment varies among different types of tumors. The cell in the proliferative cycle is more sensitive to antitumor drugs or radiotherapy, while the G0 phase may contribute to recurrence due to insensitivity to antitumor drugs or radiotherapy. For example, high growth fraction tumors (such as highly malignant lymphoma) are more sensitive to radiotherapy and chemotherapy. However, tumors with low growth fraction and in non-proliferating phrase (such as gastric cancer) are less sensitive to radiotherapy and chemotherapy. To treat the latter class of tumors, it is advisable to perform surgery to remove most of the tumors. After surgery, the residual G0 stage cells can enter into the proliferative phase, thereby increasing sensitivity of the remaining tumor to radiotherapy and chemotherapy.

There are two main classes of drugs to treat tumor cells, the first class is a cyclical nonspecific drug which works at every phase of cell cycle, the second class is a cell cycle-specific medicine which works during certain phases of the cell cycle; for example, 5-FU mainly works during the S phase. Tumor therapy may target cell cycle regulation in various ways, such as inhibiting tumor cell overgrowth by inhibiting CDKs and cyclin activity. Detecting and targeting cell cycle checkpoint defects to accelerate tumor cell death is the main mode of action for this class of drugs.

4.1.2.2　Apoptosis and the growth of the tumor cells

Dysregulation of apoptosis results in many diseases; more than 50% of the tumor cells have defects in pathways leading to apoptosis. Abnormal apoptosis may contribute to tumor formation by allowing cells with mutations in cell cycle regulating components to excape death, thereby leading to uncontrolled proliferation. Therefore, to some extent, it can be said that tumors are a type of disease with characterized by abnormal apoptosis.

(1) Apoptosis

Apoptosis is a process of programmed cell death which occurs in multicellular organisms. Apoptosis is characterized by cellular/nuclear blebbing, cell shrinkage, nuclear fragmentation, chromatin condensation, chromosomal DNA fragmentation, and global mRNA decay. Apoptosisis distinct from necrosis. Its biological significance is to remove excess, dysplasia, reduce to presence of mutated cells.

(2) Regulatory mechanism of apoptosis

During the development of malignant tumors, abnormal apoptosis may be the result of mutations to any components of the apoptotic signaling pathway. Below are examples of the most characterized mutations that lead to aberrant apoptosis.

1) Bcl-2 and malignancies

The Bcl-2 family protein is an important regulator of apoptotic signaling. The expression of Bcl-2 is significantly increased in many tumor cells such as breast cancer, lung cancer, colon cancer and prostate cancer. Bcl-XL is another family protein which is highly expressed in many blood tumors. Bcl-2/Bcl-XL inhibits apoptosis through Bcl-2 gene rearrangement, which disrupts the normal apoptosis and confers insensitivity to apoptotic signaling in tumor cells. This also confers resistance to conventional chemotherapy and radiotherapy in tumor cells. A high level of Bcl-2/Bcl-XL is also related to poor prognosis.

2) *TP53* and malignancies

DNA damage is one of the most widely studied inducers of apoptosis. An important gene involved in the induction apoptosis is the *TP53* gene. Many stress signals such as DNA damage, abnormal increased activity of telomerase, oncogene activation and hypoxia are involved in the development, invasion, and metastasis of tumor cells. Any of the previous cellular stresses can activate *TP53* expression. The *TP53* gene plays a pivotal role in preventing tumorigenesis by regulating the growth and survival of cells in response to stress. *TP53* gene deletion or mutation can be detected in more than 50% of malignancies. Importantly, wild-type *TP53* also exists in other tumors. *TP53*-deficient tumors do not undergo apoptosis have increased resistance to chemotherapy and radiotherapy.

3) Apoptosis and cancer treatment

Research into the molecular mechanisms of tumor cell apoptosishas provided new insights that may lead to the development of novel, highly specific anti-cancer drugs. Activation and blocking of apoptotic signaling pathways may be targets for antitumor medicine development. For instance, targeting intracellular Bcl-2/Bcl-XL in tumors may lead to induction of apoptosis and sensitivity to chemotherapy and radiotherapy.

4.2 Tumor angiogenesis

Angiogenesis is not only a prerequisite for tumor growth, but also an important factor in promoting tumor metastasis. In 1945, Algire first proposed the concept of tumor angiogenesis. In 1971, Folkman further suggested that angiogenesis is closely related to tumor growth and metastasis. Therefore, if angiogenesis can be inhibited, the tumor growth would also be inhibited.

4.2.1 The concept and basic process of tumor angiogenesis

4.2.1.1 Angiogenesis

Angiogenesis refers to the process of new capillary growth in the existing capillary networks. Angiogenesis in tumor tissue is a pathological state and its biological characteristics including low reactivity, high permeability and low oxygen supply. Tumor vessels provide tumor cells with nutrients and additional metabolic conditions that contribute to tumor growth. At the same time, their structural defects of high permeability contribute to tumor metastasis.

4.2.1.2 The basic processes of tumor angiogenesis

- Endothelial cells are activated by growth factors to produce the phenotype of angiogenesis.
- The extracellular matrix of the vascular sites is altered, the basement membrane is degraded, and the endothelial cells bud, proliferate and migrate.
- Neonatal endothelial cell cord form tubular capillaries and lumen.
- Pericytes stabilize the newly formed capillary network and eventually form a mature blood vessel.

4.2.2　Regulatory mechanism of tumor angiogenesis

Angiogenesis is regulated by a series of angiogenic regulators, including angiogenic factors and angiogenesis inhibitors. The imbalance of angiogenic factors and inhibitory factors keeps blood vessels in a state of continuous growth and remodeling, eventually forms a distorted vascular system.

4.2.2.1　Angiogenenic factors and tumor angiogenesis

So far, dozens of endogenous molecules with the angiogenesis activity have been isolated and identified; however, only a few molecules, such as vascular endothelial growth factor (VEGF) and angiopoietin (angiopoietin) can directly affect the receptors on the surface of endothelial cells, causing their proliferation and activation. Most angiogenic factors, such as fibroblast growth factor and platelet-derived growth factor can promote angiogenesis by stimulating the expression of vascular endothelial growth factor or by recruiting related cells.

(1) VEGF and its receptor family

1) VEGF family

VEGF is mainly produced by perivascular cells and plays an important role in promoting angiogenesis and inhibiting the apoptosis of endothelial cells. VEGF is a mitogen inducible factor with the highest specificity to endothelial cells and the strongest angiogenesis ability. At the same time, it is the activator and inhibitor of fibrinogen which further regulates the degradation of basement membrane matrix during angiogenesis. VEGF can also increase the permeability of blood vessels and increase the ability of endothelial cells to accept stimulating factors. The family members identified so far include VEGF-A, VEGF-B, VEGF-C, VEGF-D, VEGF-E, and placenta growth factor (PlGF). These VEGF family members are secreted proteins and exist ashomodimers.

2) VEGF receptor family

VEGF receptors can only be activated by the binding of VEGF family members, thus triggering a series of signal transduction processes. So far, the VEGF receptors that have been identified include VEGFR 1, VEGFR 2 and VEGFR 3, all belonging to Fms like tyrosine (Flt) kinase family. VEGFR 1, also known as Flt-1, exists in hematopoietic stem cells, macrophages and mononuclear cells, and is related to the migration of these cells. VEGFR 2, also known as fetal liver kinase 1 (fetal liver kinase 1, Flk-1), is mainly present in vascular endothelial cells and lymphatic vascular endothelial cell surface, and can promote the proliferation and migration of endothelial cells and increase permeability of blood vessels. VEGFR3, also called Flt-4, can maintain the integrity of the endothelial cells and participate in tumor angiogenesis, and is essential for the development of embryonic vessels. In adults, Flt-4 mainly exists in lymphatic endothelial cells, and participates in maintaining the survival of lymphatic endothelial cells and promoting their proliferation and migration.

(2) Angiopoietin and TIE-2 receptor

Angiopoietin (Ang) is the first identified protein family which has angiogenic activity in human tumor tissue; the Ang family is composed of Ang-1, Ang-2, Ang-3 and Ang-4. These proteins can bind to tyrosine kinases with immunoglobin-like and EGF-like domains 2 (TIE-2) on the endothelial cell surface. Of all the Ang-family members, Ang-1 and Ang-2 are the most closely related to angiogenesis. Ang-1 is mainly synthesized by para-vascular support cells, and can bind specifically to the TIE-2 receptor on the membrane of the endothelial cells, causing receptor activation and subsequent signal transduction. Unlike VEGFR, the activation of TIE-2 cannot lead to the induction of endothelial cell proliferation, but its activation regulates the interaction between endothelial cells and perivascular interstitial cells, thereby maintaining vascular stability.

Ang-2 has similar structure with Ang-l, and can also bind with TIE-2. It is present at low levels in normal adult tissues, but its expression is significantly increased under hypoxic conditions or in response to VEGF stimulation. Under these conditions, Ang-2 and Ang-1 bind competitively with TIE-2, leading to the degradation of endothelial cells by the extracellular matrix, thereby promoting angiogenesis.

(3) Fibroblast growth factor family

The fibroblast growth factor (FGF) family is the most important family of angiogenic factors aside from the VEGF family. Basic fibroblast growth factor (bFGF) and acid Fibroblast Growth Factor (aFGF) have been extensively studied. Currently, four kinds of FGF receptors (FGFR) have been identified: FGFR1, FGFR2, FGFR 3 and FGFR 4. FGFR and VEGFR belong to the Tyrosine kinase receptor family, and their binding to FGF leads the activation by homologous or heterologous auto-phosphorylation, which further results in endothelial cell proliferation, migration and differentiation, and angiogenesis.

(4) Matrix Metalloproteinase

Matrix metalloproteinase (MMPs) are a class of Zn^{2+} dependent endogenous proteolytic enzymes, which are important angiogenesis factors that are responsible for promoting angiogenesis and extracellular matrix degradation. More than 20 MMPs have been discovered, and new members are continuing to emerge.

According to the structure and main substrates, this family can be divided into several types: collagenase, type Ⅳ collagenase, stromal lysin, matrix metallo proteinases, interstitial lysin and other MMPs. Among them, type Ⅳ collagenase and matrix metalloproteinase are the most important, which can directly regulate angiogenesis and play a key role in the degradation process of ECM, which is an essential component of angiogenesis under pathological and physiological conditions.

4.2.2.2 Angiogenesis inhibitor and tumor angiogenesis

Angiogenesis inhibitors can be divided into 7 categories: large molecule fragment of protein precursor enzyme, cytokines, protease inhibitors, angiogenesis inhibitor including TSP type 1 repeat motif, tissue inhibitors of metalloproteinases, tumor suppressor genes and other angiogenesis inhibitors.

(1) Large molecule fragment of protein precursor enzyme

1) Angiostatin

Angiostatin is one of the first discovered endogenous angiogenesis inhibitors and is a proteolytic product of plasminogen. It was first isolated from serum and urine of Lewis lung cancer mice. Angiostatin specifically inhibits the proliferation and migration of endothelial cells and induces apoptosis in endothelial cells.

2) Antiangiogenic antithrombin Ⅲ

Antiangiogenic antithrombin Ⅲ (aaAT) is a member of the serine protease inhibitor family. aaAT is an anti-thrombin with the hydroxyl end ring resected, and can specifically inhibit the proliferation and angiogenesis of endothelial cells, but not affect other normal cells or tumor cells.

3) Endostatin

Endostatin is an angiogenesis inhibitor isolated from the supernatant of rat angioma in 1997. It inhibits the proliferation and migration of endothelial cells and induces endothelial cell apoptosis.

(2) Cytokines

Interferon (IFN) is a regulatory cytokine with many biological functions. Its members IFN-α, IFN-β and IFN-γ can inhibit angiogenesis by downregulating the growth factors such as VEGF and bFGF in tumor cells.

(3) Serine protease inhibitor superfamily

Serine protease inhibitor (Serpin) superfamily is a protein family composed of a series of homologous proteins, some members of which, such as pigment epithelium derived factor (PEDF), MASPIN and angiotensinogen, have functions of inhibiting angiogenesis.

(4) Tissue inhibitor of metalloproteinase

Tissue inhibitor of metalloproteinase (TIMP) is an inhibitor of metalloproteinases naturally occurring *in vivo* including TIMP-1, TIMP-2, TIMP-3 and TIMP4. TIMP inhibits MMP in two stages; in the stage of activation of MMP zymogen, TMP binds to MMP to form stable complexes and inhibits its self-activation; in the stage of post-activation, TMP binds to MMP with the proportion of 1 : 1 to inhibit its activity.

4.2.2.3 Pericytes and angiogenesis

Pericyte (PC) refers parietal cells located at outer side of endothelial in the capillary. Pericytes can interact with endothelial cells through direct contact and paracrine pathway. A pericyte can interact with multiple endothelial cells at the same time to integrate and coordinate adjacent endothelial cells.

Pericytes and endothelial cells co-regulate angiogenesis and maturation through the main regulatory pathways including PDGF/PDGFRβ which regulates cell proliferation and migration of pericytes, TGFβ which regulates the differentiation of pericytes, as well as the Ang/TIE-2 and SIP/Edg signaling pathway which regulates vascular stability. Among these pathways, PDGF/PDGFRβ signaling pathwaysplay an important role in the regulation of angiogenesis and tumor metastasis.

4.2.2.4 Proto-oncogenes, tumor suppressor genes and tumor angiogenesis

Tumor angiogenesis is a multi-stage process that is contingent upongenetic changes in tumor cells (proto-oncogene activation, tumor suppressor gene inactivation) as well a shost response; each factor plays an indispensable role in tumor development.

(1) Proto-oncogene and tumor angiogenesis

1) Regulation of VEGF activity

The proto-oncogene *RAS* can directly up-regulate VEGF expression in tumor cells, and increase VEGF expression in adjacent stromal cells through the stimulation of cyclooxygenase-2 (COX-2), thus promoting angiogenesis. Like *RAS* gene, more than 20 proto-oncogenes promote tumor angiogenesis by inducing the expression of VEGF. *TP*53 protein, encoded by the tumor suppressor gene *TP*53, is a transcription factor that can down-regulate intracellular HIF-1α expression by inhibiting transcriptional activation of HIF-1α and by promoting ubiquitination and proteasome degradation of HIF-1α mediated by MDM2, further inhibiting the expression of HIF-1 targeted VEGF gene and angiogenesis

2) Regulation of scatter factor activity

In vivo, scatter factor (SF) is a potent angiogenic factor; in vitro, SF can stimulate endothelial cell proliferation, migration, differentiation and protease production. The activity of SF is mediated by the proto-onco gene c-MET, and the activity of MET kinase in endothelial cells is sufficient to stimulate angiogenesis.

3) Activity regulation of other proteases

In tumor cells, proteases stimulated by proto-oncogene protein products play important roles in establishing and maintaining of angiogenesis phenotype, and the activation of endothelial cells can mediate proteolytic degradation of matrix proteins. This is an important step in the initiation of neovascularization in human tumors and connective tissue.

(2) Tumor suppressor gene and tumor angiogenesis

The tumor suppressor gene *TP*53 can inhibit the angiogenesis by regulating the transcription of the downstream genes and stimulating the expression of *SMAD*4. The mutation of *TP*53 gene can lead to angiogenesis, which is beneficial to the rapid growth of the tumor and is often occurs late during tumor development.

4.2.3 Tumor angiogenesis and tumor treatment

Angiogenesis is an important pathological feature of tumorigenesis, and the inhibition of angiogenesis is of great significance in the treatment of tumors. Compared with traditional treatment methods (radiotherapy and chemotherapy) targeting tumor cells, angiogenesis inhibitors are broad-spectrum compounds that target tumor vascular endothelial cells; they are advantageous due totheir low toxicity, board-spectrum and hard to-produce drug resistance.

In February of 2004, the first tumor angiogenesis inhibitor in the world—bevacizumab was approved by the U.S. Food and Drug Administration (FDA), followed by many anti-angiogenesis drugs for different targets for tumor therapy. There are many drugs that are used to target VEGF, VEGFR and their signal transduction pathways in research. In addition, a variety of small molecule drugs targeting other growth factors and MMP have been developed, some of which have entered into the clinical trial stage.

Although several angiogenesis inhibitors are currently in clinical trials, the anti-tumor effect in human is not the same as that in animal experiments, implying that the angiogenesis is a complex process involving multiple factors and signaling pathways and blocking a signal pathway alone may not completely prevent angiogenesis. A combination of several angiogenesis inhibitors with different mechanisms of action should achieve a better outcome. Additionally, the combination of antiangiogenic therapy and radio-and chemotherapy may enhance the sensitivity of tumor cells to radiotherapy and chemotherapy, is expected to be more efficacious.

4.3　Progression and heterogeneity of tumor

4.3.1　Tumor progression

4.3.1.1　Tumor progression

Malignant tumors become more invasive during tumor growth. This phenomenon is called tumor progression, which includes accelerated growth, tumor infiltration of adjacent tissues and distant metastasis.

4.3.1.2　The Pathogenesis of Tumor Progression

The pathogenesis of the tumor progression includes: ①uncontrolled cellular proliferation; ②cell adhesion destabilization; ③enhancement of tumor matrix enzymolysis; ④increased tumor cell mobility; ⑤escape from immune surveillance; ⑥function change of mismatch repairing system; ⑦chromosomal instability.

4.3.2　The heterogeneity of tumor

4.3.2.1　The heterogeneity of tumors

Tumor heterogeneity describes the observation that different tumour cells can show distinct morphological and phenotypic profiles, including cellular morphology, gene expression, metabolism, motility, proliferation, and metastatic potential. This phenomenon occurs both between tumours (inter-tumour heterogeneity) and within tumours (intra-tumour heterogeneity). A minimal level of intra-tumour heterogeneity is a simple consequence of the imperfection of DNA replication: whenever a cell (normal or cancerous) divides, a few mutations are acquired-leading to a diverse population of cancer cells. The heterogeneity of cancer cells introduces significant challenges in designing effective treatment strategies. However, research into understanding and characterizing heterogeneity can allow for a better understanding of the causes and progression of disease. In turn, this has the potential to guide the creation of more refined treatment strategies that incorporate knowledge of heterogeneity to yield higher efficacy.

4.3.2.2   The pathogenesis of tumor heterogeneity

Because genetic instability, cancerous cells can mutate spontaneously due to the loss of *TP*53 gene and mutation of genes controlling DNA repair proteins. When these mutations accumulate to a certain extent, tumor cells will exhibitaltered biological characteristics. During the incubation period of the tumor, the cancerous cells proliferate many times. Therefore, the heterogeneity of the tumor cells occurs prior to clinical discovery. Some tumors, such as osteosarcoma, already contain potentially metastatic subsets at the time of diagnosis. Others, such as mixed salivary adenomas, rarely produce invasive subsets, and will only have such activity at its late stage even if at all.

4.3.3   Stem cell of cancer tumor

4.3.3.1   Stem cells

Stem cells (SC) area class of pluripotent cells with the ability to self-renew and/or differentiate into functionally specialized cell types. They are categorized into embryonic stem cells and adult stem cells according to the developmental stage of the organism. According to the developmental potential of stem cells, they can be divided into 3 categories: totipotent stem cell (TSC), pluripotent stem cells (pluripotent stem cell) and single stem cells (unipotentste cell).

4.3.3.2   Cancer stem

Cancer stem cells (CSCs) are cancer cells (found within tumors or hematological cancers) that possess characteristics associated with normal stem cells, specifically the ability to give rise to all cell types found in a particular cancer sample. One CSC can generate two heterogeneous cells by asymmetric division. One daughter cell would possess the same "stem-like" potential as the mother cell, while the other differentiates into a common non-tumorigenic cancer cell that make up most of the tumors. The consequence of this asymmetric type of division is the maintainance of two distinct cellular populations that contribute to tumor growth. CSCs may generate tumors through the stem cell processes of self-renewal and differentiation into multiple cell types. Such cells are hypothesized to persist in tumors as a distinct population and contribute torelapse and metastasis by giving rise to new tumors. Therefore, development of specific therapies targeted CSCs holds hope for improvement of survival and quality of life of cancer patients, especially for patients with metastatic disease.

4.3.3.3   The difference and similarity between CSC and SC

(1) The similarity between CSC and SC

①Having the characteristics of unlimited proliferation and differentiation;②similar signal transduction pathways regulating self-renewal;③showing different phenotypes and heterogeneity;④ terminal roughening enzyme activity;⑤ being able to transfer to different tissues and having similar homing as well as transferring pathways.

(2) The difference between CSC and SC

①The negative feedback mechanism of self-renewal signal transduction pathway has been compromised;②lack of ability to differentiate into mature cells;③tendency to accumulate errors of cell replication.

From the similarities and differences between CSC and SC, it is simple to hypothesize that CSC may be derived from the mutation of the corresponding normal stem cells.

4.3.3.4 Cancer stem cell and drug resistance

CSCs have many properties of normal stem cells. Stem cells have been able to divide indefinitely (under controlled conditions) due to many unique properties such asactive DNA repairing capacity, high expression of three phosphate adenosine binding cassette (ATP binding cassette, ABC) transporter, drug resistance, anti-radiation, and anti-apoptotic properties. As a result, cancer stem cells may also have drug resistance. The drug resistance of cancer stem cells may be related to the following factors: firstly, cancer stem cells are mostly in the G0 stage, and rarely proliferate; therefore they are not sensitive to many anti-cancer drugs, especially the cell-cycle specific drugs. Secondly, amutation or overexpression of the drug target causes the drug to lose its activity and to reduce its intracellular concentration.

4.3.3.5 Cancer stem cell and cancer therapy

Evidence suggests that CSCs area small group of cells that causes drug resistance and insensitivity to radiotherapy as well as chemotherapy. Drug resistance due to CSCs has been reported in leukemia, malignant melanoma, glioma and breast cancer. Targeted therapy for CSCs may improve the therapeutic effect of tumor therapy and reduce the risk of recurrence and metastasis. Strategies for targeting CSCs in order to treat cancer tumors include: elimination of CSCs using specific targeting molecules, reversing drug resistance due to the CSC phenotype, and inducing CSCs differentiation.

(1) Eliminating CSCs by specific targeting molecules

In human glioma, CD133+ glioma stem cells often express L1 cell adhesion molecule (L1CAM). In vitro studies, it was discovered that the capacity of forming nerve bulb decreased significantly after down-regulating L1CAM expression by RNAi in tumor cells. Marian and coworkers used Telomere terminal transferase inhibitor, GRN163L, for targeted cancer therapy to treat malignant glioblastoma (GBM) stem cells, which can shorten the telomere of GBM stem cells and reduce the cellular proliferation rate, leading to stem cell death. GRN163L can play a synergistic effect with the combined use of Temozolomide and radiation therapy to inhibit the growth of GBM stem cells more effectively.

(2) Reversing the drug resistance of CSCs

Clinical research shows that, in many kinds of malignant tumors, inhibiting the drug resistance of cancer stem cells can positively impact cancer chemotherapy regimens. For example, inhibition of resistance to a variety of drugs mediated by the ABC transporter family can reverse the tolerance of tumor stem cells to chemotherapy. In malignant melanoma stem cells, targeting of the ABCB5 transporter, which is largely responsible for drug efflux, by both monoclonal antibody inhibitors and siRNA have been shown to reverse drug resistance to Adriamycin in vitro.

4.4 Invasion and metastasis of tumor

Invasion and metastasis are the most important biological characteristics of malignant cancers that endanger life. Invasion describes the process utilized bytumor cells to destroy the surrounding normal tissue in various ways contributing to the expansion and distribution of the tumor cells into adjacent tissues. A preliminary sign that invasion has occurred can be observed due to the destruction of the basement membrane. Metastasis is a pathogenic agents spread from an initial or primary site to a different or secondary site within the host's body; it is typically spoken of as such spread by a cancerous tumor. The newly pathological sites, then, are metastases. Invasion happens during the whole process of metastasis and is the prelude to metastasis；metastasis is the result of invasion.

4.4.1　The main process during the invasion and metastasis of tumors

Invasion and metastasis are comprised of multiple steps，which can be figuratively called the multistep waterfall process. The main processes of the invasion and metastasis of various tumors are similar，and they include the following steps. A picture of invasion and metastasis.

4.4.1.1　The hyperplasia of tumor cells

The proliferation of tumor cells is the precondition and basis of tumor invasion. Tumor cells lack the ability to produce growth inhibitors，which can activate adenylate cyclase to form cAMP. The decrease of cAMP affects cell contact inhibition. The loss of contact inhibition，the proliferation of tumor within a close range，and the significant increase of internal pressure，all facilitate the invasion and metastasis of tumor cells to low pressure.

4.4.1.2　Angiogenesis

When the diameter of the tumor reaches 1–2 mm，the nutrients provided by micro-environment infiltration do not guarantee the growth of the cancer cells. At this point，the new blood vessels are formed via the process of angiogenesisin order to provide nourishment to the tumor. The entireprocess is under the common regulation by various antigenic factors and angiogenesis inhibitors.

4.4.1.3　Tumor cells sloughing and cell matrix invasion

Some tumor cells can secrete a substance that inhibits the expression of adhesion factors，thereby increasing the movement ability of tumor cells，and cause sloughing from the tumor body. The sloughed tumor cells break down the extracellular matrix by secreting a variety of proteolytic enzymes，thus facilitating cell matrix invasion.

4.4.1.4　Tumor cells enter circulation system

The tumor cells closely contact with the local capillaries or capillary endothelial cells，and thereby penetrate the wall of the tube. Neovascularization induced by the tumor is not only related to the growth of primary tumor，but also a basic condition for the invasion of free tumor cells into the circulatory system.

4.4.1.5　The formation of cancer embolus

Most of the cancer cells that enter the circulatory system are killed during transport. Only a few highly metastatic cells survive to form tiny tumor thrombus.

4.4.1.6　Tumor cells escape circulation system

When cancer cells adhere to vascular endothelium，endothelial cell retraction may be induced，thereby exposing extracellular matrix. Cancer cells can be attach to and digest the extracellular matrix to promote tumor metastasis to the secondary organ.

4.4.1.7　Tumor cells grow at secondary location

When tumor metastasis cells are in contact with secondary organ cells，they can induce multiple autocrne，paracrine or endocrine signaling cascades. These tumor cells proliferate and grow under the actions of various factors，and eventually form metastases tumor.

4.4.1.8　Metastatic carcinoma continues to spread

As the primary tumor，when the volume of the metastases increases to a certain extent，the newborn capillary network thus forms and connects the cancer tumor. The tumor cells of the metastatic tumor can also produce a secondary metastatic tumor by sloughing away and entering the circulatory system.

4.4.2　The main route of tumor invasion and metastasis

4.4.2.1　Invasion

(1) Interstitial

After tumor cells invade the surrounding tissue, they tend to grow in tissues which have minimum pressure and become irregular masses(Aka "Direct spread"). This phenomenon usually occurs in blood vessels and lymphatics surround the tumor. In addition, tumors also may grow in gaps surrounding nerve fibers.

(2) Lymphatic

Sometimes tumor cells invade the lymphatics and spread along the tubes; this circumstance usually take place at the final stage of cancer with lymphatic reflux disorder. Dilated lymph vessels full of tumor cells resemble white thin nets which are called "lymph vessel tumoremboli".

(3) Serous membrane

Tumor cells can invade the serous and lacunas beneath it, for example, in the case of uterine cavity metastasis of cervical cancer. However, one must distinguish between serosal involvement and metastasis as well as multicentric occurrence. In general, serosal involvement usually acts as continuous growth while multicentric occurrence is rare.

4.4.2.2　Metastasis

(1) Lymph node metastasis

Lymph node metastasis is a common pathway of metastasis, especially for epithelial malignant tumors. First, tumor cells that grow in stroma invade lymphatic through gaps between endotheliocytes. After invasion, tumor cells grow and move to the lymph nodes. Tumor cells subsequently grow in the marginal sinus before invading the parenchyma through endothelial and basilar membrane.

(2) Hematogenous metastasis

Hematogenous metastasis occurs astumor cells pass through the gaps between vascular endothelial cells and grow into tumor thrombi within the vessels. Together with blood cells, tumor cells are transported to other organs, pass through the vessel wall and basilar membrane, and eventually grow into metastatic tumors.

(3) Implantation metastasis

Besides lymph node metastasis and hematogenous metastasis, there is another metastasis pathway known as implantation. Tumor cells slough off the serous crevasse and then land on surface of serous, mucosa or other organs. After landed, tumor cells grow into metastatic tumors.

4.4.3　Molecular biology mechanism of tumor invasion and anti-metastasis

Tumor invasion is a complex process and involves tumor cell genetic code, surface structure, antigenic characteristics, adhesion ability, angiogenesis/coagulation factor generation ability, secretion and metabolic function and interaction between tumor cells and host cells as well as with stromal cells.

4.4.3.1　Genetic regulation and tumor invasion/metastasis

Tumor invasion and metastasis involve regulation of multiple oncogenes and tumor suppre. ssor genes. Studies have shown that dozens of oncogenes can promote tumor invasion or metastasis, such oncogenes include Bcl-2, MYC, MOS, RAF, FES, FMS, SER, FOS, TP53(mutation), ErbB-2 etc. Tumor suppressor genes such as NM23, TIMPs, KISS-1 have become a hot spot of cancer research.

4.4.3.2   Cell adhesion and tumor invasion/metastasis

Cell adhesion maintains tissue integrity. Adhesion is mediated by cell adhesion molecules (CAMs). There are many types of CAMs; however, cadherins and integrins are indispensable for tumor invasion and metastasis.

(1) Cadherins

Cadherins belong to a transmembrane protein family which form connections between homologous cells. There are 3 types of cadherins: E-cadherins are mainly distributed in epithelial tissue; P-cadherins are distributed in epithelial tissue and basal line of placenta; N-cadherins are mainly distributed in nervous, hearts, skeletal muscle and corneal. There is evidence suggesting that E-cadherins are most commonly associated with tumor invasion and metastasis. E-cadherins suppress tumor cells invasion or metastasis. Deficiency of E-cadherins accelerate tumor invasion and metastasis while up-regulation of E-cadherins suppress the spread of tumor cells.

(2) Integrin

Integrins area type of membrane mosaic glycoprotein. Integrins contain an α and β subunit. Variation of these subunits generate many subtypes of integrin. Integrins play an important role in mechano-transduction signaling to the nucleus. Aside from directly mediating adhesion and regulation of extracellular environment, integrins also help to alter cell morphology, movement, proliferation and cell longevity by regulating pathways of signal transduction, cytoskeleton and energy metabolism. Integrin signaling may also mediate cell escape from apoptosis.

Other CAMs such as immunoglobulin superfamily, selectin etc. are also involved in tumor invasion and metastasis.

4.4.3.3   Protein degradation and tumor invasion/metastasis

(1) Extracellular matrix (ECM)

Major components of ECM include collagen, glycoprotein, proteoglycan and glucosamine. ECM exists largely in the basal part of the cell in the form of the basement membrane. Collagen is the main component of ECM; there are at least 12 types of collagens while type I, E, E and W are the most widely characterized. Type I, E, E collagens are the main components of Interstitial connective tissue while type W collagen mainly exists in inner basement membrane.

Tumor invasion and metastasis are dynamic process which includes protein synthesis and degradation. Basement membrane collagen degradation is an important early events of tumor invasion. This process does not just rely on the type and amount of protease, but also the balance between protease and their respective inhibitors.

(2) Matrix metalloproteinase and inhibitor

As mentioned above, ECM degradation requires protease enzymes. Protease is a super family made up of many components. MMPs and their inhibitors play an important role in tumor invasion and metastasis.

Based on their structure and function, MMPs are divided into 4 different types: collagenase, gelatinase, matrix lysozyme, and Membrane-type matrix metalloproteinases. MMPs can degrade different types of ECM depending upon their type. Activity of MMPs is related to the tumor invasion and metastasis, that is to say, enhanced activity of MMPs accelerate tumor invasion/metastasis.

(3) Lysosomes and their regulators

Fibrinogen becomes fibrinolytic enzyme under the action of plasminogen activator. Fibrinolytic enzyme can degrade most matrix components and it can induce collagenase to become active and participate in ablation. These processes are important for tumor angiogenesis, tumor cell exfoliation, matrix invasion, invasion/

escape circulatory system, secondary organ metastasis and microenvironment transformation. plasminogen activator promotes these processes while plasminogen activator inhibitor suppress them. These processes are depended on the balance between PA and PAI.

(4) Angiogenesis and invasion/metastasis

When tumor size reaches a specific level, it requires angiopoiesis to receive oxygen and key nutrients, as well as to transport waste away from the tumor site. Angiogenesis is essential for tumor growth and invasion and is needed through the whole process of tumor metastasis.

(5) Tumor stem cells and invasion/metastasis

Some researchers believe that CSCs might be the primary cause of tumor metastasis, and propose the theory that CSCs are the "seed" of tumor metastasis. Studies show that metastasis of the same primary tumor expressing the same karyotype and may came from single cell cloning process. CSCs retain powerful proliferation potential; once a distant tissue is reached after exiting the circulatory system, CSCs can trigger hyperplasia of cloning while non-CSCs usually cannot.

(6) Immunity and invasion/metastasis

In the past thirty years, the relationship between the immune system and tumor metastasis has attracted much attention. Key issues that are actively being researched include the heterogeneity and metastasis of tumor cells, the internal immunogenicity of tumor cells and the identification and killing ability of host. Hosts' immunity includes NK cell, T cell, macrophage, TIL cell and cytotoxic T lymphocyte etc. Human immune system can be divided into systemic and local immunization. Tumor cells must avoid every one of these systems before they can reach and grow on the secondary organ. Very few tumor cells possess the necessary traits to escape immune surveillance and give rise to a metastatic tumor.

Immune editors are a new concept that summary the interaction between the immune system and the tumor. Immune editors includes 3 processes: rejection, balance and escape. Through immune editing, tumor cells change their immunogenicity to escape from host's immune systems and form clinically observed tumors. Through the immune editing process, the invasion and metastasis of tumor cells are enhanced and increases tumor develoment.

(7) Tumor microenvironment and tumor invasion/metastasis

The microenvironment is the complex internal environment of the tumor. Multiple matrix cells are involved, for example, fibroblasts, immune/inflammatory cells, adipocytes, glial cells, smooth muscle cells, and some types of vascular cells. These cells can be induced by tumor cells, and produce a large number of growth factors, chemokines and matrix degrading enzymes around them, which is conducive to the proliferation and invasion of tumor cells.

The proliferation of the tumor requires the establishment of an external environment suitable for its own growth. As tumor growth progresses, the nutritional conditions of the tumor environment cannot meet the growth needs of the tumor. However tumor cells can continuously construct new nutritional and metabolic networks by inducing tumor angiogenesis that subsequently promote the growth of tumor cells. This underlying behavior fuels tumor progression, and is the basis for the malignant change and metastasis of the tumor.

4.4.3.4 Tumor invasion and metastasis and tumor treatment

It is a lengthy process for tumor cells to distantly metastasize from the primary tumor. If metastas is meets obstacles, metastasis cannot continue. At present, there are various therapies for tumor invasion and metastasis, including gene therapy, cell adhesion factor inhibitors, matrix metalloproteinase inhibitors, angiogenesis inhibitors, etc.

The US Food and Drug Administration have approved a number of anti-tumor angiogenesis drugs to enter the clinical, Bevacizumab, for example, binds to VEGF to prevent its binding to the endothelial cell surface receptor, inhibit the mitosis of endothelial cells and reduce the formation of neovascularization. Through these processes, Bevacizumab plays anti-tumor role by blocking blood, oxygen and other nutrients that are needed for tumor growth, thereby preventing tumor, growth, invasion, and metastasis.

Ma Wang, Guan Chengnong

Chapter 5

Tumor Pathology

5.1 Definition and role of pathology

Pathology is the study of the essential nature of diseases and especially of the structural and functional changes produced by them. In medical terms, pathology is the analysis of the histological and physiological deviations from the normal that constitute disease or characterize a particular disease. Among medical disciplines, pathology plays a critical role in understanding of disease and in decision-making for quality patient care. Particularly, pathology is one of the essential clinical components in management of cancer.

Tumor, or more precisely neoplasia (Latin, new growth), is an abnormality of cellular differentiation, maturation, and control of growth. Dr. Rupert Willis, a British pathologist, defined in early 1950 that "A neoplasm is an abnormal mass of tissue, the growth of which exceeds and is uncoordinated with that of the surrounding normal tissues and persists in the same excessive manner after cessation of the stimuli that evoked the change". His definition of neoplasm is still one of the best to for understanding the complicated features of this unique entity. Neoplasms are commonly recognized by the formation of masses of abnormal tissue. Though tumor could be applied to any swelling, it is used most commonly to denote suspected neoplasm (Figure 5-1).

Neoplasms can be roughly divided into two categories: benign or malignant depending on nature of the neoplasms. Among other features, the most distinctive parameter of the malignant neoplasms is their ability of to spread from the site of origin, namely metastasis. In contract, benign neoplasms grow but remain localizcd. Some tumors, however, have tendency to recur but rarely metastasize, and belong to so-called borderline tumor.

Biologically, all malignant neoplasms possess certain common characteristics, such as the capacity for uncontrolled continuous growth. Morphologically, they display enormously varied gross and microscopic features. Furthermore, biological and phenotypical features of the neoplasm are determined by the underlying molecular abnormalities of tumor cells. These biological and histological variations as well as genomic derivations are foundations for their diverse clinical presentation, behavior, effects, response to therapy, andprognosis.

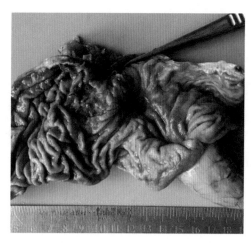

Figure 5-1   Uicerative mass on the gastric flexure

Morphologically, malignant cells display great variability in the size and shape, or pleomorphism. Particularly, the variability of nuclei is the landmark changes of malignant tumor. Typically, the cancer nuclei is two to three or more bigger in the counterpart of normal cells, leading to higher nuclei to cytoplasm ratio. In addition, the quality of nuclei is changed, with thickened nuclear membrane, tortured nuclear groves and enlarged nucleoli. Furthermore, the architecture of cell arrangement is changed in malignant tumor. In normal colon mucosa, for example, the epithelial cells lining on the mucosal surface is single layer with regular nuclei proximal to the basement membrane. In colon cancer, the neoplastic cells can arranged to two or more cellular layer with irregular arranged nuclei. Though it is a feature characteristic of malignant neoplasms, pleomorphism could also be seen in non-malignant cell types e. g. , neuroendocrine cells, Arias-Stella reaction. Therefore, to make a malignant diagnosis, other morphological features should be considered.

Other morphological features of malignant cells are increased mitotic figures, presence of atypical mitotic figures, increased single cell necrosis (apoptotic body), massive necrosis, lymphovascular invasion.

5.2   Classification of malignant neoplasms

Cancers may be classified in different ways. Traditionally cancers have been grouped by their primary site of origin or by their histological or tissue types. Based on tissue types cancers may be classified into eight major categories.

5.2.1   Carcinoma

This type of cancer originates from the epithelium that forms the linings of internal organs, such as pancreatobillary system and gastrointestinal tract, and the external linings of the body, such as skin(Figure 5-2).

Carcinomas have two major types-adenocarcinoma and squamous cell carcinoma. Adenocarcinoma develops in an organ with columnar epithelium or gland, such as endometrial and urothelial mucosa. Squamous cell carcinoma originates in squamous epithelium, such as oral cavity, esophagus and skin. Rarely, a cancer can consist of the above two epithelial types, and it is called adenosquamous carcinoma(Figure 5-3).

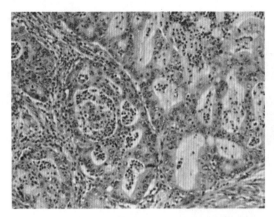

Notice the pleomorphic enlarged tumor cells with abnormal arrangement and necrosis, the land-markers of malignant tumors.

Figure 5-2　Adenocarcinomain Gastric body

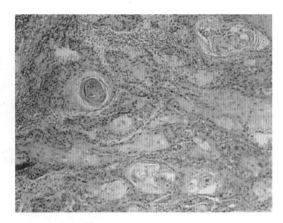

It is well to moderately differentiated, due to remaining some morphological features of normal squamous epithelium.

Figure 5-3　Squamous cell carcinoma in esophagus

5.2.2　Neuroendocrine carcinoma

Neuroendocrine carcinoma is a specialized malignant epithelial tumors, arising in the neuroendocrine cells throughout the body, such as in the gastrointestinal tract and pulmonary system.

5.2.3　Sarcoma

Sarcomas, malignant neoplasms of mesenchymal tissue, originate in connective tissues such as muscles, bones, cartilage and fat. Sarcoma affects the young most commonly. Sarcomas appear like the tissue in which they grow.

Terminology of common sarcomas. Bone cancer is one of the sarcomas termed osteosarcoma. Other examples include liposarcoma (adipose tissue), leiomyosarcoma (smooth muscles), fibrosarcoma (fibrous tissue), rhabdomyosarcoma (skeletal muscles), chondrosarcoma (of the cartilage), angiosarcoma or hemangioendothelioma (blood vessels), Glioma or astrocytoma (neurogenic connective tissue of the central nerve system), and myxosarcoma (primitive embryonic connective tissue). Rare mesenchymal tumors can consist of two or more connective tissues, such as mixed mesodermal tumor (mixed connective tissue types).

5.2.4　Malignant melanoma

Melanocytes in the skin and mucosal surface give rise to melanoma. A brown pigment called melanin, which gives the skin its tan or brown color, protects the deeper layers of the skin from some of the harmful effects of the sun. Long exposure of ultraviolet light from sun is the major cause of malignant melanoma.

5.2.5　Malignant mesothelioma

Malignant mesothelioma, a special neoplasm, arises in the membranous lining of pleural and peritoneal cavities. It is known that asbestos exposure could result in malignant mesothelioma.

5.2.6　Lymphoma

These are cancers of the reticuloendothelial system, or lymphomas are "solid cancers" of hematopoietic system. These may affect lymph nodes throughout the body, bone marrow, and lymphoid tissue at specific sites like stomach, brain, intestines etc, the latter is referred to as extranodal lymphomas.

Lymphomas consist of two major types-Hodgkin's lymphoma and Non-Hodgkin's lymphomas. In Hodgkin lymphoma there is characteristic presence of Reed-Sternberg cells in the tissue samples which are not present in Non-Hodgkin lymphoma. Non-Hodgkin lymphomas are sub-classified into a number of special lymphomas, depending on morphology, genetic abnormalities identified byfluorescence in situ hybridization (FISH) and molecular tests, and clinical characteristics. For example, T cell lymphoma and B cell lymphoma can be identified by characteristics of differential cell membrane receptors and gene arrangement.

5.2.7　Leukemia

Contract to lymphomas, the solid form of hematopoietic system, leukemia is a group of cancers that are liquid components of hematopoietic system. These cancers affect the bone marrow which is the site for blood cell production, due to that the bone marrow produce excessive immature white blood cells, or blastic cells, that fail to perform their usual actions and the patient is often prone to infection.

Common types of leukemia include:

1) Acute myelocytic leukemia (AML)-these are malignancy of the myeloid and granulocytic white blood cell series commonly seen in childhood.

2) In contrast, chronic myelocytic leukemia (CML)-this is usually seen in adulthood.

3) Acute lymphatic, lymphocytic, or lymphoblastic leukemia (ALL)-these are malignancy of the lymphoid and lymphocytic blood cell series seen in childhood and young adults.

4) Chronic lymphatic, lymphocytic, or lymphoblastic leukemia (CLL)-this is seen in the elderly.

5) Myeloma: a type of blood cancer, due to neoplastic proliferation of the plasma cells of bone marrow.

Based on morphology, flow cytometry, genetic tests and molecular profiling, AML is further sub-classified into several types, which are differently managed clinically.

5.2.8　Mixed neoplasms

These have two or more malignant components, such as teratocarcinoma consisting of three cancerous elements. Other examples include mixed mesodermal tumor, carcinosarcoma, and adenosquamous carcinoma.

(1) Pathology grade of cancer

By comparison of cancer with its original normal counterpart, cancers can be graded into three or four groups. In other words, the neoplastic proliferative cells with respect to surrounding normal tissues determines the grade of the cancer. Morphologically, the abnormal features of cancer consist cellular abnormal and architectural abnormal, when compared with normal cells. Increasing abnormality increases the grade, from 1–4.

Cells that are well differentiated closely resemble normal specialized cells and belong to low grade tumors. Cells that are undifferentiated are highly abnormal with respect to surrounding tissues. These are high grade tumors.

1) Grade 1: well differentiated cells with slightly abnormality.

2) Grade 2: cells are moderately differentiated and slightly more abnormal.

3) Grade 3: cells are poorly differentiated and very abnormal.

4) Grade 4: cells are immature and primitive and undifferentiated.

(2) Pathology stage of cancer

Stage of Cancer is essential part of oncology, and pathology plays a key role in staging cancers. There are several types of staging methods. The most commonly used method uses classification in terms of tumor size (T), the degree of regional spread or node involvement (N), and distant metastasis (M). This is called the TNM staging.

For example, T_0 signifies with no evidence of tumor, T_{1-4} signifies increasing tumor size and involvement and Tis signifies carcinoma in situ or limited to surface cells. Similarly N_0 signifies no nodal involvement and N_{1-4} signifies increasing degrees of lymph node involvement. N_x signifies that node involvement cannot be assessed. Metastasis is further classified into two-M_0 signifies no evidence of distant spread while M_1 signifies evidence of distant spread.

Stages may be divided according to the TNM staging classification. Stage 0 indicates cancer being in situ or limited to surface cells while stage I indicates cancer being limited to the tissue of origin. Stage II indicates limited local spread, Stage II indicates extensive local and regional spread while stage IV is advanced cancer with distant spread and metastasis.

5.3   Methodologies used in tumor pathology

5.3.1   Intraoperative pathology diagnosis

Intraoperative pathology diagnosis, or rapid frozen section diagnosis is a common perioperative process to help decision-making for management of cancer patient. Such as to assess resection margins of a head and neck squamous cell carcinoma. The College of American Pathologists requires the frozen section diagnosis be done within twenty minutes.

Though a zero error rate is not realistic, given the limitations of frozen tissue, pathologist sampling, and the technique itself, among other factors, all efforts should be made to efficient communications between the surgeon and pathologist. Often times, it is helpful for the surgeon to come to the pathology frozen suite to review the frozen section tissue, orientate the specimen, and discuss relevant issues regarding the case.

5.3.2   Immunohistochemistry

Immunohistochemistry (IHC) one of the most common techniques used in tumor pathology, is a special technique for localizing protein expression visualized at a light microscopic level. It is based on the specific antigen-antibody reaction in the tissue. Although IHC was developed in early 1940s, the method has only found general application in surgical pathology since late 1980s after the IHC technique became applicable to routinely formalin-fixed and paraffin-embedded sections. In the meantime, a number of technical developments in IHC have created sensitive detection systems, from the simplest one-step direct conjugate method to multiple-step detection techniques such as the avidin-biotin conjugate(ABC), peroxidase antiperoxidase, and biotin-streptavidin techniques as well as the highly sensitive polymer-based labeling methods. Furthermore, the hybridoma technique has revolutionized IHC and facilitated the manufacture of abundant, specific monoclonal antibodies. In addition, the antigen retrieval technique has simplified pretreatment procedures, and dramatically increased the intensity of IHC staining. Since it also demonstrates a higher level of reproducibility compared to the traditionally enzyme digestion pretreatment, the antigen retrieval technique, to some extends, ensures consistency of IHC staining results. Though the details of these techniques are beyond the scope of our discussion, one should be familiar with all steps in the "total IHC test" in order to detect, reduce and correct deficiencies in IHC. Equally important, in order to achieve a successful result, one should be familiar with the antigen under investigation before performing IHC staining, particularly being familiar with the subcellular localization of the antigen and detailed information regarding the primary antibody and detection system(Figure 5-4).

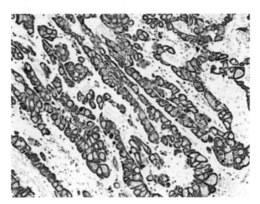

Figure 5-4   CK20 positively expressed in
gastric adenocarcinoma

5.3.3   Applications of immunohistochemistry in pulmonary lung neoplasms

Based on clinicopathologic features and biologic properties,the heterogeneous spectrum of lung carcinomas are roughly separated into two major groups:non-small cell lung cancers (NSCLCs) and small cell lung cancers (SCLCs). Separating these groups of neoplasms is critically important for treatment purposes, while specific histologic categorization of NSCLCs is less important. Although diagnosis and classification of lung cancer are mainly based on histopathological features,immunohistochemistry (IHC) is frequently used to confirm or eliminate a pathologic diagnosis due to the existence of overlapping morphology between examples of NSCLC and SCLC,lung carcinomas and low grade pulmonary neuroendocrine neoplasms,lung carcinomas and malignant mesotheliomas, and primary and other metastatic extrapulmonary malignancies. In fact,a broad spectrum of antibodies has been increasingly applied for resolution of these differential diagnostic questions.

In addition to features intrinsic to the neoplasms,the pathologist is also increasingly challenged by the quality of the samples submitted for diagnosis. Small bronchoscopic biopsies and cytology samples,and fine needle aspirates (FNAs),have become the preferred media for diagnosis due to the obvious patient care advantages of bronchoscopy and fine needle aspiration over operative procedures. In order to maximize the information one can derive from these samples,ancillary tests including IHC are frequently ordered. By working closely with the clinician who performs a careful clinical history and assessment,the pathologist should develop a working differential diagnosis based on tumor location, radiological characteristics of the tumor and tumor morphology. This information is essential to utilizing IHC as a cost-effective tool in patient care. No doubt,when applied selectively and judiciously,IHC is a powerful tool for the accurate pathologic classification of neoplasms in the lung.

Among "specific" markers studied for pulmonary epithelium, thyroid transcription factor-1 (TTF-1) has received the most attention. TTF-1,a 38 kD nuclear protein and a member of the Nkx2 homeodomain transcription factor family,was originally characterized as a promoter of thyroid-specific transcription of the thyroglobulin and thyroperoxidase genes. TTF-1 was subsequently detected in the fetal lung as well as within certain areas of the diencephalon. In normal lung tissues,TTF-1 has been observed primarily in the nuclei of alveolar cells,particularly type Ⅱ alveolar pneumocytes,non-ciliated bronchiolar cells (Clara cells), and basal cells. Among NSCLCs,up to 94% of adenocarcinomas have been reported to express TTF-1. Immunoprofiles of primary lung adenocarcinomas vs. metastatic adenocarcinomas is summarized in Table 5-1.

Table 5–1 Immunoprofiles of primary lung adenocarcinomas vs. metastatic adenocarcinomas

Tumor site	TTF-1[a]	CK7	CK20	ER	PSA	GCDFP	INHB	HEP	CD10
Lung	+[b]	+	--	--	---	--	--	---	---
Colorectal	---	---	+	--	---	--	--	---	--
Breast	---	+	--	+	---	+	--	---	--
Prostate	---	+/-	+/-	--	++	+	--	---	--
Ovary	---	+	--	+	--	--	+	---	--
Hepatocellular	---	+/-	+/-	--	---	--	--	++	--
Kidney	---	+/-	--	--	---	--	--	--	+
Adrenocortical	---	--	--	--	---	--	++	---	--

[a] TTF-1: thyroid transcription factor-1; ER: estrogen receptor; PSA: prostate specific antigen; GCDFP: gross cystic disease fluid protein; INHB: inhibin; HEP: hepatocyte-related antigen.

[b] ++, almost always diffuse, strong positive; +, mostly positive with variable staining; --mostly negative with variable staining; --, almost always negative.

5.3.4　Fluorescence in *situ* hybridization

Fluorescence in *situ* hybridization (FISH) is a test that "maps" the genetic material in a person's cells. This test can be used to visualize specific genes or portions of genes. For example, HER_2 receptors receive signals that stimulate the growth of breast cancer cells, and HER_2 gene amplifications have been found in several malignant tumors. Specifically, HER_2/neu overexpression and/or gene amplification is currently the major criterion for selection of patients with breast cancer for HER_2/neu-targeted therapy with the recombinant humanized anti-p185 HER_2/neu antibody trastuzumab. Therefore, FISH testing is routinely done on breast cancer tissue removed during biopsy or resection to see if the cells have extra copies of the HER_2 gene. The more copies of the HER_2 gene that are present, the more HER_2 receptors the cells have.

Generally, the FISH test is not as widely available as another method of HER_2 testing, called immunohistochemistry. However, FISH is considered more accurate and golden standard to assess the HER_2 status of tumor. In many cases, a lab will do the IHC test first, ordering FISH only if the IHC results don't clearly show whether the cells are HER_2 positive or negative (Figure 5–5).

In addition, FISH is widely used in diagnosing sarcomas, and in classifying leukemias and lymphomas.

5.3.5　Electron microscopy

There are two types of electron microscopes(EM), transmission electron microscope and scanning electron microscope.

The transmission electron microscope (TEM) uses a high voltage beam of electrons to create an image of a specimen. The electrons emitted by an electron gun are accelerated, focused and transmitted through a partially transparent specimen. The beam then emerges from the specimen and carries information to the objective lens where magnification occurs. Photographic recording of the image can also occur by exposing film directly to the beam. TEMs can yield information about the morphology including size, shape and arrangement of particles. They can also relay crystallographic information for example the arrangement of atoms and their degree of order, compositional information (relative ratios of the elements and compounds or defects in areas as small as a few nanometers).

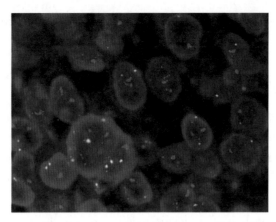

The red dots represent the *HER2* genes, and the blue dots are centromere. Notice the ratio of HER2/centromere: greater than 2.2.

Figure 5-5   FISH results showed *HER2* gene amplification in breast cancer

Unlike the TEM, the scanning electron microscope (SEM) makes an image by using the electron beam that scans the specimen across a rectangular area. While an SEM produces an image with a slightly lower resolution, it can analyze larger specimens and can produce great representations of 3D shapes. Like the TEM, a SEM can present information about morphology, composition and crystallography. However, they are limited to looking at composition in areas of one micrometer and degrees of order on single-crystal particles of greater than 20 micrometers. In addition, a SEM can also yield information about topography, the surface features and texture, down to a few nanometers.

Due to many new techniques and tools used in tumor pathology, such as IHC, FISH, flow cytometry, molecular tests and next generation sequencing (NGS), EM has not been used as frequently as thirty years ago. However, EM, particularly TEM still plays a role in assessment of ultrastructural abnormalities of rare tumor and in diagnosis of undifferentiated malignancies.

5.4   Molecular diagnosis used in tumor pathology

Although the future of molecular diagnostics is likely to be shaped by current trends and technologies, this field is evolving rapidly in ways that we can hardly predict with accuracy beyond a few years. One certainty is that the use of molecular diagnostics will become far more routinely established in clinical practice. This will be particularly true for tests using technologies or platforms that have established robust performance characteristics identifying molecular alterations directly paired with targeted therapeutics forming companion diagnostics. We can forecast the changing landscape in terms of evolving newer techniques or methods, paradigm shifts in the use of targeted therapies and companion diagnostics, and other ancillary viewpoints such as how enhancing the assessment of quality, clinical utility, and health economic effects may bear upon decisions related to clinical practice guidelines, regulatory approval, and reimbursement for these tests. From each of these perspectives, a broader view of novel molecular therapeutics emerges in which we are continually adapting new technology, improving clinical utility, and evaluating costs vs. benefits for the patient, laboratory and healthcare systems.

5.4.1   Evolving targets and techniques in cancer diagnostics

Molecular diagnostic assays in oncology have expanded rapidly in the last decade following the earlier development of diagnostic assays based on immunohistochemistry (IHC), cytogenetics, flow cytometry, fluorescent in situ hybridization (FISH), PCR, and more recently real-time PCR (RT-PCR), dideoxy (Sanger) sequencing, and other techniques. Many of these techniques have been incorporated into assays that are routinely ordered in the work-up of various hematolymphoid disorders and some solid tumors. In many cases they are used to determine prognosis, monitor response to treatment, identify recurrence, and for other purposes. Newer technologies such as massively parallel pyrosequencing (454 sequencing), competitive genomic hybridization SNP arrays, methylation or gene expression assays, microRNA expression levels, and mass spectrometry-based proteomic analysis offer tantalizing glimpses into what might be used in future diagnostic assays and what challenges these tools might present. Examples of novel applications today include dual in situ hybridization (DISH) assays for HER2 that merge chromogenic in situ hybridization (CISH) with IHC to better identify gene amplification and genetic heterogeneity in breast, gastric, and ovarian carcinomas and help avoid false-negative results on small biopsies. High resolution SNP arrays pinpoint copy number changes such as small deletions or gains as well as features of allelic imbalance (loss of heterozygosity) or uniparental disomy associated with Beckwith-Wiedemann syndrome and cancer predisposition.

Both FISH and SNP arrays can detect chromosomal alterations not visible by conventional karyotyping and have also been used to identify the origins of chromosomal fragments such as double minutes and homozygous staining regions which can provide clues to gene amplification or deletion that are important to tumorigenesis and tumor behavior. SNP arrays have identified deleted tumor-suppressor or regulatory genes associated with aggressive forms of hepatocellular carcinoma and genes associated with key oncologic drivers such as MYCN amplification. They have also been used to distinguish neoplasms that are morphologically similar but prognostically different (e.g., renal tumors or brain tumors) or to distinguish tumor from reactive tissue such asgliosis. A significant topic of interest for SNP microarrays are small copy number variations (CNVs), which are common but may have no known or established clinical relevance. Interpreting such findings requires considerable experience to put them into proper context.

5.4.2   Next generation sequencing the cancer genome

Dideoxy (Sanger) sequencing was initially introduced into the clinical laboratory for determination of HIV genotypes associated with drug resistance, but the procedure has more recently become commonly used for determination of EGFR mutations, KRAS mutations, and other single-base pair substitutions and frameshift deletions, such as those responsible for loss of p53 function in Li-Fraumeni syndrome-related sarcomas. However, major limitations of Sanger sequencing relate to sensitivity in detecting minority allelic variants, need for relatively high DNA input (up to 150 ng per exon typically) and there is a possible error of interpretation requiring a high degree of training and experience for the proper use of this technique.

Massively parallel high throughput pyrosequencing (454 sequencing) and bead-based microarrays have proven to be highly sensitive methods that create opportunities to perform high-resolution DNA analysis, to evaluate gene expression and methylation, analyze exome sequences, and to sequence very complex and polymorphic gene structures such as HLA. High throughput sequencing also provides a powerful way to evaluate amplified disease-specific regions from mononuclear cell subclones to quantify minimal residual chronic lymphocytic leukemia (CLL) after therapy.

Various direct gene sequencing assays have generated a paradox similar to that for SNP microarrays: is the information gained useful or is it unnecessary information that may be misleading or without benefit? Despite promises of a new era of personalized medicine based on whole genome sequencing, there are lingering concerns about how to generate truly useful clinically "actionable" reports with such techniques based on the results of "expected" potential mutations and "unexpected" genetic abnormalities. In the cancer genome, passenger alterations may vastly outnumber the driver events, leading to considerable confusion at best and to unnecessary worry and concern for patients or liability for physicians at worst.

Most of these neoplastic genetic changes are somatic, but answers to uncertainties about inherited colon cancer, prostate cancer, and breast cancer risk will also undoubtedly lie in the use of high throughput sequencing to initially identify panels of known target genes in both normal and cancer cells, followed by advanced bioinformatics to rapidly evaluate small changes or SNPs and compare them with established clinical laboratory databases, similar to what is currently practiced in HIV genotyping, but vastly expanded with the use of Genome Wide Association Studies (GWAS). These relational databases of genomic information will grow substantially over the next decade. As disease markers and their associations are refined, management of patient care and outcomes will improve. These technologies introduce new levels of data complexity and cost that will have to be optimized to bring them into routine use in the clinical laboratory. In short, NGS is now widely used in clinical oncology for decision-making and precision cancer medicine. As an example, the targeted NGS of colorectal adenocarcinoma is summarized in Table 5-2.

5.4.3　Combining technologies in oncology reporting

Despite rapid advances, it remains likely that traditional and novel diagnostics will be combined and used in a complementary way for the foreseeable future. Hematopathology reports currently feature morphologic descriptions, flow cytometry, cytogenetics, and molecular genetics on a single summary report. We can imagine future oncology reports combining many different DNA targets and assay modalities. For instance, PathFinderTG integrates LOH analysis near tumor-suppressor genes, KRAS mutations, cytology, DNA quantity and quality, and protein markers to identify pancreatic cysts as mucinous or non-mucinous and to evaluate the risk of malignancy. Reports can or soon could also define hepatitis B virus mutants (HBx) associated with hepatocellular carcinoma, HLA subtypes associated with ovarian cancer prognosis, and HPV genotypes associated with highest risk of cervical cancer, among others. Imagine a report predicting recurrence of HBV-related hepatocellular carcinoma after liver transplantation based on evaluation of plasma DNA for allelic variants matched to the original tumor DNA. This has already been described using matrix-assisted laser desorption ionization-time of flight (MALDI-TOF) mass spectrometry (on plasma DNA) paired with SNP microarray profiling of tumor DNA extracted from formalin-fixed, paraffin-embedded (FFPE) tissues (Figure 5-6).

5.4.4　"Liquid biopsy": from tissue to blood

Various diagnostic needs require the use of many sample types such as nasal, cervical and buccal mucosal swabs, fine needle aspiration cytology, liquid-based cytology media (for cervical cancer screening), and FFPE tissue. Whereas infectious or germline disorder assays are usually performed using fresh tissue DNA sources such as whole-blood lymphocytes, the vast majority of oncology-related defects are acquired or somatic changes seen only in tumor cells. For laboratories, this presents challenges as they need to work with FFPE or limited sample sizes of rather precious tumor procured from CT-guided needle biopsies, aspirates, and other invasive procedures. More recent whole genome amplification (WGA) techniques such as multiple displacement amplification (MDA) have enabled genomic characterization of single cells from early

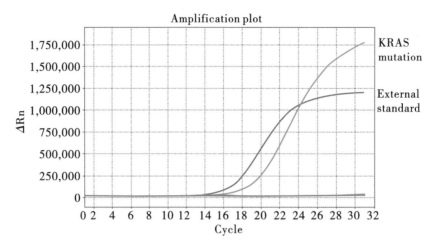

Figure 5-6　KRAS mutation in colon cancer

stage embryos for preimplantation genetic diagnosis of fragile X syndrome and other disorders, prefacing techniques aimed at the cancer genome using very limited sample sources such as circulating DNA or tumor cells.

　　With innovative technologies and continuing improvements, the molecular diagnosis of cancer will perhaps become routine like many blood tests. Larger high throughput instruments with integrated software and optimized reagents will reduce laborious steps, run failures, and reporting variations, driving "costs per test" lower over time. At the opposite end of spectrum, point-of-care testing (POCT) has the potential to reduce turnaround time and eliminate some of the pre-analytic costs such as sample packaging, handling, and shipping. POCT devices today can assay a few analytes in a short period of time, usually within an hour, and recent advances in lab-on-a-chip technologies could make POCT for nucleic acids practical in settings such as the physician office clinic or even a patient's home. These uses and necessary performance characteristics are still to be fully defined but might first encompass recurrence monitoring for established malignancies (e.g., re-staging) or other targeted clinical applications.

　　Determining whether a specific molecular drug target is present in metastatic tumor cells could influence future cancer care and have predictive value; however, it has yet to be established whether molecular analysis of circulating tumor cells (CTCs) or circulating cell-free tumor DNA would predict drug response more accurately than analysis of a primary tumor biopsy specimen. Monitoring genetic variation over time is a potential application. Illustrating this point, there are reports of HER2 positive CTCs in patients with a HER2 negative primary tumor, which might affect the selection of trastuzumab (Herceptin) in advanced disease. There are also descriptions of discordant PIK3CA mutations in metastatic breast cancer, EGFR mutations detected in plasma DNA, BRAF mutations found in circulating melanoma cells, and ERG, AR and PTEN alterations found in circulating prostate cancer cells in patients non-responsive to castration. Whether or not treatment is initiated or changed with this information, such assays have potential value as a noninvasive means of identifying and confirming recurrent or metastatic disease when biopsy is not possible. Genetic monitoring for disease recurrence is already commonly used in chronic myelogenous leukemia, where relatively abundant leukemic cells provide much more tumor DNA than can be found in relatively rare circulating solid tumor cells or cell-free serum or plasma DNA.

5.4.5　Companion diagnostics：predicting response to specific therapies

The last few years have seen growing recognition that nearly all future therapeutic targets will derive from specific molecular defects that can be identified with companion diagnostic tests，predicting response to those therapies. Pathologists and other diagnostic experts recognize that we can no longer simply classify tumors as to origin and subtype. Today we must consider a plethora of commonly altered epithelial membrane receptors，cell cycle regulatory proteins，signal transaction pathways，and non-random chromosomal alterations. In nearly all tumors，deletions，gains，inversions，translocations，and mutations affecting key cellular components and pathways are driving oncogenesis. Understanding these pathway alterations has become critical to novel pharmaceutical development and will soon become our major diagnostic focus.

Following notable examples such as HER2，BCR-ABL and PML-RARA，in 2008 key evidence from several studies presented at ASCO showed that resistance to cetuximabtherapy in metastatic colorectal cancer could be predicted by the presence of activating KRAS mutations. These mutations have been identified in codons 12，13，and 61 in varying frequencies，leading to important differences between tumors and between methods for KRAS assays. In the last few years，several other single-gene targets in non-small cell lung cancer（EGFR，ALK）and malignant melanoma（BRAF）have become important companion diagnostic targets，with results of assays closely linked to success or failure of particular targeted therapies. More recent clinical trials for established targeted therapies，initially used for relapsed or refractory metastatic disease，are demonstrating their value as first-line agents，such as erlotinib（Tarceva）in EGFR-mutated non-small cell lung cancer（NSCLC）. Furthermore，well-established assays such as HER2 have found expanded use in advanced gastric and GE junctional adenocarcinoma to predict response to targeted therapy with trastuzumab（Herceptin）. Hundreds of compounds are now being investigated in various pre-clinical and clinical trials，most of them in conjunction with a molecular diagnostic assay for a specific target（Figure 5–7）.

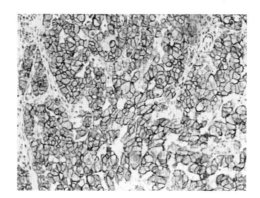

This patient could benefit from Herceptin treatment.

Figure 5–7　HER2 positively expressed in gastric adenocarcinoma（+++）

Studies of multiple genes in panels，such as Genomic Health's OncotypeDx，have been evaluated in relation to breast cancer for prognostic and predictive use in making decisions about chemotherapy or in relation to stage Ⅱ colon cancer where such a panel was shown to be prognostic（for recurrence risk）but not predictive of chemotherapy benefit. For some patient populations，germline rather than somatic defects have been evaluated to identify patients predisposed to cancer or more likely to respond to a particular cancer therapy. Examples include the evaluation of mismatch repair protein defects（microsatellite instability or MSI-H）in suspected hereditary non-polyposis colorectal cancer（HNPCC or Lynch syndrome），germline *p*53 defects (Li-Fraumeni syndrome), hereditary medullary thyroid cancer, and BRCA1/BRCA2 for breast cancer and ovarian cancer patients and their families. Of note, MSI-H colorectal cancer, which can occur in either inherited or sporadic forms, has been characterized as clinically and genetically distinct from other forms of colorectal cancerwith chromosome instability or microsatellite and chromosome stability. MSI-H colorectal cancer shows better stage-specific prognosis despite a propensity to less well-differentiated subtypes, higher stage at diagnosis, and lack of 5-fluorouracil monotherapy benefit compared with microsatellite-stable (MSS) tumors. BRCA1/2 mutation carriers with ovarian carcinoma frequently show durable responses to PEGylated liposomal doxorubicin (Doxil) and poly(ADP)-ribose polymerase (PARP) inhibitor therapy owing to defective homologous recombination DNA repair.

The programmed death-1 (PD-1) pathway is a negative feedback system that represses Th1 cytotoxic immune responses and that, if unregulated, can damage the host. It is up regulated in many tumors and in their surrounding microenvironment. Pembrolizumab could block PD-1 or its ligands has led to remarkable clinical responses in patients with many different types of cancer. A recent study found that the immune related objective response rate and immune related PFS rate in dMMR CRCs were 40% and 78% respectively, while 0 and 11% in pMMR CRCs. The median PFS and OS were not reached in the cohort with dMMR CRC, but were 2.2 and 5.0 months, respectively, in the cohort with pMMR CRC. The comparison of the cohorts with dMMR and pMMR showed hazard ratios for disease progression or death and for death that favored patients with pMMR CRC. This study showed that MMR status predicted clinical benefit of immune checkpoint blockade with pembrolizumab.

5.4.6 Target profiles: molecular testing in an information age

The versatility of gene sequencing has offered a broader glimpse of SNPs and small indels associated with cancer risk, treatment sensitivity or resistance, and identification of genes not previously known to be associated with cancer. New techniques such as allele-specific PCR, high resolution melting curve analysis (HRM), and high throughput next generation sequencing (e.g., 454 sequencing) have been used to determine the status of EGFR, KRAS, and BRAF genes (for example, as a reference method for a targeted PCR assay) but can also simultaneously evaluate multiple gene targets for tumor profiling. Increasingly, attention in clinical research has turned from single targets as first-line choices to entire signal transduction pathways, profiling large numbers of potential targets and assessing molecular pathways in terms of likely pharmacological response or resistance to various agents. Combination therapies in clinical trials are looking to overcome pathways of pharmacological resistance, similar to current triple therapy approaches to HIV infection.

In such a treatment paradigm, the value of molecular diagnostics has significantly increased and a premium is placed on diagnostic accuracy and turn-around time. Until recently the high cost of certain molecular assays and other conventional cytogenetic or FISH techniques favored the use of a sequential algorithmic approach. As targeted therapies move from being used primarily in the metastatic setting into a more prominent role as first-line adjuvant therapies, similar to the role for trastuzumab (Herceptin), the assays will also evolve from ancillary or adjunct tests into a more prominent role as an essential part of the initial diagnostic work-up. In this role the expense of molecular assays is offset by the clinical advantage of more effective therapeutic choice, reduced complications, and collectively reduced pharmaceutical and medical care expenses.

Piloting such a personalized medicine approach, Dr. Daniel Von Hoff has used advanced diagnostic test panels in oncology trials and clinical practice in Phoenix, Arizona, while colleagues at MD Anderson Cancer Center in Houston, Texas, have established complex diagnostic panels as part of a treatment triage strategy for clinical trial selection in the BATTLE program. Other centers around the world have quickly moved to establish similar studies using molecular diagnostic tests to qualify patients for various trials. In this research setting, unique or novel assays such as high throughput sequencing can be used, but for most patients once a histologic diagnosis of malignancy is established the use of specific *in vitro* diagnostic (IVD) tests proven to be predictive of response to a particular agent is required for optimizing safety and efficacy and for reducing unnecessary complications or expenses related to non-effective therapy choices.

5.5 Tumor pathology in clinical practice, using colorectal cancer as an example

To summarize the role of tumor pathology in oncology, we would like to use colorectal cancer, as an example, to illustrate the role of tumor pathology in clinical oncology.

Colorectal cancer (CRC) is a complex collection of genetic diseases. Based on the distinct patterns of genetic instability, CRC can roughly be classified into three groups. Approximately 70% of CRCs are associated with chromosomal instability (CIN) due to allelic imbalance of chromosomal foci, chromosome amplification, or translocation. About 15% of CRCs have microsatellite instability (MSI), i. e., frameshift mutations and base-pair substitutions that commonly arise in short, tandemly repeated nucleotide sequences. The remaining 15% of CRCs do not show CIN or MSI. CIN CRCs are aneuploid and are associated with intrinsic drug resistance and poor prognosis, whereas most MSI CRCs are near-diploid, with better overall survival. Based on epigenetic characteristics, about one third of CRCs have the CpG island methylator phenotype (CIMP). Overlap exists between MSI and CIMP tumors, because about 60% of CIMP-H tumors have methylation of the *MLH*1 promoter, which leads to MSI. Molecular classification of genetically heterogenetic CRC will potentially have significant impact on clinical practice of personalized medicine of CRC. Molecular tests for CRC are being increasingly used in clinical practice where they have significant implications for the risk assessment, diagnosis, prognosis, and treatment of this common malignancy.

5.5.1 Risk assessment

Approximately 20% of CRC cases are associated with familial colorectal neoplasms, that is, two or more first-degree relatives with colorectal adenomas and carcinomas. First-degree relatives of patients with newly diagnosed familial colorectal neoplasms are at increased risk of CRC. Genetic susceptibility to CRC mainly occurs in inherited colorectal syndromes such as Lynch syndrome and familial adenomatous polyposis. The common hereditary syndromes and incidences of CRC are listed in Table 5-2. It is recommended that all CRC patients be queried about their family history and considered for risk assessment as detailed in the National Comprehensive Cancer Network (NCCN) Colorectal Cancer Screening Clinical Practice Guidelines.

Table 5-2　Targeted nextgen sequencing (NGS) of colorectal adenocarcinoma

Targeted Gene	Significance
APC (Exon 1–16)	Familial adenomatous polyposis syndrome
BRAF (Exon 15,16)	Resistance to anti-EGFR monoclonal antibody treatment Prognosis
KRAS (Exons 2,3)	Resistance to anti-EGFR monoclonal antibody treatment
*MLH*1 (Exons 1–19)	Lynch syndrome; 5-FU therapy response
*MSH*2 (Exons 1–16)	Lynch syndrome; 5-FU therapy response
*MSH*6 (Exons 1–10)	Lynch syndrome; 5-FU therapy response
MUTYH (Exons 1–16)	Familial adenomatous polyposis syndrome
NRAS (Exons 2,3)	Resistance to anti-EGFR monoclonal antibody treatment
PIK3CA (Exons 9,20)	Resistance to anti-EGFR monoclonal antibody treatment
*PMS*2 (Exons 1–15)	Lynch syndrome; 5-FU therapy response
PTEN (Exons 7,8)	Resistance to anti-EGFR monoclonal antibody treatment
*STK*11 (Exons 1–10)	Peutz-Jeghers syndrome

5.5.2　Hereditary cancer syndrome

Individuals with Lynch syndrome—including those with existing cancer and those who have not yet developed cancer—have a predisposition to CRC and certain other tumors. Lynch syndrome is the most common form of genetically determined colon cancer predisposition, accounting for 2% –6% of all CRC cases and usually displays distinctive clinical features.

5.5.3　MSI assay

In the clinical MSI assay, DNA is usually extracted from microdissected paraffin-embedded tumor and non-neoplastic tissue. The extracted DNA is subsequently analyzed by a polymerase chain reaction (PCR)-based method. Revelation of PCR amplification products is usually carried out by either capillary electrophoresis or polyacrylamide gel electrophoresis (PAGE)-silver staining. Because defective MMR genes do not affect all microsatellites in a given neoplasm, multiple microsatellites that are frequently affected by instability are needed in order to study MSI. Repeats with units ranging from two to hundreds have been used to classify microsatellites. Although there is no consensus on the minimum number of repeated nucleotide units required to define a microsatellite, the U. S. National Cancer Institute (NCI) proposed a panel of five markers (BAT25, BAT26, D2S123, D5S346, and D17S250) as a standard test panel for MSI. This "NCI panel" has been recently expanded to include other markers, such as BAT40, BAT34c4, MycL, and TGFBR2, based on evidence that MSI sensitivity can be enhanced by including more markers, particularly mononucleotide markers, in the testing panel. Therefore, a recent pentapplex of 5 quasimonomorphic mononucleotide repeats has been described; this panel, consisting of BAT25, BAT26, NR21, NR24, and NR22 or NR27, has two potential advantages: does not need the corresponding normal control germline DNA and has higher (nearly 100%) specificity and sensitivity. It has been reported that analysis of MSI of the same tumor samples using the pentaplex panel in several different testing facilities had the same results with no discrepancies.

Regardless of whether five, seven, or more markers are used, if 40% or more of the markers tested are abnormal (for example, when at least three of seven markers are abnormal), the CRC specimen is categorized as high-level MSI (MSI-H). When no abnormality is detected in the tested microsatellite markers, the specimen is called MSI-stable (MSS). If one marker or less than 40% of the markers tested show abnormalities, the specimen is categorized as low-level MSI (MSI-L). The biologic significance of MSI-L is not entirely clear, and MSI-L tumors have clinical features of MSS tumors (Figure 5-8).

For external quality assessment and evaluation of inter-laboratory reproducibility, proficiency testing for MSI was introduced by the College of American Pathologists.

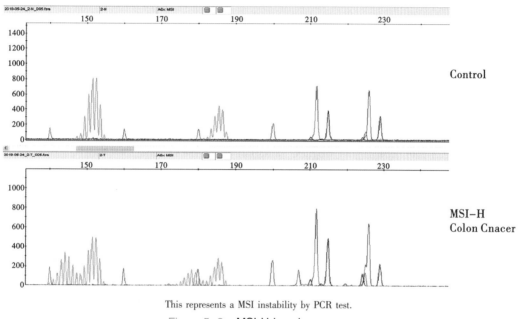

This represents a MSI instability by PCR test.

Figure 5-8   **MSI-H in colon cancer**

5.5.4   Assessment of MMR proteins

Compared with the PCR-based MSI assay, IHC analysis is more convenient and inexpensive. More importantly, IHC analysis directly detects the MMR gene that is likely to be mutated.

MMR proteins function in heterodimer pairs. MLH1 and MSH2 are the obligatory dimers. PMS2 can form a heterodimer only with MLH1, and MSH6 can form a heterodimer only with MSH2; however, MLH1 and MSH2 can form heterodimers with other MMR proteins, such as MSH3 and PMS1. In general, mutations in MLH1 and MSH2 result in subsequent proteolytic degradation of the secondary partners, PMS2 and MSH6, respectively. On the other hand, mutations in PMS2 or MSH6 may not result in proteolytic degradation of its primary partner. Also, important to note that MSH6 can be lost as a result of defective mismatch repair because MSH6 gene itself contains a microsatellite, or it can be lost as a result of germline mutation. Accordingly, the use of a two-antibody panel consisting of PMS2 and MSH6 for screening for Lynch syndrome has been proposed. Studies of two-antibody panels for examining colonic and extracolonic Lynch syndrome-related tumors have shown fairly consistent results compared with results for four-antibody panels, indicating the potential value in reducing the cost of MMR protein IHC analysis.

In general, IHC analysis to interpret MMR protein is straight forward since all MMR proteins are readily recognizable on nuclear staining. It is always helpful to carefully assess the expression of MMR proteins, first in non-neoplastic cells and then in tumor cells. Cases are classified with loss of expression when there is a lack of expression in tumor cells in the presence of internal positive controls (lymphocytes, stromal cells). However, it should be noted that immunostaining of MMR proteins can be heterogeneous throughout the tumor, and difficult cases with patchy, weak immunoreactivity, particularly with MLH1 and MSH6, are encountered. Any equivocal staining should be repeated, or even red one with a different antibody clone. It has also been reported that a subset of cases with loss of MMR protein were initially misinterpreted as tumors exhibiting intact MMR protein by individuals without knowledge of the potential pitfall of frequently present intratumoral lymphocytes, underscoring the important role of experienced pathologist in assessing MMR proteins. Furthermore, partial expression of MSH6 has been reported in colorectal carcinoma after neo-adjuvant treatment; in general a low percentage of tumors with intact expression of the mismatch enzymes can have microsatellite instable genotype. Therefore, concurrent testing for both mismatch enzymes and PCR testing for microsatellite markers are advocated.

5.5.5   MLH1 hypermethylation and BRAF mutation in sporadic MSI CRC

Approximately 19% of all colorectal tumors have MSI, and most CRCs with MSI are sporadic. One of the characteristic features of sporadic CRCs with MSI is biallelic methylation of the *MLH1* promoteR. In addition, sporadic CRCs with MSI display frequent mutation of the *BRAF* gene.

Because of the significant clinical implications between the two subsets of MSI-associated CRCs, it is essential to distinguish them. Several workup algorithms have been proposed, although currently there is no consensus on the approach or workflow to distinguish Lynch syndrome from sporadic CRCs with MSI. One cost-effective way is to perform a *BRAF* gene mutation test when MLH1 immunoexpression is absent in the tumor. The presence of *BRAF* mutation indicates that *MLH1* expression is down-regulated by somatic methylation of the promoter region of the gene and not by a germline mutation, ruling out Lynch syndrome. If no *BRAF* mutation is detected, the sample should further undergo a hypermethylation test of *MLH1*. If no *MLH1* hypermethylation is detected, the case is most likely a Lynch syndrome, requiring an *MLH1* mutation test for confirmation and subsequent genetic counseling.

5.5.6   Predictive and prognostic markers

Predictive biomarkers indicate the likelihood of treatment benefit, allowing the identification of patients who will or will not benefit from the use of a particular therapy; prognostic biomarkers, independent of the treatment effect, provide information about the natural history of the disease and are associated with patient survival. We have little knowledge of why some CRC patients respond to therapy, yet others do not, or why some experience disease relapse, whereas others do not. However, progress has been made by using various techniques to refine prognostic and predictive information.

5.5.7   MSI and chemotherapy—predictive power

MSI status is important to consider during the decision-making process for the use of adjuvant chemotherapy in CRC patients. On a molecular level, evidence has shown that patients would need intact MMR gene function to induce apoptosis of 5-fluorouracil (5-FU)-modified DNA. There is evidence that MSI has decreased benefit or even a detrimental effect from adjuvant therapy with a fluoropyrimidine alone in patients with stage Ⅱ disease.

5.5.8   MSI and clinical outcomes—prognostic power

MSI status is closely associated with patient prognosis. A recent prospective evaluation of 1,852 colon cancers demonstrated that MMR deficiency has prognostic value for stages Ⅱ and Ⅲ colon cancer. The NC-

CN CRC panel recommends that MMR gene testing, as well as planned adjuvant therapy with a fluoropyrimidine alone, be considered for patients with stage Ⅱ disease.

Due to the significant impact of MSI on the treatment and prognosis of CRC, both on the patient and possibly on the patient's family members, it has been recommended that all patients with newly diagnosed CRC be screened for MSI by MSI testing or IHC analysis. In fact, some centers now perform both IHC and MSI testing on all colorectal tumors to determine which patients should have genetic testing for Lynch syndrome. The cost-effectiveness of this so-called reflex testing approach has been confirmed for CRC, and this approach was endorsed by the EGAPP Working Group at the Centers for Disease Control and Prevention.

Assessment of biomarkers in colorectal cancer is summarized in Table 5–3.

Table 5–3   Assessment of biomarkers in colorectal cancer

Biomarker	Function	Alteration	Consequence
MSIDNA	nucleotide mismatch repair	MSI-H	Improved prognosis
		Need to rule out Lynch syndrome	
MLH1	DNA nucleotide mismatch gene	Hypermethylation	Rule out Lynch syndrome
CIMP*	CpG island methylator	Hypermethylation	Improved prognosis
KRAS	key player in the RAS/RAF/ MAPK pathway	Mutation	Resistance to anti-EGFR mAB
BRAF	RAS/RAF/ MAPK pathway	Mutation	Resistance to anti-EGFR mAB
		Confirmation of sporadic MSI-H CRC	
NRAS	RAS/RAF/ MAPK pathway	Mutation	Resistance to anti-EGFR mAB
PIK3CA			
PI3K-AKT-mTOR	pathway	Mutation	Resistance to anti-EGFR mAB
PTEN	regulator of the PI3KCA/AKT	pathway	Loss/MutationResistance to anti-EGFR mAB
TS	thymidine generation	TSER 28 bp (2R)/(3R) tandem repeats 5 'UTR	Reduced response to 5-FU
	thymidine generation	TSER 3R G>C SNP	Increased response to 5-FU
ERCC-1	DNA excision repair	High mRNA expression	Resistance to platinum-based therapy
18q	LOH or loss	Poorer prognosis	

* CIMP: CpG island methylator phenotype. mAB: monoclonal antibody. TS: thymidylate synthase. bp: base pairs. 2R: two tandem repeats. 3R: three tandem repeats. UTR: untranslated region. TSER: TS enhancer region. SNP: single nucleotide polymorphism. ERCC-1: excision-repair cross-complementing-1.

5.6   Role of pathology and pathologist in multidisciplinary term approaches to cancer management

Cancer is a group of complex and serious disease. Traditionally, during the course of treatment, the patient will encounter many different physicians with different specializations. A patient is likely to either work with or be evaluated by: a radiologist, a surgeon, nurse, a radiation oncologist, general practitioner, pathologist, psychologist, social worker, clinical oncologist, hemato-oncologist, and medical technologists. From later 1990s, MD Anderson Cancer Center, Texas, USA, has started multidisciplinary team (MDT) approach to comprehensively manage the patients, and offered one-stop service by a group of physicians for each challenging case. Each patient is personalized managed to maximize the modern oncology has to offer. For examples, eight MDT groups in the gastrointestinal cancer clinical services at MDACC, and each week, at least eight MDT conferences for the gastrointestinal cancers. Five to eight cases are discussed in each conference, where a group healthcare professionals including radiologist, surgeon, radiation oncologist, general practitioner, pathologist, medical oncologist, psychologist, social worker, medical genetic counselor, and clinical trial nurse discuss the cases thoroughly, and come up a consensus to how comprehensively and efficiently manage the patients in a personalized manner. The outcome of MDT at MDACC has been successful and made contributions to improve quality of life and reduce mortality rate for cancer patients. Now, MDT has become a universe practice in big cancer centers throughout the world.

5.7   Future of tumor pathology

Advances in molecular oncology diagnostics promise many new avenues for future care improvement, some of which likely will remain investigational while others may become well-established standards of care. Realizing the dream of targeted therapies and companion diagnostics in oncology will require a concerted long-term effort by commercial manufacturers, healthcare providers, governmental agencies, professional societies, and academic institutions to achieve objective improvements in care. These parties have a shared interest in working together to advance the quality of care for unmet medical needs. Recognizing valuable contributions of each party is essential to building dialogue and forming strategies that will pave the way for the future development of effective molecular diagnostic assays.

Zan Likun, Tan Dongfeng

Chapter 6

Application of Imaging Medicine in Oncology

Tumor has always been the top killer of human life, and its diagnosis and treatment is a major challenge in the medical field. Imaging examination technology plays an important role in the diagnosis and treatment of tumor diseases. For decades in clinical application, imaging technology has been progressing with relevant scientific development. Nowadays, imaging technology has been used in all stages of tumor diagnosis and treatment. The common imaging techniques used in clinic include X-Ray, CT, MR, ultrasound and nuclear medicine. Different imaging techniques have their own characteristics in diagnosis and treatment of tumor. They are described in the following.

6.1　The application of X-ray in oncology

X-ray examination is widely used in the diagnosis of tumors. It is one of the most effective methods for early clinical diagnosis and differential diagnosis of tumors. With increasing experience in X-ray examination and diagnosis, the continuous improvement of equipment and the application of new technology, X-ray examination has become an indispensable tool in the diagnosis and treatment of tumors.

X-ray examination includes fluoroscopy, radiography, angiography, and etc. It can not only locate and characterize the lesions, but also analyze the size, quantity, scope and the relationship with the surrounding tissues or organs, thus providing reliable basis for the selection of clinical treatment, the observation of curative effect and the estimation of prognosis. As long as all kinds of X-ray examinations are used reasonably, combined with analysis of clinical history, physical signs and other examinations, the designated goal of diagnosis can be achieved.

Take the diagnosis of mammography in breast cancer as an example. Mammography is the most simple, convenient and accurate method for the examination of breast diseases, which is recognized internationally. Its major characteristic is that it can detect breast masses which doctors might have missed by touching. Its diagnostic accuracy is as high as 95%. The diagnostic criteria of mammography for breast cancer include: ①the presence of a mass in the breast, and the size, shape and borderline of the mass; ②the number, shape and distribution of calcifications in the breast; ③the presence of structure disorder; ④other indirect signs (Figure 6-1).

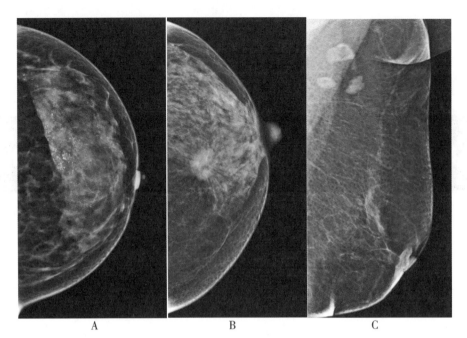

A. the asymmetric, dense and fine calcification in the upper outer quadrant of the left breast, with regional distribution. B. a high-density mass in the deep part of the left breast central area, with a size of about 16 mm×14.5 mm, rough edge, uneven density, and clustered surrounding glands. C. the asymmetric dense change of the gland in the posterior region of the left papilla. The skin of the nipple was thickened and the nipple was sunken. Enlarged lymph nodes can be seen under the armpit. The imaging diagnosis results of the above three cases were all BI-RADS 4, and they were confirmed to be breast invasive carcinoma by patholog.

Figure 6-1   Mammography of breast carcinoma

X-ray is helpful for the early diagnosis of central lung cancer. The general manifestations are: ①hilar mass, with lobulated; ②obstructive atelectasis, hilar mass and atelectasis in the upper lobe of the right lung can form a typical "S" pattern; ③obstructivepneumonia; ④obstructive emphysema (Figure 6-2).

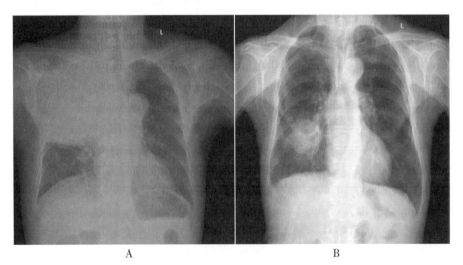

A. shows an enlarged shadow and blurred structure in the right hilum of the lung. The transmittance of the middle lobe and upper lobe of the right lung was reduced, indicating obstructive atelectasis of them. B. shows the patchy density mass of the right lung with unclear boundary. Both cases were proved to be squamous cell carcinoma by pathology.

Figure 6-2   X-ray picture of central lung cancer

Osteosarcoma has distinctive X-ray manifestations. Most of the tumors are located at the metaphyseal end of the long bone. It has the characteristics of new bone formation and bone destruction, unclear edge, bone trabecular destruction, high tissue density around the tumor, and as can be seen in the Codman triangle (Figure 6-3).

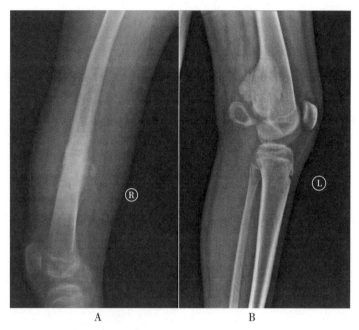

A. uneven density in the medullary cavity of the middle and lower part of the right femur, and local thickening of the bone cortex. Tumor bone was seen in the surrounding soft tissue. B. an increase in mass density in the lower segment of the left femur. Periosteum reaction can be seen at the edge, with local triangular changes. Both cases were pathologically confirmed as osteosarcoma.

Figure 6-3   Codman triangle of osteosarcoma

With the continuous development of interventional radiology, X-ray examination has evolved from simple disease diagnosis to disease treatment. At present, interventional therapy of tumor can be executed via various methods. With future technology development, there will be more extensive application of X ray examinations.

6.2   The application of CT in oncology

computed tomography (CT) is widely used in clinics because it has high resolution for detecting lesions especially in the early detection of small lesions. Enhanced CT scanning using contrast media can help obtain functional information about tissues, estimate the relationship between lesions and surrounding tissues, and detect the lesions with more sensitivity compared to routine CT scan. CT makes diagnosis of tumor mainly based on the imaging features of the lesions, for example, lobulated or speculated margin can be observed in lung cancer (Figure 6-4A, B). Hepatocellular carcinoma is characterized by "fast in and fast out" in the enhancement scanning, that is, the lesion is obviously enhanced in the arterial phase, and quickly cleared in the portal vein phase (Figure 6-4C, D, E).

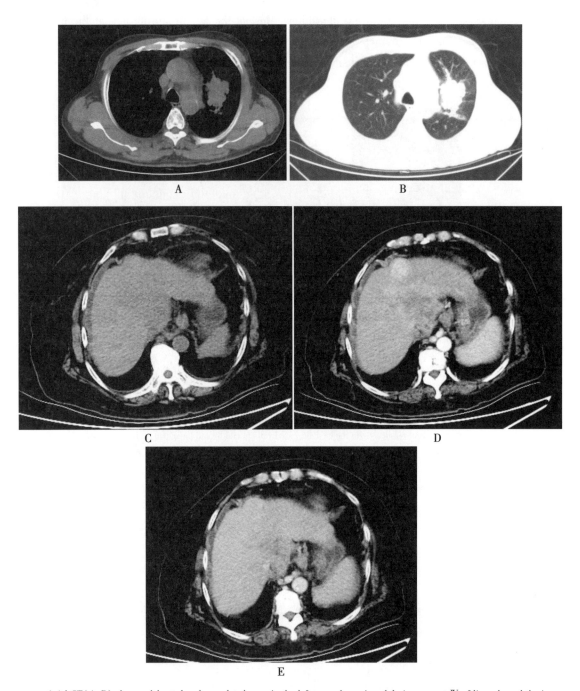

Axial CT(A,B) shows a lobuated and speculated mass in the left upper lung. A nodule in segment Ⅳ of liver showed the iso-density lesion on plain CT (C), obvious enhancement on arterial phase of CECT (D) and relative iso-density on portal venous phase (E).

Figure 6-4   CT findings of lung cancer

With advances in technology, the application of various post-processing software (such as 2-dimensional and 3-dimensional reconstruction, etc.) makes it possible for CT examination to cover almost every system of the body beyond the traditional axial images, especially for the localization and staging of tumor, for example, CT staging of gastrointestinal tumors is helpful for the choice of follow-up treatment (Figure 6-5).

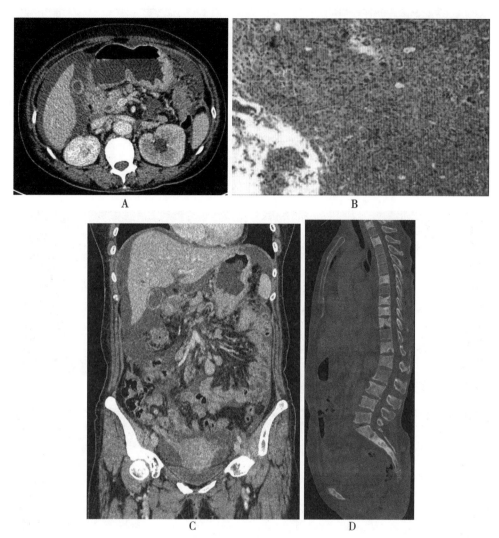

A (axial image) and C (coronal image) showed thickening of the gastric gastric body wall, and pathology (B) confirmed signet ring cell carcinoma. Multiple enlarged lymph nodes can be seen between liver and stomach, retroperitoneum and abdominal cavity. Effusion can be seen in the pelvic cavity and abdominal cavity. D (sagittal) bone window shows multiple abnormal changes in bone density, with bone metastasis being considered.

Figure 6-5   CT findings of gastric carcinoma

With improving CT technology, the diagnostic information of CT moves beyond the morphology of the lesions, to include the functional performance. It provides a new basis for accurate diagnosis.

CT perfusion is a functional imaging, which can reflect the changes of blood perfusion in tissues and lesions, and is conducive to the qualitative diagnosis of lesions. For example, more lesions can be found by pancreatic perfusion than conventional non-enhanced and enhanced CT scan(Figure 6-6).

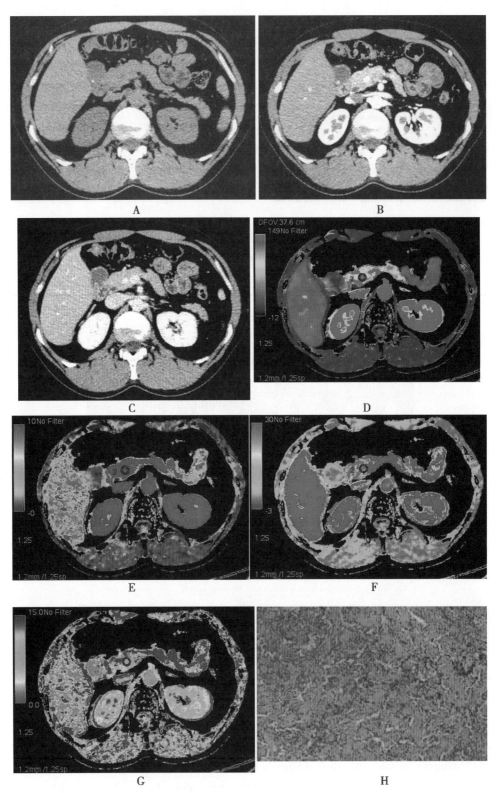

Slightly low-density nodule can be seen on plain scan of the head of pancreas(A) ,with unclear boundary. The degree of nodular enhancement was the same as artery in the arterial phase (B) and was significantly reduced in venous phase (C). Pancreatic perfusion showed a nodular high perfusion area in the head of pancreas, with increased blood flow (BF) (D) ,slightly increased blood volume (BV) (E) ,increased permeability surface (PS) (F) ,and shortened mean transit time (MTT) (G). It was pathologically (H) confirmed as insulinoma.

Figure 6-6   CT findings of pancreas mass

The new generation of CT spectrum imaging which represents the direction of future tumor CT diagnosis, has specific strengths in the early diagnosis of tumor, the evaluation of tumor blood supply, tissue origin, degree of malignancy, and the differentiation diagnosis of neoplastic and non-neoplastic diseases by multi-parameter imaging model. One example is the differential diagnosis of benign and malignant pulmonary nodules(Figure 6-7).

The clinical application of CT-guided puncture biopsy can obtain a few tissue specimens for diagnosis by pathology to guide further treatment of the tumor. In addition, the methods of tumor therapy, such as radiation particle implantation and radiofrequency ablation, which are based on CT-guided puncture, are increasingly widely used in clinical practices.

However, there are still limits of CT in the examination of tumor, for instance, CT is not sensitive enough to detect small lesions and mucosal changes of gastrointestinal tract. CT also has limitations to the qualitative diagnosis of disease to a certain extent.

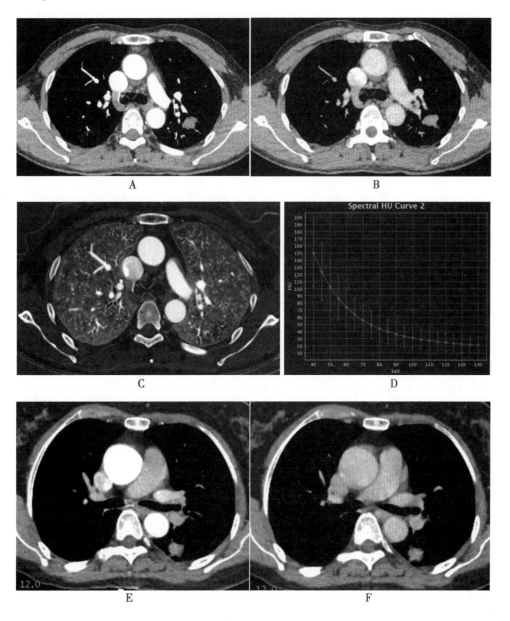

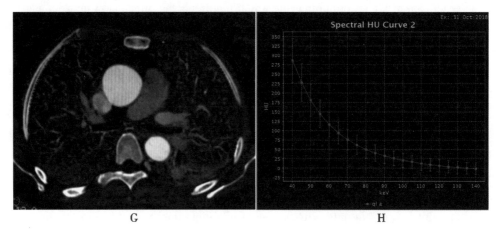

A-D show a 52-year-old male with dual stage CT enhanced image (A,B) to diagnose the left upper lobe occupying lesion, which is considered carcinoma. The arterial iodinogram (C) and energy spectrum curve of focus (D) show that the iodine concentration in arterial phase (IC-AP) was 14.45 (100 mg/L) and the slope of 40－70 keV horizontal energy spectrum curve (K1) was 3.13, both of which were lower than the threshold value, so it was considered as benign lesion. The final pathology confirmed chronic lung inflammation and focal pneumonia. E-H show a 60-year-old female with dual stage CT enhanced image (E,F). Nodules in the lower lobe of the left lung were diagnosed. The arterial iodinogram (G) and energy spectrum curve of focus (H) show that the iodine concentration in arterial phase (IC-AP) was 37.38 (100 μg/ml) and the slope of 40－70 keV horizontal energy spectrum curve (K1) was 7.13, both of which were higher than the threshold value, so it was considered as malignant lesion. Lung adenocarcinoma was confirmed by pathology.

Figure 6－7　The differential diagnosis of benign and malignant pulmonary nodules

6.3　The application of MRI in oncology

MRI (magnetic resonance imaging) is a tomographic technique that can display anatomical structures. It is based on the principle of magnetic resonance. Through the detection of hydrogen atoms in water or fat in human tissues, the electromagnetic signal is obtained from the human body, which is converted into human tissue information.

MRI has many advantages in the diagnosis of tumor. It has no ionizing radiation, no contrast agent, or high sensitivity, and can obtain three-dimensional or even four-dimensional images. It is used to detect various tumor diseases such as brain tumor, internal tumor of spinal canal, primary liver cancer, uterine fibroids and prostate cancer, etc. MRS (magnetic resonance spectroscopyanalysis) is developed on the basis of MRI and has a greater advantage in tumor imaging. It can detect the metabolites of tumor cells and normal cells to determine their differences.

MRI has the feature of high soft tissue resolution, multi-parameter and multi-azimuth imaging, which can clearly show the anatomical position, size, shape and signal characteristics of the tumor. The difference of MRI imaging signals is based on the relaxation time of different tissues. In clinical practice, various weighted images are mainly collected to diagnose the lesions according to the signal differences of the images. Longitudinal relaxation time T1, and transverse relaxation time T2 are basic physical quantities of MRI, which can provide information about tumor size, invasion, and lymph node metastasis, etc, so as to improve the level of detection and evaluation of prognosis of tumor.

6.3.1   MRI in diagnosis of brain astrocytoma

In traditional clinical pathology, the degree of brain astroncytoma diagnosis are differentiated into grades Ⅰ-Ⅳ. Grade Ⅰ is benign astrocytoma; Grade Ⅱ is benign and malignant transition type; Grades Ⅲ and Ⅳ are malignant astrocytoma. For MRI diagnosis, the MRI signal of benign is generally more uniform, when the T1-weighted image is mostly low signal, and the T2 weighted image is slightly higher than the irregular slice. Enhancement scanning, tumor enhancement is not obvious or mild enhancement. There are few qualitative signs of MRI. The Anaplastic astrocytoma (malignant), equivalent to Ⅲ level, between tumor andmalignant degree is higher. The T1-weighted image in the nonenhanced scan showed a mixed signal with uneven signal and other signals, while the T2-weighted image was an uneven high signal, indicating that the high signal was more obvious in the edema region. Tumor had different degrees of enhancement in the enhanced scanning. When there exists a small amount of tumor hemorrhage, small patchy high signal appears in the T1-weighted image and T2 weighted image. Glioblastoma is the same like the previous case with the highest tumor malignancy, the T1 weighted image and T2 weighted image show all unevenly mixed signals. There is often hemorrhage, necrosis and cystic signal in the lesion. The tumor morphology is irregular, the boundary is clear, and the oedema and occupying effect are obvious. After enhancement, the tumor displays inhomogeneous and irregular ring reinforcement.

6.3.2   MRI in diagnosis of primary liver cancer

Liver cancer includes primary liver cancer and metastatic carcinoma from other organs. Primary hepatic carcinoma is one of the most common malignant tumors in China, with high morbidity and mortality. It is closely related to hepatitis B and cirrhosis, and when detected many patients are already in advanced stage. Therefore, early examination and diagnosis have important influence on treatment and prognosis. The diagnosis of liver cancer is more and more dependent on imaging diagnosis. In MRI the tumor in T1 weighted imaging is mostly low signal, and the center has hemorrhage, and thebad dead are high and low mixed signals. In T2 weighted imaging, the lesions were mostly high signal, accounting for more than 90% of the lesions. The boundary maybe clear or unclear, the signal is uniform or uneven within the linear low signal, and arterial phase shows obviously homogeneous or inhomogeneous enhancement, with no obvious enhancement of liver parenchyma, and portal venous phase and parenchymal phase has significantly improved, exiting of contrast agents and low density lesions. Conventional dynamic contrast enhancement MRI has certain sensitivity and specificity in the diagnosis of liver cancer, but it still has a deficiency in the diagnosis of small liver cancer. With the development of MRI technology, more and more contrast agent are used in clinical, cell specificity enhanced magnetic resonance contrast agent for different components of focal liver lesions, which can not only improve the specificity and accuracy of diagnosis of liver cancer, but also can overcome the deficiency of the conventional dynamic contrast-enhanced MRI in the diagnosis of small hepatocellular carcinoma limitations of low positive rate, and improve the diagnosis accuracy of small liver cancer.

Pummelian for the new type of MRI contrast agents, from histological level to reflect the nature of the lesion, because the phagocytosis of benign nodular cirrhosis exist in normal liver cells, the liver image signal is the same as the normal liver tissue. For cirrhosis of the liver cancer nodules, because of its normal phagocytosis in liver cell damage, and, in comparison with normal hepatic tissue, lesion area's Pummelian show significantly lower intake, thus liver parenchyma phase is no signal or low signal phase images, and the surrounding liver parenchyma of contrast is very obvious, therefore, it can improve the lesions diagnostic accuracy and sensitivity.

6.3.3 MRI in diagnosis of prostate cancer

MRI has been recognized as one of the best imaging diagnostic techniques for prostate cancer based on its high resolution in three-dimensional space and soft tissue contrast and multi-sequence and multi-parameter imaging. MRI has the advantage of multi-sequence and multi-azimuth imaging, which can clearly show the anatomical structure of prostate. More importantly, through the DWI (diffusion-weighted imaging), MRS (magnetic resonance spectroscopy), DCE-MRI (dynamic contrast enhanced magnetic resonance) imaging and other imaging techniques, MRI can also provide functional imaging and metabolic imaging of prostate, thereby better evaluate tumor location, tumor size, tumor invasion and its scope and aggressiveness. The results show that the signal intensity distribution of the prostate gland in T1WI was relatively uniform, and the dissection of the anatomic regions was not clear. On T2WI images, relative to the normal prostate central zone and transition zone of low signal intensity, peripheral zone displays as obviously high signal, and in the region of the prostate, MRI signal is significantly reduced. In the surrounding of high signal intensity in the peripheral zone of carcinoma tissue contrast shows better. In the early dynamic enhanced phase, cancer significantly quickens reinforcement uniformity. Prostate cancer has high signal on imaging, and the signal is higher than the surrounding normal tissues, and decrease of Cit peak and the rise of Cho peak is MRS changing characteristic of prostate cancer.

In conclusion, MRI has excellent resolution of soft tissue and can clearly show the anatomical structure and morphology of the lesion. Multi-dimensional imaging facilitates to display anatomic structures and pathological changes in the body of the spatial location and mutual relationship. It can be a functional imaging and sublimation metabolic analysis, and can comprehensively illustrate the tumor of anatomical position, size, shape and signal characteristics. However, the scan time of the MRI is longer, and the chest and abdomen examination is limited. Patients with cardiac pacemaker or ferromagnetic substance in the body cannot be examined, and the display of calcification is far less than that of CT. In addition, it is difficult to make a diagnosis of lesions characterized by pathological calcification(Figure 6-8, Figure 6-9).

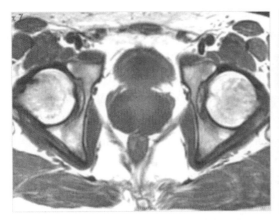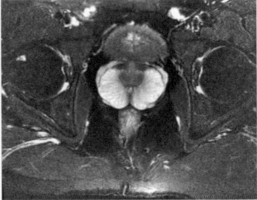

Figure 6-8 T1WI and T2WI was medium signal in the central and peripheral zone, and T2WI was high signal in peripheral zone, and the horizontal axis was the best position to observe the prostate

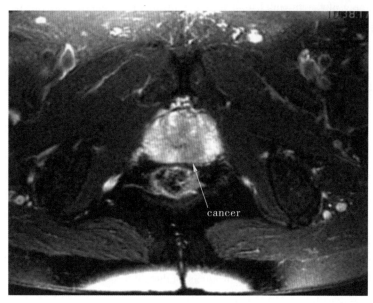

Figure 6-9   On the left side of the peripheral zone, there is a low signal nodule of prostate cancer

6.4   The application of ultrasound in oncology

The principle of medical ultrasonic diagnosis is that ultrasound will reflect at the interface of two layers with different acoustic impedances. The echo signal contains information such as the position, shape, and hardness of the interface. Then the ultrasonic probe with transducer receives the echo signal and form the ultrasound imaging which contains the internal details of the media, shows the structure and characteristics of the lesions to achieve the purpose of diagnosis of disease.

The echo strength of the ultrasound image depends on the acoustic impedance difference of the two media, the angle of the incident ultrasound and the interface, and is related to the tissue composition. Substantial organs such as liver, spleen, thyroid and other tissues show uniform and weak echoes; organs containing liquid such as eyeball, gallbladder, bladder, and heart show echoes on each interface and no echo in the cavity. Gas-bearing organs such as the lungs and intestines show strong echoes due to total gas reflexes; while bone tissue expresses strong echoes.

The sonographic appearance of the tumor is related to the composition of the tumor tissue. Benign tumors which mostly contain envelopes, often manifest as clear boundaries, more uniform internal echoes, and less or no blood flow signals. Malignant tumors which mostly contain no envelopes grow rapidly and infiltrates to the periphery. Small tumors are mostly tumor cells, while large neoplasms may be with necrosis and hemorrhage. Ultrasound shows that the tumor border is unclear or pseudopodia extension. Small tumors are mostly hypoechoic and the larger ones have different internal echoes and more abundant blood flow signals. Fluid-containing organs such as gallbladder and bladder will protrude into the cavity when tumors develop.

Ultrasound has unique advantages in diagnosing neoplastic diseases because of its features of safety, non-invasiveness, repeatability, etc. It can not only visualize the size, shape, margins, internal echo, but also the internal blood supply of the tumor. It can measure blood flow velocity and the resistance index. Ultrasound has unmatched diagnostic value for thyroid occupancy, breast occupancy and cardiac cavity occupancy in particular.

New ultrasound technologies such as ultrasound elastography, contrast-enhanced ultrasound, B-flow technology, and three-dimensional ultrasound imaging have been developed rapidly in recent years and have been gradually applied in clinical practice. They can be used to evaluate the hardness, enhancement patterns, neovascularization, internal micro-calcification and the three-dimensional shape of the tumor tissue to comprehensively evaluate the tumors, benign or malignant.

With the maturation of ultrasound-guided biopsy techniques, this method has become the preferred method for the diagnosis of tumors and their classification. Ultrasound-guided biopsy of the tumor is safe, reliable, simple and easy to carry out. So it is of great significance to judge the pathological type, especially for the pathological diagnosis of superficial organs with irreplaceable value. Ultrasound-guided biopsy provides minimally invasive safety, so older and critically ill patients can tolerate it. Ultrasound-guided fine needle aspiration has a high early diagnostic value for some malignant lesions, and is helpful for early detection, early diagnosis and early treatment of malignant lesions.

With the rapid development of ultrasound technology, ultrasound has been applied not only to the diagnosis of tumors but also to their treatment. Interventional ultrasound has become one of the most important supporting techniques for minimally invasive treatment. Its clinical application is extensive. The advantage of interventional ultrasound is that it is real-time imaging with good accuracy, light and flexible operating. Because of these advantages, it cannot be surpassed by other surgical methods. Ultrasound ablation including radio frequency ablation, microwave ablation, cryoablation, and high-intensity focused ultrasound play an important role in the treatment of liver cancer and thyroid cancer. Interventional ultrasound is also useful for some benign lesions such as uterine fibroids. Interventional ultrasound can reduce the surgical trauma and improve quality of life for the patients(Figure 6-10, Figure 6-11).

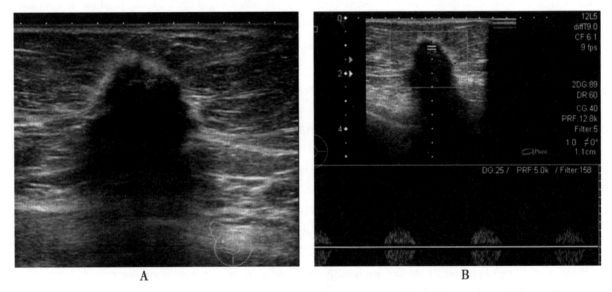

A. Two-dimensional ultrasound showed hypoechoic nodules in the mammary gland with unclear border, irregular morphology, and crescent-shaped limbs on the edges, the echo internal and posterior attenuated. B. Spectral Doppler shows high-resistance blood flow in the mass.

Figure 6-10   The ultrasound image of breast cancer

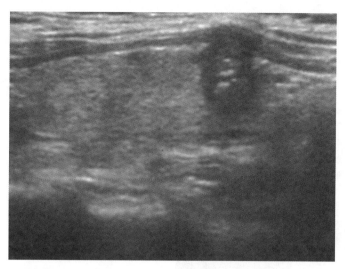

Two-dimensional ultrasonography showed hypoechoic nodules in the thyroid gland with no capsule, unclear and burr-like borders, irregular morphology and visible sand-like calcification.

Figure 6–11   Ultrasound image of thyroid cancer

6.5   The application of nuclear medicine in oncology

In recent years, with the progress of medical technology, nuclear medicine plays an increasingly important role in the diagnosis and treatment of tumors. The detector receives and records the radiation emitted by radioactive tracers that are introduced into the body's target tissues or organs, and displayed in the form of images. This method can not only show the anatomical structure of organs or lesions, such as location, shape and size, but also provide information about blood flow, function, metabolism and even molecular level of organs and lesions. So it helps early diagnosis of disease. The most commonly used instruments for diagnosing tumor related diseases are position emission tomography (PET) and single photon emission computed tomography (SPECT). They can be combined with CT and MRI to show not only the metabolism, but also the location of the lesion. Functional metabolism imaging of nuclear medicine is currently the most widely used in clinical practice. It is one of the most prominent advantages of nuclear medicine, and also one of the most mature technologies in molecular nuclear medicine. ^{18}F labeled deoxyglucose (^{18}F-FDG) imaging is the most common use. Generally, the higher the malignancy of the tumor, the higher metabolism of glycolysis, and the more aggregation of ^{18}F-FDG (Figure 6–12). Therefore, nuclear medical examination has unique advantages in detecting metastatic lesions.

Bone scanning is a preferred method for bone metastasis because of its high sensitivity. Changes in bone metabolism often occur before morphological changes. The concentration of imaging agents in bone lesions is often higher (Figure 6–13) suggesting that the blood supply of bone tissue is abundant, and metabolism is vigorous and osteogenesis is active. But its specificity is poor. The most extensive application of nuclear medicine in the treatment of cancer is taking ^{131}I for thyroid cancer. ^{131}I can scavenge residual thyroid tissue and small metastatic lesions that are difficult to detect. Thereby the recurrence rate and metastasis rate of thyroid cancer were reduced. Another treatment is to implant ^{125}I radioactive particles into the tumor tissue. The radiation released by ^{125}I decay is used to kill tumor cells. ^{125}I particle implantation has a certain local control effect, and can improve the patient's survival time and quality of life. Nowadays, nuclear medicine related techniques can be used to diagnose and treat tumors at the molecular and gene level, and will be more widely used in the future.

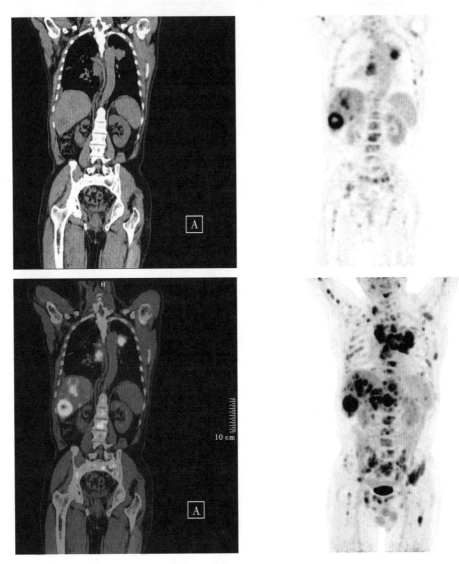

It is more sensitive than CT in showing metastatic tumor.

Figure 6-12   PET-CT showed multiple organs, lymph nodes and bones and other metabolic areas

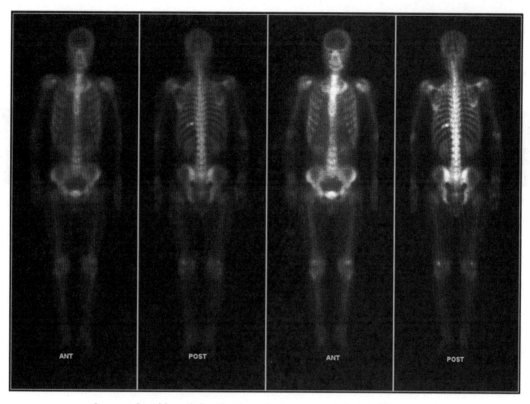

It was confirmed by pathology that it was the bone metastatic lesion of lung cancer.

Figure 6-13   The bone scan showed that the left 10th posterior costal imaging agent was aggregated

Zhang Yonggao

Chapter 7

Laboratory Examinations of Tumor

7.1 Summary of key points

Tumor is a group of cells in local tissues that lose the normal regulation of their growth at the gene level and form abnormal proliferation or differentiation under the action of various carcinogenic factors. Early detection of tumor, small volume, less metastasis, such as timely surgical treatment can thoroughly clear the focus, can effectively control the development of the tumor, and receive twice the result with half the effort. The World Health Organization (WHO) estimates that the cure rate of early tumors can reach 833. Therefore, the study of early detection, diagnosis and early treatment of tumors has been actively carried out. It is very important to prevent and control cancer. At present, laboratory examination is mainly based on tumor markers as an index of observation. Tumor markers have great practical value in the clinical diagnosis of tumor, detection of tumor recurrence and metastasis, evaluation of tumor therapeutic effect and prognosis, and group follow-up observation. It also opens up a new prospect for early detection of tumor and systematic study of its occurrence, development mechanism, treatment, and prognosis monitoring. In addition, the emergence of new experimental techniques provides a more accurate and effective method for the detection of tumor in laboratory.

7.2 Tumor markers

7.2.1 The basic concept and history of tumor markers

Tumor markers were proposed by Herberman in 1978 at the National Cancer Institute (NCI) meeting on human and tumor immunological diagnosis. It was confirmed the following year at the 7th British Conference on Oncogenesis Biology and Medicine. With the development of biotechnology and the further study of tumor pathogenesis, many new tumor markers have been found in recent years, especially the screening and detection of tumor markers by proteomics.

Tumor markers are proteins, oncogenes, tumor suppressor genes and their related products that are usually increased in quantity in the form of antigens, enzymes, receptors, hormones or metabolites with the appearance of tumors. These components are generated and secreted by tumor cells, or part of the tumor cell structure that is released, not only in tumor cells but also frequently in serum or other body fluids, which can respond to the presence of tumors in vivo to a certain extent.

From the cellular level, tumor markers are expressed the surface of cell membrane, cytoplasm or nucleus, so various components of the cell can be used as tumor markers. In particular, various components of the cell membrane include membrane antigens, receptors, enzymes and isozymes, glycoproteins, adhesion factors, carcinoembryonic antigens secreted in the cytoplasm, tumor-related antigens. Enzymes and transporters are associated with genes in the nucleus. These substances can be secreted into circulating blood and other body fluids or tissues, through immunology, molecular biology, proteomics and other techniques and methods to determine the level or content of their expression, so as to be used in clinical. As the auxiliary diagnosis of tumor, the therapeutic effect and prognosis of tumor were monitored. In addition, with the development of molecular biology and cancer genome, changes in chromosome level, including transcriptome and micRNA, can be used as tumor markers. It is believed that the study of DNA level and RNA level will enrich the theory and application of tumor markers.

7.2.2 Classification of tumor markers

The ideal tumor markers should accord with the following conditions: ①high sensitivity; ②strong specificity; ③tumor markers and tumor metastasis, the degree of malignancy is related. It can assist in tumor staging and prognosis judgment. The concentration of tumor markers is related to tumor size, the half-life of tumor markers is short, and the tumor markers decrease quickly after effective treatment. It is easy to detect tumor markers in the body fluid, especially in blood.

According to the source, distribution, biological characteristics, and basic principles, tumor markers are generally classified into five categories.

7.2.2.1 Enzyme tumor markers

The enzyme is one of the earliest tumor markers to be studied and used. Before the discovery of carcinoembryonic antigen and monoclonal antibody, enzymes have been used in tumor diagnosis. This is also the second stage of the development of tumor markers. Abnormal changes in the activity or expression of enzymes occur during tumor development. With the necrosis of tumor tissue or the change of membrane permeability of cancer cells, enzymes were released into the peripheral circulation. Increased enzyme activity is also found in pancreatic duct or bile duct obstruction and renal dysfunction. The localization of enzyme in the cell may determine the release rate of enzyme. When the enzyme is released into the peripheral circulation, it often means the appearance of malignant tumor. The increase of enzyme level may indicate the metastasis of the tumor(Table 7-1).

Table 7-1   The relationship between enzyme and tissue type of tumor

Name of enzyme	Assay method	Tissue type of tumor
Alcohol dehydrogenase	Activity	Liver
Aldolase	Activity	Liver
Alkaline phosphatase	Activity	Bone, liver, leukemia, sarcoma
Alkaline phosphatase-placenta	Activity	Ovary, lung, trophoblast, gastrointestinal tract, seminoma, hodgkin's lymphoma

Continue to Table 7-1

Name of enzyme	Assay method	Tissue type of tumor
Amylase	–	Bladder
ARB	Activity	Colon, breast
Creatine kinase	Activity	Prostate, lung (small cell carcinoma), breast, colon, ovary
Esterase	Activity	Breast
Galactoside transferase	Activity	Colon, bladder, stomach, etc.
γglutamine transferase	Activity	Liver
Hexokinase	Activity	Liver
Lactate dehydrogenase	Activity	Liver, lymphoma, leukemia, etc.
Leucine aminopeptidase (LAP)	Activity	Pancreas, liver
Neuron-specific enolase	RIA	Lung (small cell tumor, neuroblastoma, benign tumor, melanoma, pheochromocytoma, pancreas
5-nucleotidase	Activity	Liver
PAP	Activity/immunity	Prostate
PSA	Activity	Prostate
Pyruvate kinase	Activity	Liver
Ribonuclease	Activity	Multiple tumors (ovary, lung, large intestine)
Sialyltransferase	Activity	Breast, colon, lung
Terminal deoxynucleotide transferase	Activity	Leukemia
Thymidine kinase	RIA/activity	Multiple tumors, leukemia, lymphoma, lung (small cell)

7.2.2.2 Hormone tumor markers

Hormones have been seen as tumor markers for half a century. During tumorigenesis, the endocrine tissue reacts to increase or decrease hormone secretion or abnormal hormone secretion from the tissue site of the tumor and begin to secrete hormones (Table 7-2) (often called ectopic hormone, such as small cell lung cancer secreting adrenocorticotropic hormone (ACTH)). Because the specific RIA method for the detection of specific hormones has little cross-reactivity with natural hormones, this method can be used to monitor the treatment of cancer patients.

Table 7-2 The relationship between hormone and tissue type of tumor

Hormone	Type of tumor
Adrenocorticotropin	Cushing's syndrome, lung (small cell) cancer
Antidiuretic hormone	Lung (small cell) carcinoma, adrenal cortical tumor, pancreatic tumor, duodenal carcinoma
Bombesin	Lung (small cell) carcinoma
Calcitonin(CT)	Medullary carcinoma of thyroid gland

Continue to Table 7–2

Hormone	Type of tumor
Gastrin	Glucagonoma of pancreas
Growth hormone	Pituitary adenoma, renal carcinoma, lung cancer
Human chorionic gonadotropin	Embryonic carcinoma, choriocarcinoma, testicular carcinoma (non-seminoma)
Human placental prolactin	Trophoblastic cell carcinoma, reproductive adenocarcinoma, lung cancer, breast cancer
Neurophysin	Lung (small cell) carcinoma
Parathormone	Liver cancer, kidney cancer, breast cancer, lung cancer
PR	Pituitary adenoma, renal carcinoma, lung cancer
Vasoactive intestinal peptide	Pancreatic cancer, bronchial lung cancer, pheochromocytoma, neuroblastoma

7.2.2.3 Embryonic antigen tumor markers

The alpha-fetoprotein (AFP) and carcinoembryonic antigen (CEA), discovered in the 1960s, are still commonly used as tumor markers. AFP and CEA are both embryo antigens, which are the only proteins in the fetal life that gradually decline and disappear as adults. These embryonic antigens reappear in cancer patients. There are few tumor markers of embryonic antigens, but they are important markers commonly used in clinical practice(Table 7–3).

Table 7–3 The relationship between antigen and tissue type of tumor

Name of antigen	Type of tumor
AFP	Hepatocellular carcinoma, germ cell carcinoma (non-seminoma)
β carcinoembryonic antigen	Colon cancer
Carcinoembryonic ferritin	Liver cancer
Carcinoembryonic antigen	Colorectal cancer, gastrointestinal cancer, pancreatic cancer, lung cancer, breast cancer
Pancreatic cancer embryo antigen	Pancreatic cancer
Squamous cell antigen	Lung cancer, skin cancer, head and neck cancer
Tissue polypeptide antigen	Breast cancer, colorectal cancer, ovarian cancer, bladder cancer, etc.

7.2.2.4 Glycoprotein tumor markers

Glycoprotein tumor markers are glycoprotein antigens on the surface of tumor cells or glycoproteins secreted by tumor cells. Glycoprotein-bound carbohydrates are a class of nitrogen-containing polysaccharides (mucopolysaccharide), and the more common ones are sialic acid and fucose. There are abundant glycoproteins on the surface of normal cell membrane. When normal cells are transformed into malignant cells, the glycoproteins on the surface of cells mutate and form a special antigen different from that of normal cells. People use a monoclonal technique to detect these antigens, so it is called glycoprotein antigens. It is a new generation tumor marker which is different from enzyme and hormone, and is far more sensitive and specific than enzyme and hormone markers. The study of glycoprotein tumor markers has promoted the development and clinical application of tumor markers(Table 7–4).

Table 7-4　The relationship between glycoprotein antigens and tissue type of tumor

Name of tumor marker	Antibody	Auxiliary diagnosis of cancer
CA125	OC125	Breast cancer
CA15-3	DF3,115D8	Breast cancer, ovarian cancer
CA549	BC4E549, BC4N154	Breast cancer, ovarian cancer
CA27-29	B27-29	Breast cancer
MCA	b-12	Breast cancer, ovarian cancer
DU-PAN-2	DU-PAN-2	Pancreatic cancer, ovarian cancer, gastrointestinal cancer, lung cancer
CA19-9	19-9	Pancreatic cancer, liver cancer, gastrointestinal cancer
CA195	19-5	Pancreatic cancer, ovarian cancer, gastrointestinal cancer
CA50	C50	Pancreatic cancer, rectal carcinoma, gastrointestinal cancer
CA724	B27.3, cc49	Gastrointestinal cancer, pancreatic cancer, ovarian cancer
CA242	C242	Gastrointestinal cancer, pancreatic cancer

　　Glycoprotein antigens can be divided into two categories: one is macromolecular mucin, such as CA125、CA15-3、CA549、CA27-29, which is mainly secreted by mammalian epithelial cells, and is called epithelial mucin. CA15-3, CA549, CA27-29 are identified in the test experiment with the similar antigen determinants, but the antibodies used are different. A large number of studies have shown that mucin, as a tumor-associated protein, is highly abnormal expressed in breast cancer, which is an important biological index of breast cancer. CA15-3, CA27-29, MCA, BCM all come from mucin, and its antigenic determinant is only slightly different. In many kinds of tumors, such as breast cancer, mucin has the following changes. ①High expression and positive correlation with malignant degree of tumor. ②The polarity distribution of cell surface was lost, and the whole cell surface and cytoplasm were able to express mucin. ③The structure changes, the new peptide chain and the sugar chain epitopes appear. This qualitative and quantitative change makes mucin a marker for tumor recurrence and metastasis. The other is the tumor marker of blood group antigens, such as CA19-9, CA195, CA50, CA724, which is a derivative of sialidase and is often used as a marker of digestive tract tumor and pancreatic cancer. At present, these important glycoprotein antigens are detected by corresponding antibodies and can be used to assist in the diagnosis of specific tumors.

7.2.2.5　Receptor tumor markers

　　(1)Androgen receptor

　　Androgens, namely testosterone, and dihydrotestosterone participate in the growth and maintenance of the prostate gland. Testosterone and dihydrotestosterone act through the androgen receptor(AR), a typical nuclear steroid hormone receptor. Androgen receptors activate the transcription of genes that contain androgen response elements, thus regulating the growth and development of prostate cancer. The role of androgen receptors in the development of the prostate is based on the fact that anti-androgen therapy works well but is short-lived. In addition, antiandrogen therapy can be seen in antiandrogen therapy to stimulate prostate cancer cells. Many mutations have been found in androgen receptors. These mutations can cause estrogen, progesterone, glucocorticoids, and androgen that can stimulate the growth of prostate cancer cells to inappropriately activate AR, suggesting that these mutations play a role in the development of cancer and the development of drug resistance.

(2) Estrogen receptor

Progesterone and estradiol levels did not change in breast cancer patients, but in some patients, progesterone receptor (PR) and estradiol receptor (ER) increased. Because progesterone receptor synthesis is dependent on estrogen, progesterone receptor testing is complementary to estrogen receptor assays. If breast cancer metastases are positive for both receptors, endocrine therapy is 75% efficient; for patients with positive estrogen receptor and negative progesterone receptors, the effective rate is 40%; for those with negative estrogen receptor and positive progesterone receptors, the effective rate is 25%. According to the results of receptor assay, the patients with endocrine therapy had longer survival time and better prognosis.

(3) Hepatocyte growth factor receptor

Hepatocyte growth factor receptor(HGFR), also known as c-Met, is a major oncogene tyrosine kinase receptor, mainly expressed in healthy epithelial cells. The natural ligand of c-Met is the hepatocyte growth factor(HGF). After being activated by its ligands, it can produce a wide range of cell responses, including proliferation, survival, angiogenesis, wound healing, invasion of organs, and so on. Overexpression of c-Met in prostate cancer, colorectal cancer, breast cancer, malignant melanoma, hepatocellular carcinoma, and cervical cancer is associated with tumor staging, metastatic potential, and poor prognosis. The increase of mRNA copy number of c-Met in colorectal cancer is related to the depth of invasion. In addition, the increase of its expression in breast cancer is associated with short survival time, and it is an independent prognostic indicator compared with Her-2 EGFR and hormone receptor status.

(4) Epithelial growth factor receptor

Epithelial growth factor receptor(EGFR) is a prototype of tyrosine kinase receptor family. The natural ligands of EGFR are epithelial growth factor EGF and transforming growth factor TGF-α. These growth factors may promote growth in tumor tissues by paracrine and autocrine. Overexpression of EGFR has prognostic value in many tumors. EGFR is an effective prognostic marker in head, neck, ovary, cervix, bladder, and esophagus.

7.3　Clinical application and prospect of tumor markers

The change of tumor markers is a biological signal reflecting the change of biological behavior of tumor cells. The combined detection of multiple tumor markers can even diagnose and discover tumors earlier than routine examination (X-ray, CT, MRI, B-mode ultrasound and cytopathology), and win valuable time for clinical treatment. Tumor markers can not only be used for screening of healthy population or high-risk population, but also can be used as a reliable basis for early diagnosis, differential diagnosis, treatment detection, curative effect evaluation, recurrence and metastasis, prognosis judgment, and finding a therapeutic target in clinic. Sometimes tumors can even be detected early in asymptomatic conditions. Here are some common tumor markers and their clinical applications.

7.3.1　Lung cancer tumor markers

The incidence and mortality of lung cancer are the highest among urban residents in China. Lung cancer is divided into two cell types: small cell lung cancer (SCLC) and non-small cell lung cancer (NSCLC). SCLC is highly invasive and has a poor prognosis, accounting for about 20% of the total number of lung cancer. Chemotherapy and radiotherapy are effective, and the total remission rate of combined chemotherapy can reach 80%. NSCLC includes squamous cell carcinoma, adenocarcinoma, and large cell carcinoma, accounting for about 75% of lung cancer. Radical resection is the only chance for patients with NSCLC to be cured. The tumor markers of lung cancer are a valuable tool that can be used in clinical diagnosis and treatment of lung cancer.

7.3.1.1   Neuron-specific enolase

Neuron-specific enolase(NSE) is a useful index for the diagnosis and monitoring of SCLC. Studies on SCLC and NSCLC suggest that the high expression of serum NSE is an important characteristic of SCLC. Its sensitivity in SCLC is 55% –99% and in NSCLC it is only 5% –21%. At present, serum NSE is the most sensitive to SCLC in known tumor markers, followed by serum LDH level. In addition to SCLC, hemolysis, small intestine and lung carcinoid, pheochromocytoma, adenocarcinoma, and melanoma may also have elevated NSE. Elevated NSE in NSCLC suggests an extremely poor prognosis, which may be due to the heterogeneity of tumor cells or neuroendocrine subtypes.

7.3.1.2   Keratin 19 fragment and CYFRA21–1

Keratin 19 (CK19) is a kind of protein intermediate metabolites, which exists in the cytoplasm of epithelial tumor cells, including lung cancer, and is an acidic cytoplasmic protein. CYFRA21–1 is a fragment of CK19 with a serum concentration of 1.8 ng/ml in normal volunteers. CYFRA21–1 is a valuable marker of NSCLC. Smoking has no effect on serum concentration. CYFRA21–1 was increased in all types of lung cancer, especially in squamous carcinoma and adenocarcinoma. CYFRA21–1 also has high sensitivity and specificity. CYFRA21–1 is one of the reliable methods for the diagnosis of squamous cell carcinoma.

7.3.1.3   Carcinoembryonic antigen

The normal reference value of carcinoembryonic antigen(CEA) is< 5 μg/L. Serum CEA levels in patients with NSCLC were elevated, including adenocarcinoma, large cell carcinoma, and squamous cell carcinoma. On the other hand, 13.6% was increased in heavy smokers and 1.8 % in non-smokers. Patients with chronic obstructive pulmonary disease (COPD) and pulmonary infection, including pulmonary tuberculosis, also have increased CEA, but they are far less frequent than those of malignant tumors.

7.3.1.4   Lactate dehydrogenase

Lactate dehydrogenase(LDHs) can be expressed in SCLC cells, but its high expression has traditionally suggested liver involvement and liver metastasis in nearly 25% of patients with SCLC. The patients with normal LDH had an obvious survival advantage. The patients with elevated LDH were less sensitive to treatment and had a low probability of complete remission. Continuous detection of LDH can dynamically observe the clinical efficacy. The level of LDH in patients with bone metastasis is almost significantly increased, so it is suggested that patients with normal blood LDH should not undergo traumatic bone marrow staging.

7.3.1.5   Progastrin releasing peptide

Progastrin releasing peptide (ProGRP) is a precursor of gastrin releasing peptide. It is found in human gastrointestinal cells, bronchoalveolar cells, and neurons. ProGRP is a specific tumor marker of SCLC. In NSCLC patients, the increase of ProGRP is rare (< 3%). If the serum concentration of ProGRP in patients with NSCLC is more than 100 pg/ml, it should be suspected clinically whether it is a mixture of small cell components, neuroendocrine subtypes or renal dysfunction.

7.3.1.6   Tissue polypeptide antigen

Tissue polypeptide antigen(TPA) is a chain polypeptide that can be isolated from the cell membrane and smooth endoplasmic reticulum of malignant tumors. In some benign diseases, such as hepatitis, cirrhosis, diabetes, and cholecystitis. Serum TPA >100 U/L in patients with NSCLC, suggesting a shorter survival period. The rise of TPA is often earlier than the recurrence and progression of clinically visible diseases.

7.3.1.7　Squamous cell carcinoma antigen

It is a glycoprotein secreted by NSCLC. In 95% healthy controls, its normal value is below 1.5 ng/ml. The serum level of squamous cell carcinoma antigen (SCCA) was increased in some pathological types of NSCLC, and it also increased when the liver and kidney function was poor, but smoking did not affect the serum concentration. Serum SCC-Ag levels increased in 35% of patients with squamous cell carcinoma and only 17% in non-squamous cell carcinoma patients.

7.3.2　Breast cancer tumor markers

Breast cancer is one of the most common malignant tumors among women. Every year, about 1.2 million women worldwide suffer from breast cancer and 500,000 people die from breast cancer. In developed countries, such as Europe and America, the incidence of breast cancer occupies the first place in female malignant tumors. In recent years, the incidence of breast cancer in China has also increased year by year, which seriously threatens the physical and mental health of women. Therefore, the early diagnosis, treatment, and prevention of breast cancer have been the focus of domestic and foreign researchers.

7.3.2.1　Combined application of CEA and CA15-3

CEA is not specific for the diagnosis of breast cancer, but CEA can be detected in the serum of most patients with breast cancer metastasis, so it can be used as a prognostic marker in patients with advanced breast cancer. CA15-3 is a good index for monitoring postoperative recurrence of breast cancer patients. For breast cancer patients, the sensitivity of single detection of CEA or CA15-3 is only 10%, and positive results can be detected in benign tumors of breast cancer and normal people. So, both of them have no practical significance for the early diagnosis of breast cancer. Therefore, combined use of CEA and CA15-3 can increase the sensitivity of detection of metastatic breast cancer and have a good clinical value for the prognosis of breast cancer.

7.3.2.2　HER2/neu

HER2/neu is one of the oncogenes that have been studied deeply in breast cancer in recent years. It is a prognostic factor for breast cancer. It plays an important role in development, metastasis, curative effect observation and prognosis of breast cancer. HER2/neu is a proto-oncogene, which is a member of human epidermal growth factor receptor family and has the activity of endogenous tyrosine kinase. The rate of amplification and overexpression of HER2/neu gene was about 90 in breast cancer patients, 20%-30% in primary invasive breast cancer and nearly 100% in acne type ductal carcinoma in situ. This shows that HER2 plays an important role in the natural occurrence of breast cancer. HER2 is mainly expressed in breast, gastrointestinal tract, respiratory tract, and genitourinary epithelium. After over-expressed HER2 protein is self-activated by polymerization on the cell surface, it leads to malignant transformation through different signal transduction pathways such as MAPK/PI3K-AktAMP and so on. Overexpression of HER2 protein is often found on the surface of breast cancer cells, but the expression of HER2 protein is very low on the surface of normal cells.

7.3.2.3　Tissue polypeptide specific antigen

Tissue polypeptide specific antigens (TPS) is a carcinoembryonic protein with no organ specificity. The mortality rate of patients with TPS<80 U/L was 3% and had no significant difference compared with that of women of the same age, while the mortality rate of patients with TPS increased by 19% and 72% at 80–400 U/L or >400 U/L respectively. Therefore, TPS can be used as a prognostic marker for breast cancer. In addition, the combination of TPS and CA15–3 will obtain the best results in the evaluation of prognosis and treatment.

7.3.2.4   Breast cancer susceptibility gene1 and breast cancer susceptibility gene2

20% of breast cancer patients have a family history, which is associated with two breast cancer susceptibility genes, breast cancer susceptibility gene(BRCA)1 and BRCA2. The BRCA1 and BRCA2 proteins are similar, both of which are nuclear proteins regulated by the cell cycle. They are highly expressed in adult testis, thymus, mammary glands, and ovaries, all of which contain transcriptional activation domains. It can act as a common regulator through direct interaction with sequence-specific transcription factors to participate in the repair of DNA damage. BRCA1 and BRCA2 are tumor suppressor genes, which encode tumor suppressor protein and inhibit tumor growth. Although mutations in BRCA1 and BRCA2 can lead to breast and ovarian cancer, not every carrier can be diagnosed. If both BRCA1 and BRCA2 have mutations, then from birth to age 70, the risk of developing breast cancer is the same. For women, the risk rate can increase from 38% to 86%.

7.3.3   Gastric cancer tumor markers

The morbidity and mortality of gastric cancer are still high in China. Compared with liver cancer, prostate cancer, and other tumors, a tumor marker has not been found to be independent in the diagnosis of gastric cancer or to judge the prognosis of gastric cancer. However, the detection of different tumor markers will be reasonably organized and combined with other relevant clinical examinations. It is still of great significance to improve the positive rate of early diagnosis and the accuracy of prognosis of gastric cancer.

7.3.3.1   Carcinoembryonic antigen

CEA is generally regarded as the digestive tract tumor markers. The positive rate of CEA in clinical primary gastric cancer was only about 25%, but the serum level of CEA was significantly increased when gastric cancer metastasized, especially liver metastasis, which was related to the degree of metastasis. Dynamic observation of serum CEA level is an important index for clinical evaluation of curative effect and recurrence.

7.3.3.2   CA19–9

The content of CA19–9 in serum is significantly increased in digestive system tumors, so it is also called digestive tract tumor-associated antigen. In the benign lesions of the digestive tract, CA19–9 also increased, but the extent was small. The increase of CA19–9 in serum of pancreatic cancer was the most obvious, and it was the first marker of pancreatic cancer. The positive rate of CA19–9 in gastric cancer is about 35%, and the clinical significance of detecting CA19–9 alone in gastric cancer is limited. However, if combined with CEA, it will be helpful to diagnose gastric cancer and judge the survival time of patients.

7.3.3.3   CA724

CA724 can be increased in all kinds of gastrointestinal tumors and ovarian cancer. Compared with other tumor markers, the increase of CA72 4 is also more common in gastric cancer and is the preferred marker for gastric cancer. In gastric cancer, the combined detection of CA724 and CEA can significantly improve the sensitivity of gastric cancer diagnosis. Detection of CA724 alone cannot be used as an indicator of gastric cancer recurrence.

7.3.3.4   Alpha-fetoprotein

Alpha-fetoprotein(AFP) is an important index in the diagnosis of liver cancer. It can also be detected in the gastric cancer of some tissue types. However, it is different from the AFP produced by liver cancer and has a gastrointestinal specificity, with the lectin reflect is characterized by AFP-C1 increase. Patients with elevated AFP are more likely to have liver metastasis and poor prognosis and are more common in the advanced stage of gastric cancer. In very few cases of early gastric cancer, if AFP is elevated or AFP continues to rise after chemotherapy, it is proved that gastric cancer is prone to liver metastasis or chemotherapy-insensitive. Therefore, the detection of AFP in gastric cancer is helpful to judge the prognosis and the curative effect of chemotherapy.

7.3.3.5   CA125

CA125 is the preferred marker for ovarian cancer, but it is also highly sensitive in other tumors, mainly in digestive tract tumors. The distant metastasis of gastric cancer, especially the abdominal metastasis, is often accompanied by the elevation of CA125. CA125 combined with laparoscopy is a good index to judge the abdominal metastasis of gastric cancer.

7.3.4   Liver cancer tumor markers

The value of tumor markers of liver cancer in clinical application are: ①diagnosis of primary liver cancer; ②general survey of high risk population of liver cancer; ③monitoring of recurrence and metastasis of liver cancer; ④differential diagnosis of liver cancer; ⑤observation of curative effect and prognosis of liver cancer; ⑥judgement of the degree of development of liver cancer; ⑦treatment of liver cancer. The tumor markers of liver cancer should have the above clinical value, which should be characterized by strong specificity, high sensitivity, and the expression or serum concentration correlate with tumor tissue size and disease course.

7.3.4.1   AFP

AFP is the first liver cancer marker to be discovered. In China, AFP is higher than normal in 60% to 70% of primary liver cancers. AFP has been the first marker of liver cancer for more than 30 years. The accuracy of diagnosis of hepatocellular carcinoma is second only to pathological examination. The criteria for the diagnosis of hepatocellular carcinoma by single AFP index were as follows: AFP≥500 μg/L for 1 month or AFP≥200 μg/L for more than 2 months, and can exclude pregnancy, active liver disease, and gonad embryonal tumors. The diagnostic accuracy rate was 98%, and the remaining 2% false positive rate mainly came from benign liver disease and yolk sac, and a few malignant tumors related to endoderms such as gonads and gastrointestinal tract. It is worth noting that the dynamic changes of serum AFP should be emphasized in the diagnosis and treatment of clinical liver cancer, and combined with image localization examination. This will contribute to the early diagnosis of liver cancer and the diagnosis and differential diagnosis to reduce the missed diagnosis.

AFP is currently recognized as the best diagnostic marker for early liver cancer. It has important application value in the differential diagnosis of primary liver cancer and other liver diseases, observing the curative effect of liver cancer, the change of disease condition and the recurrence and metastasis after operation. AFP combined with ultrasound imaging has become a common, convenient, economical and effective method for monitoring postoperative liver cancer.

As a marker of liver cancer, AFP also has some problems. Firstly, it was a false positive. In physiological condition, AFP mainly existed in embryonic serum and disappeared immediately after birth. In addition to considering primary liver cancer, AFP can also be seen in yolk sac and embryogenic tumor. Therefore, AFP is also a good marker for reproductive adenocarcinoma and teratoma, such as testis, ovary and so on. AFP is also common in gastric cancer, pancreatic cancer, and cholangiocarcinoma. Inaddition, fetal congenital malformations and obstetric disorders can also have a significant increase in AFP. Secondly is a false negative. In China, 30% –40% of HCC patients have serum less than 20 μg/L, that is, the so-called false negative. The reasons may be related to the number of AFP hepatoma cells, the growth cycle of HCC cells, the size of HCC cells and the differentiation degree of HCC cells. In addition, the AFP concentration of HCC with severe denaturation and necrosis or more fibrous connective tissue components can be decreased or not increased. For the qualitative diagnosis of AFP false-negative HCC, other liver cancer markers can be used to detect it.

7.3.4.2　Enzyme and isoenzyme

(1) Abnormal prothrombin

The positive rate of abnormal prothrombin(AP) in liver cancer patients is relatively close, ranging from 55% –75% . The false positive rate of benign liver diseases is lower, such as chronic hepatitis, cirrhosis is about 10% , so it is superior to AFP in differentiating benign liver diseases. AP was not associated with AFP, and the positive rate of AP was about 60% in AFP negative or low concentration HCC. As for the diagnostic value of AP assay for small hepatocellular carcinoma, opinions are not consistent. In general, there is no diagnostic value for microscopic liver cancer with a tumor diameter of less than 2 cm, and a positive rate of 50% –60% for small hepatocellular carcinoma with 2–5 cm. As a marker of liver cancer, the change of plasma content of AP has the following characteristics: ①with the growth and development of liver cancer, the plasma content of AP increases gradually; ②the plasma content of liver cancer decreased gradually after surgical treatment, and even to be normal; ③after recurrence of liver cancer, the plasma level increased again. Therefore, the determination of AP can reflect the growth process of HCC and is helpful to evaluate the curative effect of HCC and to monitor recurrence.

(2) Ferritin

Ferritin is an important iron storage protein in human body. Most of them are found in liver, spleen, pancreas, bone marrow and blood cells. Serum ferritin is an effective indicator of iron deficiency or iron overload. The serum ferritin antibody which has more anti-L subunits is used for radioimmunoassay, and the content in a normal person is 10–15 μg/L, generally less than 200 μg/L. 50% –70% ferritin increased significantly in HCC cells, which may be due to the release of necrotic ferritin into the blood, the reduction of ferritin clearance and the increase of ferritin synthesis. However, in most benign hepatocellular diseases, the serum ferritin level is also very high, so the value of serum ferritin determination in the diagnosis of liver cancer is limited due to its low specificity.

(3) Transferrin

Transferrin(TF) is an important ferritin in the blood. The TF in HCC is slightly lower than that in the healthy control group and the bigger the tumor is, the lower the TF value is in patients with liver cirrhosis, suggesting that TF is not a marker for early diagnosis of HCC.

7.3.4.3　Serum enzymes

γ-glutamine transpeptidase isozyme Ⅱ (γ-GTP-Ⅱ) has no relationship with AFP. Both of them can be synchronized or sequentially abnormal, or they can be individually positive. It can be seen that γ-GTP-Ⅱ is one of the good markers of liver cancer. The serum detection of alkaline phosphatase isoenzyme Ⅰ (ALP-Ⅰ) was only found in hepatocellular carcinoma (HCC) and a very small number of patients with metastatic liver cancer (HCC). The sensitivity of ALP-Ⅰ is low, but the specificity is high to 96.7% , and it has nothing to do with AFP and γ-GTP-Ⅱ, so it is a supplementary method for the diagnosis of liver cancer. The activity of alpha-L-fucosidase is 7 times higher in liver cancer tissue than that in host liver. It can be used as a marker of primary liver cancer and can be used for differential diagnosis between primary and secondary liver cancer. Inaddition, the level of MMP-9 may also be used as a marker for HCC, especially in terms of invasiveness and metastasis.

7.4 Combined detection and application of hepatocellular carcinoma markers

The clinical application of markers in the diagnosis of liver cancer has its limitations. There is a problem that the positive rate is not high or the specificity is not strong when the single test is carried out. Therefore, the combined detection of multiple markers, especially with AFP, can complement each other and increase the positive rate, which is an effective way to solve the problem of false negative and false positive of AFP in the diagnosis of liver cancer. It was reported in domestic literature that the positive rate of combined detection of γ-GTP-Ⅱ、AFU and AP in the diagnosis of liver cancer was 91.7%; the positive rate of AFP combined detection of AP, hypoxia-inducible factor (HIF-1) and AFU was 84.2%, 93.2%, and 93.9%, respectively; the positive rate of AFP, ferritin, and CEA combined detection is as high as 97.3%; the positive rate of AFP, γ-GTP-Ⅱ, ALP-ⅠPA in the diagnosis of liver cancer was as high as 98%. Therefore, the combined detection increased the positive rate of the above markers in the diagnosis of liver cancer. Of course, too many joint test items are bound to affect its clinical utility. It is recommended that the combined detection of AFP and γ-GTP-Ⅱ has a positive rate of 94.4% for the diagnosis of liver cancer, which is relatively simple and practical.

7.4.1 Colorectal cancer tumor markers

Colon cancer and rectal cancer are common malignant tumors, the morbidity and mortality of digestive system cancer are second only to gastric cancer, esophageal cancer. As early colorectal cancer does not have metastasis, surgical resection can often obtain good results. Therefore, the early detection and diagnosis of colorectal cancer are very important. Up to now, no tumor markers have been found to be specific to colorectal cancer. Among the tumor markers associated with colorectal cancer, carcinoembryonic antigen (CEA) is highly sensitive.

CEA is one of the commonly used diagnostic methods and one of the main reference indexes in the clinical diagnosis of colorectal cancer, but at present, CEA cannot be used as an early detection index of colorectal cancer. If combined with cytological examination, the diagnosis rate of colorectal cancer can be improved. At present, the determination of CEA in clinic is mostly used for dynamic observation, such as maintaining CEA at a high level or increasing indicates that the possibility of malignancy increases, which has some auxiliary diagnostic value for colorectal cancer, liver cancer, pancreatic cancer and so on.

The following table includes the results of CEA CA19-9 and CA242 in patients with colorectal cancer. It shows that the combined detection of various tumor markers can improve the positive detection rate, and its sensitivity is higher than that of CEA alone, but the disadvantage is that the specificity is reduced. Combined detection can improve the positive rate, which is of great clinical significance(Table 7-5).

Table 7–5   Comparison of frontal positive rate and specificity of various markers in detecting colorectal cancer

Markers	Positive rate/%	Specificity/%
CEA	55.2	96.5
CA19–9	34.3	93.5
CA242	57.5	89.0
CEA+CA242	73.1	86.5
CEA+CA19	59.7	91.5
CA242+CA19–9	68.2	88.5
CEA+CA19–9+CA242	73.1	68.5

In addition, CEA and CA series of tumor markers (such as CA19–9 and CA242) were closely related to the staging of colorectal cancer, and the positive rates were increased with the progression of colorectal cancer (Table 7–6).

Table 7–6   Comparison of serum CEA, CA19–9 and CA242 levels in patients with colorectal cancer

Stage	Number of examples	CEA/(μg/L)	CA19–9/(U/ml)	CA242/(U/ml)
A	10	2.89±2.61	14.81±9.99	5.76±4.34
B	63	9.13±11.65	21.32±34.08	17.72±25.93
C	44	12.25±17.58	69±62.23	30.86±35.06
D	17	21.62±27.87	89.54±86.27	64.29±49.46

7.4.2   Esophageal cancer tumor markers

The early stage of esophageal cancer is relatively hidden, and most of the patients with esophageal cancer have reached the middle and late stage. These patients often have a poor prognosis, their overall 5-year survival rate is lower than 10%, and the 5-year survival rate of early comprehensive treatment of esophageal cancer can be as high as 90%–100%. Therefore, early diagnosis is the key to improve the survival rate of esophageal cancer patients, and tumor markers play an important role in the diagnosis and treatment of esophageal cancer.

7.4.2.1   Cytokeratin 19 fragment

Cytokeratin 19 fragment (CYFRA21–1), also known as cytokeratin 19 fragment, had a sensitivity of 46% and 45.5%, and specificity of 89.3% and 97.3%, respectively, when the cutoff value was 1.4 μg/L. Postoperative CYFRA21–1 levels were significantly correlated with survival rate and tumor survival. The positive rate of CYFRA21–1 in patients with esophageal squamous cell carcinoma increased with the progression of disease. After treatment, the serum CYFRA21–1 level increased significantly before operation, suggesting that it can be used to monitor the recurrence of esophageal cancer.

7.4.2.2   Squamous cell carcinoma antigen

The level of squamous cell carcinoma antigen (SCCA) is related to the tumor load and the activity of tumor cells. Continuous dynamic monitoring is helpful to monitor the therapeutic effect, especially the sensitive index for monitoring the curative effect of the operation. The biological half-life of SCCA in blood was only a few minutes. Once the radical tumor was removed, the preoperative abnormal increase of SCCA could rapidly decrease to normal within 72 hours, but after palliative resection, the level of SCCA could be decreased temporarily. But most of them are still higher than normal. SCCA can be used as an important reference index for follow-up after treatment.

7.4.2.3　Carcinoembryonic antigen

The positive rate of CEA in esophageal carcinoma is lower, which may be related to the pathological type of esophageal carcinoma. Squamous cell carcinoma is the most common in esophageal carcinoma, accounting for 90% of esophageal carcinoma, and adenocarcinoma is less. However, CEA is mainly used in the diagnosis of adenocarcinoma. Therefore, CEA may be useful in clinical staging and postoperative monitoring of esophageal cancer.

7.4.3　Tumor markers for gallbladder and pancreas

In the early diagnosis of gallbladder carcinoma and pancreatic cancer, the detection of tumor markers has been widely used in clinic. Protein antigens, enzymes, hormones, peptides and other substances synthesized and secreted in tumors are generally detected by molecular biology or immunology, as well as abnormal gene changes during tumorigenesis.

7.4.3.1　Carcinoembryonic antigen

CEA is not a specific marker for malignant tumors and has only auxiliary value in diagnosis. The most important use of CEA is to monitor the development of tumor, the observation of curative effect and the evaluation of prognosis. It has no value for the early diagnosis of tumor, but it can be used as a reference index for the diagnosis of middle and late stage tumor.

7.4.3.2　Pancreatic cancer embryo antigen and pancreatic cancer-associated antigen

Pancreatic cancer embryo antigen(POA) is a glycoprotein extracted from embryonic pancreas and can be used as a specific marker of pancreatic cancer. In some patients with liver cancer, gastric cancer, cholangiocarcinoma, and lung cancer, the serum POA level was also increased, which was difficult to distinguish from pancreatic cancer, but the concentration of POA in benign pancreatic diseases was relatively low. pancreatic cancer-associated antigen(PCAA) is a glycoprotein isolated from pancreatic cancer ascites. The serum PCAA content of normal people is less than 16. 2 μg/L. Pancreatic cancer, lung cancer, and breast cancer all had positive rates. Histochemical studies showed that PCAA existed in normal human stomach, duodenum, large intestine, liver and bile epithelium. Cancer in these tissues, especially those containing mucus, has increased significantly. The positive rate of PCAA in well-differentiated adenocarcinoma of pancreas was higher than that in poorly differentiated adenocarcinoma. At present, the tumor markers of these two kinds of pancreatic cancer have a certain specificity for the diagnosis of pancreatic cancer, and the practical application value needs to be further examined.

7.4.3.3　Carbohydrate antigenic enzyme

CA19-9 is the most sensitive, clinical and valuable tumor marker for pancreatic cancer, a radioimmunoassay was< 37 U/ml. The sensitivity and specificity were 70% -93% and 60% -85%, respectively, using 37 U/ml as the standard for the diagnosis of pancreatic cancer. Serum CA19-9 level was positively correlated with TNM stage of pancreatic cancer but negatively correlated with survival time. The clinical significance: ①in adenocarcinoma, gallbladder carcinoma, and ampullary cholangiocarcinoma, the serum CA19-9 level was significantly increased, especially in the advanced stage of pancreatic cancer, the positive rate was about 74.9% ; ②CA19-9 also increased to varying degrees in acute pancreatitis, cholecystitis, cholestatic cholangitis, cirrhosis, hepatitis, and other diseases. Although CA19−9 is valuable in the diagnosis of pancreatic cancer, it cannot be used as a separate marker for differentiating pancreatic cancer from benign diseases.

7.4.4　Prostate cancer tumor marker

At present, the primary diagnosis of prostate cancer is mainly determined by PSA and rectal finger diagnosis, and the diagnosis must be performed by prostate biopsy. The screening of prostate cancer markers PSA is a recommended method in most western countries. There are many markers related to prostate cancer, such as total PSA(t-PSA), free PSA(f-PSA), composite PSA(c-PSA), ratio of fPSA/tPSA, proPSA, benign PSA(b-PSA), prostate specific membrane antigen (PSMA), human glandular kallikrein 2(hK2), et al.

7.4.4.1　Prostate specific antigen

Prostate specific antigen (PSA) is a serine protease activity protein chain glycoprotein. PSA is mainly synthesized by prostatic epithelial cells. A large number of PSA in semen are involved in the liquefaction process of semen. The content of PSA in serum is very small. When prostate cancer occurs, the tissue barrier between prostate and lymphatic system is destroyed, the contents of prostate enter into blood circulation, and the content of PSA in blood increases. Every gram of prostate cancer tissue can make serum PSA increase about 3.5 µg/L. But prostatic hyperplasia and prostatitis can also cause a slight increase in serum PSA. Therefore, it is not tumor-specific. Although PSA has limitations in clinical use, it is still the current screening for prostate cancer. The best indicator of adjuvant diagnosis and monitoring curative effect.

(1) PSA exists in serum in two biochemical forms

Some of them(5%−40%) are in the form of free PSA(f-PSA) with molecular weight of 33 kDa, and the majority (60%−90%) is in the form of a combination of f-PSA and α1-antichymotrypsin, α2-macroglobulin, etc. and is referred to as complex PSA (c-PSA). Total clinically measured PSA (t-PSA) includes f-PSA and c-PSA in serum. The half-life of PSA is 2−3 days.

(2) Reference range of PSA

The reference range of PSA for prostate cancer detection was 0−4 µg/L. About 25% of patients with prostate cancer had normal PSA levels, while about 50% of patients with benign prostate disease had elevated PSA levels.

(3) Free PSA and compound PSA

5%−40% of PSA in serum is in unbound form, called f-PSA. Benign prostate disease has higher f-PSAs, while prostate cancer patients have lower f-PSA. The percentage of f-PSA and t-PSA can help to detect early prostate cancer. In the diagnostic gray zone with a t-PSA concentration of 4−10 µg/L, if %f-PSA is less than or equal to 25%, the detection rate of cancer can be kept at 95%, and 20% unnecessary biopsy can be avoided. Some experts also argue that f-PSA may help predict prognosis on the grounds that a lower percentage of free PSA may indicate a higher degree of malignancy in prostate cancer. 60%−90% of PSA in the blood binds to a variety of endogenous protease inhibitors to form c-PSAs. Compared with t-PSA, c-PSA can enhance the specificity of prostate cancer diagnosis, but more clinical data are needed to confirm it.

7.4.4.2　ProPSA and benign prostate specific antigen

ProPSA is one of the f-PSA components. The detection of proPSA in serum can significantly increase the specificity of prostate cancer diagnosis. The detection of proPSA in the gray area of 4−10 µg/L PSA concentration is more valuable in differentiating prostate cancer from prostatic hypertrophy. Benign prostate specific antigen (b-PSA) is a form of degradation of f-PSA, a kind of f-PSAs that is shredded or decomposed internally. B-PSA was first found in transitional nodular tissue specimens of the prostate, and later b-PSAs were found in semen and serum of men with benign prostate disease. But the amount of b-PSA in serum was much smaller than that in prostate tissue and semen. Many studies suggest that prostatic b-PSA is a special subgroup of f-PSA, which is closely related to benign prostatic hyperplasia. B-PSA is not associated with prostate cancer, and can not be used alone to distinguish prostate cancer from benign prostatic hyperplasia.

7.4.4.3   Prostate specific membrane antigen

Prostate specific membrane antigen (PSMA) is a transmembrane glycoprotein expressed on the surface of prostatic epithelial cells. It is composed of 750 amino acids and has a relative molecular weight of 100 kDa. It is a kind of membrane surface marker. PSMA appears to be expressed only in the prostate, while PSMA expression is up-regulated in prostate cancer, significantly higher than that in benign prostate specific antigen(BPH). Recently, it has been reported that the high expression of PSMA is related to the grade, pathological stage, and recurrence of prostate cancer, and the high expression of PSMA mRNA can be found in the early stage of prostate cancer. Overexpression of PSMA protein can also be seen in the metastasis of prostate cancer, so it is considered to be a good tumor marker and target antigen for tumor therapy.

7.4.5   Tumor markers of testicular malignant tumors

Approximately 95% of the malignant tumors in the testis are germ cell tumors, and the other 5% are lymphoma, testicular mesothelioma, and mesothelioma. There are two main types of germ cell tumors: seminoma and non-seminomatous germ cell cancers of the testis(NSGCT). The detection of serum tumor markers in testicular tumor patients is very important. It can be used in tumor diagnosis, evaluation of curative effect, disease monitoring and so on. The recurrence of the tumor may only show the increase of tumor marker concentration in the initial stage. The most commonly used serological markers in testicular tumors are AFP and human chorionic gonadotropin (HCG). At least one of the serum markers in most NSGCT patients is elevated, and HCG and its free β subunit are very important for the detection of seminoma. Lactate dehydrogenase (LDH) and placental alkaline phosphatase (PLAP) can be used to detect seminoma and non-seminoma.

7.4.5.1   HCG and β-HCG

HCG is a heterodimeric glycoprotein hormone containing two subunits of α and β. α-subunit contains 92 amino acids, which are the same in HCG, luteinizing hormone (LH), follicle stimulating hormone (FSH) and thyroid stimulating hormone (TSH). The β-subunit is unique to HCG. Usually, HCG is determined by measuring the biological activity of the β-chain. The single subunit had no HCG activity, but β-HCG could enhance the growth and inhibit apoptosis of tumor cells. Sandwich ELISA assay was helpful for the detection of low concentrations of HCG and β-HCG in plasma of male and non-pregnant women. 5 U/L is a recognized threshold for diagnosis of testicular neoplasms. In addition, chemotherapy resulted in inhibition of gonad function and increased HCG level. Therefore, the increase of HCG level from< 2 U/L to 5 - 8 U/L during chemotherapy does not predict the recurrence of tumor.

7.4.5.2   AFP

AFP is a very sensitive marker for yolk sac tumors in testis. AFP is also a reliable marker for tumors with yolk sac components in adults. And it is also expressed in some embryonic carcinomas. In addition, the increase in serum AFP levels is usually caused by hepatocellular tumors, and sometimes by gastrointestinal tumors. AFP derived from the liver and yolk sac has different carbohydrate components, and the combination with exogenous lectins can distinguish whether the elevated AFP is derived from testicular carcinoma or liver disease. In addition, AFP has a certain value in identifying whether it is a testicular seminoma and a non-seminoma. It is mainly considered to be a mixed embryo in the tumor.

7.4.5.3 Placental alkaline phosphatase

Placental alkaline phosphatase(PLAP) is an alkaline phosphatase isoenzyme associated with tumor, which is useful for the diagnosis of seminoma. It is higher in 60% –70% of the patients with seminoma, but the increase in its content is also common in smokers. Immunohistochemical staining of PLAP is very useful for the diagnosis of germ cell tumors(Table 7–7). It is helpful for the diagnosis of intratubular seminoma and can be used as an early diagnostic index for testicular cancer.

Because of the diversity of the location and type of testicular tumor, the distribution of tumor markers in serum has its own characteristics. The combination of the above three tumor markers is helpful to the diagnosis, prognosis and treatment evaluation of tumor types.

Table 7–7   Immunohistochemical expression of multiple markers in tumor components of different histological types

Histological type	AFP	HCG	PLAP
Seminoma	Negative	30% –50%	>95%
Yolk sac tumor	90% –95%	Negative	40%
ECC	10%	Negative	95%
Syncytial trophoblastic tumor	Negative	90% –95%	40% –50%
Dermoid tumor	20%	Negative	<5%

7.4.6   Nasopharyngeal carcinoma tumor markers

Nasopharyngeal carcinoma (NPC) has no specific tumor markers. At present, there are EB virus antibody VCA-IgA and EBV-specific DNase antibody; other tumor molecular markers such as SCCA, TPA, TPS, and CEA are also elevated.

7.4.6.1   VCA-IgA and EA-IgA

After EBV infection, LMP and EBNA were mainly expressed in the incubation period, while early membrane antigens(EMA), early intracellular antigen(EIA), EB virus capsid antigen(VCA) and advanced associated antigenwere mainly expressed in the cleavage and replication stage. The antibodies associated with these antigens can be detected in the serum of nasopharyngeal carcinoma patients. Elevated serum VCA-IgA and EA-IgA levels are common in patients with nasopharyngeal carcinoma. It has been reported that VCA-IgA is as high as 96.5% in NPC patients, while the detection rate of VCA-IgA in the serum of non-NPC patients in the control group is only 4%. In the diagnosis of nasopharyngeal carcinoma, the sensitivity of anti-IgA was higher than that of anti-EA-IgA, but the specificity of the latter was higher than that of the former. Both specificity and sensitivity will be improved by combining the two methods. The level of anti-VCA-IgA can be used as a marker for screening high-risk population and observing the prognosis of treatment.

7.4.6.2   Anti-Epstein-Barr virus specific thymidine deoxynucleoside kinase antibody

Thymidine deoxynucleoside kinase(TK) is an enzyme that catalyzes the conversion of thymidine to monophosphate deoxythymine. It plays a key role in the synthesis of DNA. Studies show that TK has a good correlation with the level of TK antibody. ELISA can be used to detect anti-TK-IgA in patients.

7.4.6.3 Lmp-1

Many experiments have proved that Lmp-1 gene is an oncogene. Lmp-1 gene can be detected from exfoliated cells of nasopharyngeal carcinoma by PCR method. The specificity and sensitivity of Lmp-1 gene are 100.0% and 94.7% , respectively. In patients with recurrence after radiotherapy, although the tumor size is very small, the Lmp-1 gene can still be detected, but in the case of radionuclide osteonecrosis (ORN) is negative. Therefore, Lmp-1 gene can be used as a marker for differentiating recurrence of nasopharyngeal carcinoma from ORN.

7.4.6.4 Anti-EB virus specific deoxyribonuclease antibody

Deoxyribonuclease(DNase) is a nucleic acid endonuclease, DNase is commonly used in clinic to judge the changes of systemic lupus erythematosus (SLE). Anti-EB virus specific DNase antibody can be used as a molecular marker for early detection of nasopharyngeal carcinoma (NPC). High level of DNase antibody may indicate the high risk of nasopharyngeal carcinoma.

7.4.7 Tumor markers of gynecological reproductive system

7.4.7.1 Ovarian cancer tumor markers

The early diagnosis of ovarian cancer has been the most challenging topic in the study of ovarian cancer. It is of profound significance to study the tumor markers in the early ovarian cancer detection. Because most ovarian malignancies are epithelial tumors (ovarian cancer), tumor marker research is mainly focused on secretory tumor markers associated with ovarian cancer.

(1)CA125

CA125 is the best tumor marker in ovarian cancer patients. The critical value of CA125 was 35 U/ml, which decreased with the increase of menopause and age. It increased during the follicular phase of menstrual cycle. It was also found that CA125 increased in 5% of benign diseases and 28% of non-gynecological tumors in 1% –2% of normal women. The increase of plasma CA125 level in non-mucinous ovarian carcinoma was significantly higher than that in other gynecological tumors, non-gynecologic tumors, and some physiological states. The level of plasma CA125 is higher than 65 U/ml, suggesting the existence of ovarian epithelial tumor. Therefore, the determination of plasma CA125 level is of great significance in the screening of ovarian cancer and its early diagnosis.

(2)Folic acid receptor

The expression of folic acid receptors in normal tissues is very low, but many tumor cells express folate receptors highly, such as skin cancer, breast cancer, and ovarian cancer. The expression of folate receptor was positive in more than 90% of ovarian cancer and negative in normal ovarian epithelium. Therefore, the expression of folate receptor could be used as a good biomarker for ovarian cancer.

(3)Estrogen and progesterone receptor

Estrogen receptor (ER) and progesterone receptor (PR) are mainly distributed in the uterus, cervix, vagina and mammary gland. A large number of studies have shown that, in the long run, a large number of hormones are closely related to the occurrence of gynecological tumors, and may be characterized by increased, decreased or lost receptor function in tumor tissues. The expression of ERP was also related to histological type. The receptor positive rate of ovarian mucinous carcinoma is lower than serous carcinoma and endometrial carcinoma, indicating that the tumors of different tissue types have different expression rates of

ER and PR, which may be affected by different levels of hormones or different responses to hormones.

7.4.7.2　Tumor markers of cervical carcinoma and endometrial carcinoma

(1) CA125 and CA19-9

CA125 is the first choice method to distinguish cervical adenocarcinoma from cervical squamous cell carcinoma. The level of CA19-9 has a certain significance in the diagnosis of cervical cancer, and CA19-9 is limited in cancer tissue, but not in normal tissue, so CA19-9 is a sign of recurrence and progression of cervical cancer.

(2) CA15-3

The positive rate of ovarian tumors was higher than that of other gynecological tumors, and the level of plasma CA15-3 in patients with gynecological tumors could reflect the progress of the disease.

(3) CEA

The level of CEA can be used to judge the invasion of cervical adenocarcinoma. The positive rate of CEA in invasive carcinoma of cervix was higher than that in carcinoma in situ. In the positive staining site of CEA, the carcinoma in situ of cervical adenocarcinoma was located in the squamous epithelium but negative in the basal layer, while the invasive carcinoma appeared in the basal layer. CEA positive staining was found in the glandular side of the cell membrane, while in the endometrial carcinoma, CEA positive reaction was found in the cell membrane and cytoplasm.

(4) Squamous cell carcinoma-associated antigen(SCC-Ag)

It is widely found in epithelial cells of normal tissues (minimal content) and malignant lesions of different organs. SCC-Ag can also be used as an index of chemotherapeutic reaction in patients with squamous cell carcinoma of the cervix. If SCC-Ag persists after chemotherapy, it means that it is insensitive to chemotherapy and should be stopped immediately; if plasma SCC-Ag is maintained at a high level, suggesting the disease may relapse.

(5) Sex hormones and hormone receptors

The pathogenesis of endometrial carcinoma is related to the long-term stimulation of estrogen. ER and PR are expressed in most endometrial carcinoma. The positive rate of ER and PR is higher in well-differentiated tumors and the survival time of the patients with a positive receptor is longer.

7.4.8　Nervous system tumor markers

We still know very little about the molecular mechanism of tumors in the central nervous system. Due to the blood-brain barrier, plasma tumor markers are rarely used in primary or metastatic brain tumors.

7.4.8.1　Brain enriched hyaluronan binding(BEHAB/brevican)

Hyaluronan(HA) is widely found in extracellular matrix of various tissues and its function is regulated by specific hyaluronan binding protein. BEHAB/brevican is a unique hyaluronic acid binding protein in brain tissue and is the most specific glioma marker. The amount of BEHAB/brevican expressed in the central nervous system was related to the activity of mitosis, and the more active the mitosis is, the more the expression of BEHAB/brevican is. BEHAB/brevican was detected in oligodendroglioma and astrocytoma. However there was no BEHAB/brevican was detected in normal cerebral cortex control specimens, intracranial metastatic breast cancer, and intracranial primary non-glial tumors.

7.4.8.2　Intermediate filament

It includes nestin and glial fibrillary acidic protein.

(1) Nestin

Nestin is a marker of neural stem cells in the central nervous system, and its expression is closely related to mitosis. Nestin can be expressed in all kinds of intracranial tumors including gliomas. From the most malignant glioblastoma multiforme to the least malignant fibroid astrocytoma, nestin expression showed a significant decrease. Therefore, nestin is of special significance in judging the malignancy of gliomas. However, it lacks the specificity of gliomas and is generally detected only by immunohistochemistry in gliomas.

(2) Glial fibrillary acidic protein

Glial fibrillary acidic protein (GFAP) is present in glial cells, especially astrocytes and astrocytomas. The content of GFAP was higher in normal astrocytes than in astrocytomas, and higher in low grade astrocytomas than in high malignant astrocytomas. A decrease in GFAP expression in gliomas may indicate the progression of the tumor.

7.4.8.3 Neuron specific enolase

Neuron specific enolase (NSE) is distributed in every system of the whole body, but 90% is concentrated in the nervous system. The order of distribution of NSE in the nervous system is brain >spinal cord > peripheral nervous system. Under normal conditions, NSE is mainly distributed in neurons and neuroendocrine cells, so NSE is considered to be a marker of neuroendocrine cells. There was a direct relationship between the NSE concentration and the degree of surgical resection. After total resection of tumor, the concentration of NSE decreased rapidly to normal, but in the subtotal resection, the concentration of NSE remained high after operation, which also indicated that malignant glioma was the direct source of NSE in serum and cerebrospinal fluid cerebrospinal fluid cerebrospinal fluid (CSF).

7.4.9 Hematological system tumor markers

In the blood system, the most common reason for the activation of tumor-related genes is chromosome translocation, especially balanced translocation, which results in changes in the expression of a gene or changes in its structure to form a new fusion gene. These genes are important genes to regulate the differentiation, growth, and apoptosis of hematopoietic cells. Some of them are associated with a specific tumor type, such as PML-RAR α and acute promyelocytic leukemia (APL), BCR-ABL and chronic myeloid leukemia (CML).

7.4.9.1 PML-RARα

Acute promyelocytic leukemia (APL or M3) has the characteristic chromosomal abnormality of t(15; 17)(q22; q11–22), which rearranges the PML gene on chromosome 15 with the RAR α of chromosome 17. PML is a phosphoprotein that is only expressed in the myeloid line and inhibits cell growth and transformation. Overexpression of PML can induce apoptosis. RAR α, a member of steroid/thyroid receptor superfamily, is an intracellular receptor that promotes differentiation and inhibits proliferation. After fusion of two genes, PML-RAR α can form heterodimer with PML and then inhibit the function of wild-type PML-RAR α, thus inducing APL. More than 95% of APL have PML/RAR α, so it is considered that PML/RAR α is the molecular marker of APL and the main cause of carcinogenesis. Routine karyotype analysis of fish and nested RT-PCR can be used for clinical detection.

7.4.9.2 BCR-ABL

The existence of the Ph chromosome is one of the characteristics of chronic myelocytic leukemia (CML). It is the translocation of chromosome 9 and 22, that is t(9;22)(q34;q11). This translocation causes the ABL gene to be translocated from chromosome 9–22. BCR was fused with BCR gene to form the characteristic Ph chromosome. This chromosome was found in 95% of CML patients and was also found in 10% –30% of adult acute myeloid leukemia (ALL), about 5% of children with ALL and a few (close to 2%) acute myeloid leukemia (AMLL), lymphoma and myeloma. BCR-ABL has tyrosine kinase activity and plays a role in signal transduction. Imatinib, a specific tyrosine kinase inhibitor, can inhibit BCR-ABL specifically and effectively.

7.4.9.3 Prospect of clinical application of tumor markers

The discovery and application of tumor markers have important clinical value. These markers are not only helpful in the diagnosis of some tumors but also have the function of predicting or monitoring the recurrence or metastasis of tumors. It is helpful to evaluate the therapeutic effect and predict the prognosis. Unfortunately, no ideal tumor marker with 100% sensitivity and specificity has been found so far. In general, early diagnosis needs a more comprehensive analysis with the combination of history, symptoms, signs, imaging examination (B-ultrasound, CT, X-ray, gastroscopy, enteroscopy). And further pathological examination is needed to make the diagnosis clear. In addition, negative tumor markers can not completely exclude the associated tumors.

In addition, abnormal tumor markers can be found in many benign diseases. For example, prostatic hypertrophy and prostatitis may have a mild or moderate increase in PSA; endometriosis may have a mild to moderate increase in CA125; acute and chronic liver disease can have CA125, CA19–9 CA50, ferritin increased in varying degrees. Thirdly, the combined use of tumor markers can improve the positive detection rate to a certain extent, and the correlation between some tumor markers is extremely high. For example, the correlation between CA19–9 and CA50 can reach 95% –98%. That is, in 95% –98% of the subjects examined, if CA19–9 is normal and then CA50 is normal; if CA19–9 is abnormal and then CA50 is also abnormal. But it is not simply believed that the more markers are tested, the more certain they are. In clinical, the application of tumor markers should be based on different conditions, different purposes or combined use, and combined with other examination and comprehensive analysis. The WHO criteria for evaluating tumor efficacy include the following normative description of tumor markers: tumor markers cannot be used for diagnosis alone. If the tumor marker is initially above the upper limit of normal levels, they must return to normal levels when all tumor lesions have completely disappeared and the clinical assessment is complete remission. This regulation indicates the clinical significance of tumor markers and confirms the value of their clinical application(Table 7–8). It is believed that with the improvement of the research methods of tumor markers and the results of genomics and molecular epidemiology, there will be more sensitive, specific and reproducible tumor molecular markers, thus providing new approaches and strategies for early warning and early diagnosis for tumors.

Table 7–8   Clinical application of different tumor markers

Number	Marker	Hint	Other factors and considerations
1	CA242	It is specific and sensitive in colorectal, stomach, ovary, uterus and lung cancer, head and neck tumors. The diagnosis of pancreatic cancer and biliary tract tumors is more specific than CA19–9	It also rises in the benign liver and gallbladder disease but is lower than the boundary value. The false positive rate of benign digestive tract diseases is low. The combination of CA242 and CEA improves the sensitivity of the diagnosis of rectal cancer by 35%

Continue to Table 7-8

Number	Marker	Hint	Other factors and considerations
2	CA19-9	CA19-9 is a sensitive marker of pancreatic cancer and cholangiocarcinoma. It is helpful for the diagnosis of gastrointestinal neoplasms combined with AFP and CEA. It also has positive rates in ovarian cancer, lymphoma, gastric cancer, lung cancer, esophageal cancer, and breast cancer	Cholelithiasis, cholangitis, cholecystitis, ovarian cyst, chronic hepatitis, chronic pancreatitis, diabetes, endometriosis, AFP negative liver cancer. Patients with gastrointestinal bleeding increased slightly
3	CA153	CA153 may be increased in breast, lung, ovarian, pancreatic and colorectal cancer. Combined with CEA, it can improve the diagnostic accuracy	Liver/bone metastasis of breast cancer, endometriosis, ovarian cyst, metastatic ovary/colon/liver/bile duct/pancreas/bronchial carcinoma, etc.
4	CA125	It is mainly found in serous ovarian cancer. It can be increased in pancreatic cancer, breast cancer, liver cancer, lung cancer, gastrointestinal malignant tumor, uterine cancer	Ovarian epithelium/fallopian tube/endometrium/mesothelial cell/cervical adenocarcinoma. Slightly increased in endometriosis/pancreatitis/cholecystitis/menstrual/hepatitis/ovarian cysts
5	CA72-4	A marker for breast, gastrointestinal and ovarian cancer	It was significantly elevated in mucinous ovarian cancer
6	MG7-Ag	MG7-Ag is increased in 55% of gastric cancer and the false positive rate is 5%	It should be observed dynamically and combined with clinical
7	NSE	Small cell lung cancer (SCLC), neuroblastoma, APUD system tumor, neuroendocrine tumor	The serum should be placed for 60-90 min before centrifugation. It also increases when the central nervous system is damaged
8	Cyfra 21-1	Non-small cell lung cancer/lung squamous cell carcinoma/bladder cancer	Cyfra 21-1 is often used to monitor the curative effect. It is mildly elevated in colon/gastric cancer, but not generally elevated in non-tumor diseases. The coincidence rate of Cyfra 21-1 combined with CEA in the diagnosis of NSCLC can be as high as 78%
9	TPA	It reflects the proliferation of tumor and is used for auxiliary diagnosis of bladder, breast, lung, colorectal, cervix, ovary and hepatobiliary carcinoma	It should be observed dynamically and combined with clinical
10	TPS	It can reflect the activity of division and proliferation of tumor cells. It can reflect tumor proliferation activity and load when combined with CA153, CA125, CA19-9 CEA, and PSA	Attention should be paid to the volume index and dynamic observation when TPS is more than 160, and when more than 250, special attention should be paid to the differential diagnosis of tumor and liver disease

Continue to Table 7–8

Number	Marker	Hint	Other factors and considerations
11	PSA	It is the best index of prostate disease. When the PSA is more than 10 μg/ml, the sensitivity of diagnosis of prostate is up to 99% and the specificity is 47%. Early prostate cancer has PSA increased earlier than clinical symptoms for more than 6 months	Prostatitis and prostatauxe. The PSA value of bone metastases from prostate cancer is higher
12	f-PSA	The ratio of f-PSA/PSA was inversely proportional to the possibility of cancer, and the ratio < 0. 1 indicated prostate cancer and >0. 25 suggested hyperplasia	The ratio of f-PSA/PSA in patients with prostate cancer was significantly lower than that in patients with prostatic hyperplasia
13	UBC	It is often elevated in bladder cancer, renal pelvis, and ureteral neoplasms	The urinary system should be examined when it is elevated
14	CEA	Preoperative serum level was correlated with recurrence time and survival time of colorectal cancer. It can also be elevated in breast, lung, pancreas and prostate cancer. CEA was increased by 100% in cerebrospinal fluid (CSF) of meningioma patients	Cervical cancer, small cell, and non-small cell lung cancer, thyroid/ENT neoplasms, smokers. CEA increased significantly in lung/mammary/bladder/ovarian cancer shows tumor invasion and metastasis. Malignant tumor pleural effusion
15	AFP	Hepatocellular carcinoma and germ cell tumor. It can be used in combination with HCG and TPS to facilitate differential diagnosis	AFP is transiently elevated in benign liver disease. It is negative or low concentrations in 35% of patients, especially in patients with small liver cancer
16	Ferritin	Lung/breast cancer. There was a significant increase in AFP-negative or low-value liver cancer in patients with hematologic diseases	Hemoglobinosis, hepatitis, etc.
17	β-HCG	Sensitivityin trophoblastic malignant tumor is 100% and in non-spermatogenic testicular carcinoma is 70% and in seminoma is 10%. Breast cancer, testicular cancer, ovarian cancer	HCG is positive in chorionic epithelioma while AFP is negative and it is the opposite in the endodermal sinus tumor. Endometriosis, ovarian cyst, etc.
18	$β_2$-MG	It is proportional to the number of plasmacytoma and is related to the stage of myeloma. Hematologic neoplasms such as chronic granulocyte, lymphoma, bile duct, liver, stomach, colorectal, lung, esophagus, bladder cancer, cervix, and other solid tumors	It can be elevated in kidney disease, hepatitis, cirrhosis, acute rejection of kidney transplantation, rheumatoid arthritis, etc. And it is elevated in cerebrospinal fluid in meningeal leukemia

Continue to Table 7-8

Number	Marker	Hint	Other factors and considerations
19	S-100	It is significantly elevated in the advanced stage of malignant melanoma, reflecting the efficacy and outcome and predicting recurrence and metastasis glioma	Acute cerebrovascular disease/multiple sclerosis/nervous system injury and increased inflammation
20	SCC	It can be used for the diagnosis, curative effect and recurrence monitoring of squamous cell carcinoma of the cervix, lung and head and neck. Esophagus, bladder tumor	Benign lesions in the flat epithelium
21	EBV-IgA	It reflects the infection and carcinogenicity of EB virus and assists in the diagnosis of nasopharyngeal carcinoma and Burkitt lymphoma	When it is positive, attention should be paid to check nasopharynx and so on
22	EBV-IgM	It can reflect the recent EB virus infection and carcinogenicity and assist in the diagnosis of nasopharyngeal carcinoma and Burkitt lymphoma	When it is positive, attention should be paid to check nasopharynx and so on
23	HGH	Pituitary adenoma/non-small cell tumor/pheochromocytoma/thyroid medullary tumor/pancreatic endocrine tumor etc.	Acromegaly, giant disease

7.5   Other laboratory tests

7.5.1   Genetic diagnosis

7.5.1.1   Overview

Gene diagnosis is based on the gene level to diagnose the disease or state of human. It is a method which uses genetic materials as objects such as DNA or RNA, and examines the structure and expression of genes to diagnose the disease by use of molecular biological techniques. The method, which mainly detects the structural change and expression of genetic materials, is chiefly used to for the diagnosis ofinfectious diseases, congenital inheritance diseases, gene mutation such as tumor, prenatal diagnosis, paternity test, and forensic evidence, etc.

Molecular biology is the principal tool of gene diagnosis. In recent years, with the rapidly developed molecular biological technique, many techniques, which are centered on nucleic acid molecule hybridization and polymerase chain reaction (PCR), are widely used in genetic diagnosis, such as single strand conformation polymorphism (SSCP), restriction fragment length polymorphism (PFLP), allele specific oligonucleotide (ASO), gene chip, reverse transcription PCR, Southern blotting, Northern blotting, dot blotting, in situ hybridization (ISH), etc.

7.5.1.2 Gene diagnosis of tumor

The formation of Tumor is the result of the interaction between genetic factors and environmental factors, with the development of tumor molecular biology, it comes to gene level in the study of cancer, and people find many tumor-related genes and have an understanding of the oncogene, proto-oncogene and tumor suppressor gene.

(1) Oncogene

It is the gene that can participate in or directly cause malignant transformation of cells. It can be divided into two categories. One is tumor non-specific oncogene, such as H-ras, K-ras, c-myc and other genes, which can be detected in many tumors such as liver cancer, lung cancer, and colorectal cancer; The other is tumor-specific oncogene, for example, c belongs to non-specific oncogene; C-sis is associated with lymph node metastasis, and c-abl is related to chronic myeloid leukemia.

(2) Proto-oncogene

It refers to the sequences of genes that can transform into oncogenes in normal cells when stimulated by certain factors. The product can be encoded in the cell membrane, cytoplasm, nucleus and extracellular.

(3) Tumor suppressor gene

It is a kind of gene that inhibits the overgrowth and proliferation of cells to contain tumor formation. The loss or inactivation of tumor suppressor gene may lead to the occurrence of tumors. For example, the wild-type P53, a tumor suppressor gene, will lose the function of tumor suppressor if the point mutation, insert mutation and deletion mutation appear. Its inactivation plays an important role in the formation of tumor. So far, mutations of P53 have been found in many tumors, such as liver cancer, gastric cancer, breast cancer, leukemia, and lymphoma. With the development of molecular biology techniques, we can apply molecular biology techniques to detect tumor-related genes, so as to make early diagnosis of cancer and to determine its histologic malignant degree.

7.5.2 Immunohistochemical technique

7.5.2.1 Overview

Immunohistochemistry (IHC) technology is a special histochemical technique which uses known antibodies or antigens to detect the corresponding unknown antigen or antibody in tissue and cells. The technology, which has sharp specificity and high sensitivity, and can combine morphology, function and material metabolism, has become the most important and indispensable conventional technique in modern diagnostic pathology.

Currently, there are thousands of antibodies used in IHC, which can be divided into two categories: polyclonal antibodies and monoclonal antibodies. Polyclonal antibodies have many advantages, they are convenient to be prepared, have a good sensitivity, can be used for the paraffin section, and some of them are highly specific to their antigens. Also, there are some shortages: the nonspecific cross reactions are common and the titer of the antiserum is not quite stable. As for monoclonal antibodies, they have strong antigen specificity, stable quality, and titer, little nonspecific cross reaction, and can be produced as required anytime; however, they have low sensitivity and some of them can only be used for frozen sections.

There are many IHC testing methods, the most common method is the peroxidase-antiperoxidase enzymatic method (PAP method) and avidin-biotin complex method (ABC method), and others like biotin-streptavidin (B-SA) method, alkaline phosphatase anti-alkaline phosphatase (APAAP) method and two-step methods for marking polymer (such as En Vision), etc.

7.5.2.2　Application

Diagnosis and differential diagnosis of malignant tumors with lower differentiation. We can differentiate cancer, sarcoma, malignant lymphoma, and malignant melanoma by the use of keratin, vimentin, leukocyte common antigen, and S-100 protein.

(1) Determine the primary site of metastatic malignant tumor

For example, the metastatic carcinoma of lymph node expressing TGB and TTF-1 suggests that tumor springs from thyroid, metastatic carcinoma of bone that expressing PSA and PAP shows that tumor comes from prostate.

(2) Diagnosis and sorting of malignant lymphoma and leukemia

If tumor cells express CD20 and CD79α, it may be B cell lymphoma; and it may be mantle cell lymphoma if gets a positive cyclinD1 after further marked. What's more, tumor cells expressing CD3 and CD45 RO may be T cell lymphoma and that expressing CD30 and ALK may be anaplastic large cell lymphoma. Classical Hodgkin lymphoma expresses CD15 and CD30.

(3) Detection of hormone and related proteins

The technique can be used to diagnose and classify neuroendocrine neoplasm or determine the abnormal function of secreting hormone of non-endocrine tumor.

(4) Determine two or more elements which make up tumors

For instance, triton tumor is comprised of Schwann cells and striated muscle cells, which can be confirmed by S-100 protein and desmin respectively.

(5) Study tumors of unknown origin

Such as soft tissue granule cell which was thought derived from myoblast. Immunohistochemistry shows tumor cells express S-100 protein, and now it is a benign tumor of peripheral nerve when we combine the evidence of leukocyte differentiation from an electron microscope.

(6) Study the relationship between pathogens and tumorigenesis

As some types of papilloma viruses (HPV16 and HPV18) have a close association with cervical carcinoma; and EB virus is related to nasopharyngeal cancer, Burkitt lymphoma, Hodgkin's lymphoma, and NK/T lymphoma.

(7) Investigate and search for markers for precancerous lesions

Agglutinin PNA, SJA and UEA-1 increase gradually in colorectal adenomas, adenoma canceration, and adenocarcinoma.

(8) Classify benign and malignant tumors and assess tumor biology behaviors

We can differentiate reactive follicular hyperplasia ($\kappa+/\lambda+$) and follicular lymphoma ($\kappa+/\lambda-$ or $\kappa-/\lambda+$). It is possible to estimate biology behaviors of malignant tumors by the use of cell proliferation activity markers (like Ki-67) or oncogene protein products (c-erbB2/p53), which can provide a prognostic indicator for tumors.

(9) Provide options of therapeutic schedule for the clinic

ER-positive or PR-positive breast cancer patients can gain the long time remission and have survival times after endocrine therapy (such as tamoxifen and letrozole). P170, a product of multi-resistant gene protein indicates that tumors are resistant to chemotherapeutics. Recently, targeted tumor chemotherapy needs the detection of relevant target spots to offer treatment options. For example, B cell lymphoma expressing CD20 can be treated with rituximab, patients with gastrointestinal stromal tumor that expresses CD117 can accept imatinib, and breast cancer patients with a higher expression of c-erbB2 can use trastuzumab.

7.5.3　Exfoliative cytological examination

7.5.3.1　Overview

Endovascular tumor that is on body surface, in body cavity or contacts with the body surface, is apt to fall off. According to the characteristic, we can take substance falling off naturally or that secreted, or suck, scrape, brush the surface cells with the help of special instruments for smear examination, we can also take flushing fluid after flushing or extract the centrifugated deposit of pleural and ascitic fluid.

Specimen that can be used for exfoliative cytological examination are as follows: sputum, urine, nipple discharge, smear of vaginal fluid, cervical smear, nasopharynx smear, esophageal netting smear, all kinds of endoscopic brush pieces, smear of pleural effusion, ascites, hydropericardium, thoracic spinal fluid after centrifugation, and smear of bronchia flushing fluid.

7.5.3.2　Application

(1) Vagina exfoliocytology

The cells which are used for smear can be sucked or scraped from cervix or vaginal vault can be stained by Pap staining or H-E staining. It is most often used for diagnosis and general investigation of squamous-cell carcinoma of cervix uteri, and the accuracy is over 90%. Moreover, it can be used to monitor the level of endocrine hormone in women.

(2) Sputum smear and bronchial brushing cytology

It's useful for the diagnosis and histological classification of lung cancer, such as squamous-cell carcinoma, small cell carcinoma, and adenocarcinoma.

(3) Exfoliocytology of pleural and ascitic fluid

Extract pleural and ascitic fluid, centrifuge them and prepare smears using precipitation, which can be used for diagnosis and differential diagnosis of lung cancer, gastrointestinal carcinoma, ovarian cancer, and malignant mesothelioma.

(4) Exfoliocytology of urine

Gather urine, centrifuge it and prepare smears by precipitation, which will be used for diagnosis of bladder tumor.

(5) Exfoliocytology of nipple discharge

It can be used to diagnose inflammation of the breast, proliferation of ductal epithelial cell, atypical hyperplasia and breast cancer.

(6) Others

Esophageal netting smear is commonly used for the diagnosis of esophageal squamous cancer and other diseases; the smear of gastric lavage fluid can be used for the diagnosis of gastric adenocarcinoma; and the centrifugation of cerebrospinal fluid and hydropericardium can be used for the diagnosis of inflammation and tumor of nervous system and pericardium of metastatic tumors and malignant mesothelioma.

7.5.4　Flow cytometry

7.5.4.1　Overview

Flow cytometry is a new technique in which flow cytometer(FCM) is applied for quantitative analysis and classified study of cells, and FCM is also called fluorescent activated cell sorter(FACS).

FCM can classify cells as fast as 5,000–10,000 cells/second, has high accuracy and sensitivity, its purity reaches 90%–99% and can measure 6–8 parameters simultaneously. We must use cell suspension for that FCM can only detect single disperse cells. As for solid tumors, we must cut tissues into pieces, then add protease to digest them into single cells for detection, and it's best to prepare cell suspension using fresh unfixed tissue.

7.5.4.2   Application

The technique can help to analysis generation cycle of tumor cells, chromosomal ploidy, rate of S phase and karyotype of a chromosome.

Monoclonal antibody indirect fluorescent staining can recognize two kinds of in distinguishable hemocytes, normal ones and clonal ones, which may be useful for the somatotype diagnosis of leukemia and malignant lymphoma.

To analysis tumor-related genes (such as *p*53) quantitatively, which can provide evidence for the prognosis.

To quantify products of genes with multidrug resistance, which can give bases for selecting chemical drugs.

To monitor curative effects and remaining tumor cells, and to determine the recurrence of tumors.

Wang Qiming

Chapter 8

Endoscopic Diagnosis of Tumor

8.1 Introduction

8.1.1 Development history of endoscopy

In 1804, Germany Dr. Philip Bozzini (May 25, 1773-April 4, 1809) first boldly put forward the idea of endoscopy and build the first internally lit device used to inspect the interior of the human body called "Lichtleiter" in 1806. This candle light source device consisting of a vase-shaped light source, candles and a series of lenses for observing the internal structure of animal's bladder and rectum. Since then, there are four major improvements in the course of nearly 200 years of development of endoscope, from the initial hard-tube endoscope (1806–1932), half-curved endoscope (1932–1957) to the fiberscope (after 1957), and nowadays electronic endoscopes (after 1983). Image quality has also undergone tremendous leaps. The clinical application of medical endoscopes is becoming more and more popular. It is moving toward miniaturization, versatility, and high image quality.

The innovation of endoscope technology never stopped. Biopsy forceps and cell brushes enable endoscope to perform pathological examinations and significantly improve the diagnostic accuracy. Camera and video technologies record various images for consultation and teaching purpose. Othercompatible accessories are forming a new field of therapeutic endoscope such as microscopic hemostasis, removal of polyps, foreign body removal, stent placement, snare ligation, etc. With the popularization of electronic technology, the electronic endoscope generally equip with a solid-state imaging device at the front end of the probe and a television monitor for in-time images observing. It changes the nature of the optical fiber endoscope by the optical fiber light guiding and peeping. The front-end micro-electronic coupling device (charge-coupled device CCD) constitutes an image sensor, which is equivalent to a micro-vacuum camera tube. After entering the gastrointestinal cavity, the in-cavity image can be clearly captured and transmitted to the image processing center through cables. Finally the image displayed on the TV screen to facilitate data storage, image acquisition, analysis and communication (Figure 8–1).

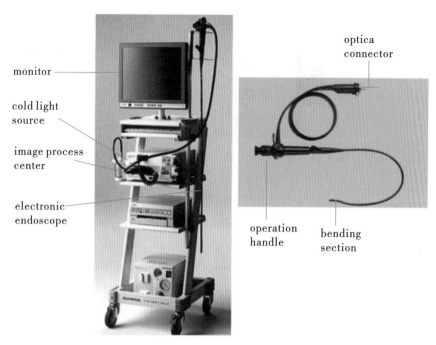

Figure 8-1   Digestive electronic gastroscope system

8.1.2   Clinical application of endoscope

The endoscope equipped with metal or fiber beams is commonly used in nasopharyngeal, laryngeal, tracheobronchial, esophagus, gastroduodenal, biliary, pancreatic, rectal, bladder, kidney, vagina, cervix and other inspections. It can also be used for abdominal cavity and mediastinum check. Most of the tumors in hollow organs and body cavities can be examined by endoscopy. The endoscope can be used to visualize the macroscopic changes of the tumor, to take pathological examination of the tissue or cells, to perform an X-ray contrast examination of the catheter into the ureter, common bile duct, and pancreatic duct. It has greatly improved the accuracy of tumor diagnosis.

At present, electronic endoscopy combined with various advanced diagnostic and treatment technologies significantly expand the clinical application of endoscope(Figure 8-2, Figure 8-3).

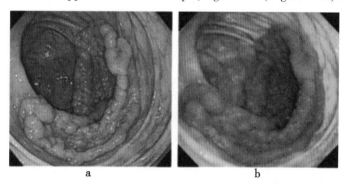

The lesion appears purple, which provides a strong color contrast with the surrounding normal mucosa shown in green.

Figure 8-2   Fluorescence endoscopy

1) confocal microendoscopy equipped with optical image technology, has enabled optical pathological diagnosis and observation of lacunae (glandular openings) and villi in the gastrointestinal mucosa. For example, itis used for judging the intestinal metaplasia of gastric mucosa and early esophageal cancer at the

cytological level with high accuracy.

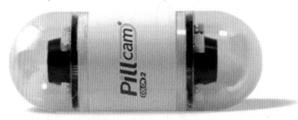

Figure 8-3　Colon capsule with two video cameras at each end of the capsule

2) Ultrasonic endoscope is based on an electronic endoscope system in which combined with ultrasound to obtain images. The ultrasonic transducer is extended into a body cavity through an electronic endoscope biopsy channel to approach a target organ. It directly visualize not only the lesion on the mucosal surface, but also obtain the whole organ and even nearby blood vessel through ultrasound scanning.

3) Fluorescence endoscopy combine endoscopy with a sensitive camera, a hybrid device and a new diagnostic photosensitizer has a high positive rate for tumors and early cancers.

4) Chromoendoscopy is the method of spraying a dye on the gastrointestinal mucosa or injecting dye intravenously followed by endoscopy. Chromoendoscopy is well usedfor morphological diagnosis, especially in selection of biopsy sites and the benign and malignant lesions. It's suitable for minor lesions detection, such as small size cancers, flat surface (Ⅱ b) early cancers, small polyps, and small erosions.

5) Capsule gastroscope is the swallowable wireless camera to provide time-lapse video images and virtual biopsy into the digestive tract.

8.2　Upper gastrointestinal endoscopy

The clinical application of upper gastrointestinal endoscopy includes esophageal, gastric, and duodenal examinations. It is the earliest and most rapidly progressing endoscopy, which is also called gastroscopy.

8.2.1　Indications

In general, all diagnoses of esophageal, gastric, and duodenal diseases can be performed. The main indications are as follows.

1) Unexplained dysphagia, post-sternal pain andheartburn, epigastric pain, discomfort andSatiety, loss of appetite and other upper gastrointestinal symptoms.

2) Unexplained upper gastrointestinal bleeding. Early endoscopic examination can do the diagnosis of gastrointestinal bleeding and microscopic hemostasis at the same time.

3) The upper gastrointestinal lesions can't be diagnosed or can't be explained by X-ray barium meal examination, especially those with mucosal lesions and suspected tumors.

4) Follow-up observation of the lesions, such as ulcer disease, atrophic gastritis, postoperative stomach, reflux esophagitis, Barrett's esophagus, etc.

5) Comparison between before and after drug treatment or postoperative follow-up.

6) Exogenousobjects remove, microscopic hemostasis, sclerosing agent injection, esophageal varices ligation, esophageal stenosis expansion, polyps of the upper digestive tract remove, and the like.

8.2.2   Contraindications

With the improvement of equipment and technological progress, contraindications have been significantly reduced compared with the past. The following conditions are contraindications.

1) Severe heart and lung diseases such as severe arrhythmia, heart failure, acute myocardial infarction, severe respiratory failure, and bronchial asthma attack. Mild cardiopulmonary insufficiency is not a contraindication, but should be conducted under guardianship conditions as necessary to ensure safety.

2) Shock, coma, and other critical conditions.

3) Unclear, insane, unable to cooperate.

4) Acute phase perforation of esophagus, stomach, duodenum.

5) Severe throat disorders, corrosive esophagitis and gastritis, giant esophageal diverticulum, aortic aneurysm, and severe cervical thoracic spine malformations.

6) Acute infectious hepatitis or gastrointestinal infections are generally suspended; chronic hepatitis B and hepatitis C or pathogen carriers and AIDS patients should have special disinfection measures.

8.2.3   Complications and treatment

General complications include throat spasm, dislocation of the mandibular joint, throat infection, parotid swelling, mallord-weiss.

Although serious complications are rare, but we should pay attention to precautions due to the severely hazardous. Serious complications include as follows.

1) Cardiac arrest: myocardial infarction, angina pectoris, etc. These cardiovascular complications are mostly caused by the vagus nerves and hypoxemia. If they occur, endoscopy should be stopped immediately, and suitablefirst aid treatment should be performed.

2) Perforation: perforation is usually caused by rough operation or blind insertion. Perforation of the esophagus generate severe upper thoracodorsal pain and subcutaneous emphysema of the mediastinum neck immediately. X-ray diagnosed and emergency surgery are needed.

3) Infection: local secondary infection may occur with microscopic treatment such as sclerotherapy, laser, and dilation. Antibiotics can be used for 3 days after surgery. In order to prevent the spread of hepatitis B and C viral hepatitis, patients are required to do the hepatitis B and virus test before gastroscopy. Special disinfect procedures such as washing, enzyme washing and drug washing are required after hepatitis B and C virus positive patients application.

4) Hypoxemia: mostly caused by endoscopic pressure on the respiratory tract, or patient's nervousness. Oxygen inhalation after endoscopic examination can generally relieve hypoxemia.

8.2.4   Endoscopic diagnosis of common upper gastrointestinal diseases

Since the use of endoscopy, the diagnostic rate of upper gastrointestinal diseases has increased significantly. The common diseases diagnosed under gastroscopy include inflammation, ulcers, and tumors, followed by polyps, esophageal varices, esophageal and gastric mucosal tears (Mallory weisis syndrome), diverticulum, exogenous objects, and parasites.

(1) Chronic gastritis

At endoscopy, the lining of the stomach looks red, irritated and swollen (inflammation), and it may also have raw, abraded areas that can bleed.

1) Chronic superficial gastritis: chronic inflammation of the lamina propria, limited to the outer third of

the mucosa in the foveolar area.

2) Chronic atrophic gastritis: the mucosa gets thicker, loss of chief and parietal cells in gastric glands.

3) Chronic hypertrophic gastritis: little inflammation, the mucosa is thinned, marked or total gland loss.

(2) Ulcers

Ulcers can locate in the esophagus, stomach, duodenum, etc. Benign ulcers have a smooth, regular, rounded edge with a flat smooth base and surrounding mucosa with radiating folds. Malignant ulcers show irregular heaped-up or overhanging margins.

(3) Tumors

1) Gastric cancer

Upper gastrointestinal tumors are quite common in China. In China, gastric cancer ranks the second most common and the second leading cause of cancer mortality. According to the infiltration depth of the cancer tissue in the stomach wall, the gastric cancer is divided into two categories, early gastric cancer and advanced gastric cancer. Gastroscopy is the best diagnosis method for early gastric cancer by observing the color (redness), surface contour, or dynamic response to air/gas insufflations. Advanced gastric cancer is divided into four types, namely, Bowman type I: mass or uplift type; Bowman type II: ulcer type; Bowman type III: infiltration ulcer type; Bowman type IV: diffuse infiltration type. Ulcerative cancers mainly occur in the antrum of the stomach, which is usually larger and more irregular than benign ulcers. The surrounding area is irregular; the bottom is uneven; the touch is hard; and the mucosa is brittle and easy to bleed. Invasive cancerous ulcers are dispensable, and the stomach wall becomes rigid, thick, limited expansion, lack of peristalsis, the formation of leather stomach, easy to be missed, should be carefully observed (Figure 8-4).

2) Esophageal cancer (Figure 8-5)

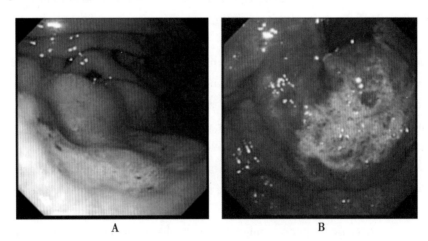

A. Endoscopic image of early gastric cancer. B. Endoscopic image of advanced gastric cancer.

Figure 8-4   Endoscopic images of gastric cancer at different stages

● Early esophageal cancer

Early esophageal cancer only invades mucosal or submucosal esophageal tissues. Regarding to the cell morphology, it can be divided into three types.

a. Surface protrude type: the mucous membrane is congested and edematized with small pieces or punctuated micro-uplift surfaces accompanied by superficial erosions that are more likely to bleed and usually have normal peristalsis and contraction of the wall.

b. Surface flat type: the mucous membrane changes to redness like a second degree burn. The surface roughness changes like a dot or a granular shape. Usually the peristalsis and contraction of the wall maintain well.

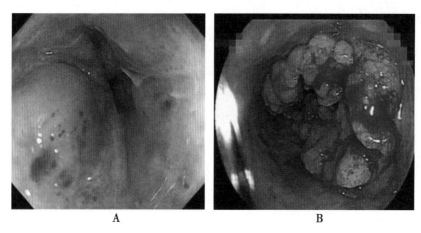

A   B

A. Endoscopic image of early esophageal cancer. B. Endoscopic image of Progressive esophageal cancer.

Figure 8-5   **Esophageal Cancer**

c. Surface depression type: a superficial erosion or a superficial ulcer is usually found in the mucosa with unsmooth edges. There is a change in the turbidity of the insects. The peristalsis of the vessel wall is poor but still shrink.

 • Progressive esophageal cancer

Progressive esophageal cancer has invaded the muscularis or exceeds the muscularis propria. The lesions mostly locate in the lower part of esophagus with a diameter larger than 3 cm. According to the endoscopic morphology, they can be divided into the following types.

a. Protrude type: bulge-like masses polypoid or cauliflower-like protrusions growth into esophageal cavity. Erosions and necrosis are found on the surface of the mucous membranes, which are easy to bleed when touching. But surrounding mucosal infiltration is not obvious.

b. Ulcer type: on the base of the ulcer, the necrotic tissue is thickly eroded, and the surface is uneven and easy to bleed. Edge organizations have irregular hyperplasia, worm-eaten or small nodular uplift.

c. Ulcer-infiltrated type: widespread infiltration of the mucous membranes around the ulcer. Esophageal lumen is usually poor expanded. Endoscopy is difficult to pass through the lesion.

8.3   Endoscopic retrograde cholangiopancreatography

Endoscopic retrograde cholangiopancreatography (ERCP) is an important diagnosis and treatment strategy for pancreatic and biliary diseases. With the development of endoscopic techniques, the clinical application of ERCP has become increasingly widespread and has become the standard method for minimally invasive endoscopic treatment of biliary and pancreatic diseases.

8.3.1   Indications

All gallbladder pancreatic diseases and suspected gallbladder pancreatic diseases are ERCP indications. It is usually applied after the abdominal ultrasound examination based on the prompted lesions. Biliary system tumors, stones, obstructive jaundice, inflammatory stenosis, chronic pancreatitis, pancreatic cancer, and ampullary lesions are all suitable for ERCP examination.

8.3.2 Contraindications

1) Non-biliary acute pancreatitis.

2) Severe biliary tract infections and bile duct obstruction without drainage conditions.

3) Severe heart, lung, kidney, liver and mental illness.

4) Other contraindications for upper gastrointestinal endoscopy.

5) Severe iodine allergy.

8.3.3 Complications

The total incidence of diagnostic ERCP complications was 1. 01% –9. 20% , operative mortality was 0. 13% –0. 50% .

(1) Hyperamylasemia and pancreatitis

Hyperamylasemia and pancreatitis are the most common complications of ERCP. The incidence of hyperamylasemia is about 20% –75% . Clinical manifestation of hyperamylasemia includes elevated serum amylase, but without apparent symptoms. If upper abdominal pain and upper abdominal tenderness occur at the same time, the incidence of pancreatitis after ERCP is about 1. 9% –5. 2% . Most of them are mild pancreatitis, but severe pancreatitis may also occur.

(2) Bile duct infection

The incidence is about 0. 33% –1. 50% , manifested as fever, abdominal pain, deepening of jaundice or jaundice, tenderness in the right upper quadrant, and even toxic shock and sepsis.

(3) Perforation

The incidence is 0. 1% . It usually occurs when the endoscope passes through the duodenal ampulla and when papilla of Vater is cut with a needle-like incision knife. Immediate surgical treatment should be performed once it occurs.

(4) Hemorrhage

The incidence is less than 0. 5% . Hemorrhage is usually seen in patients with gastrointestinal reactions due to excessive, severe nausea, vomiting caused by tearing of the cardiac mucosa, and papillary incision. Most of hemorrhage can be cured after medical treatment or endoscopic treatment.

(5) Others

Drug reactions, cardiovascular and cerebrovascular accidents, heart rate, respiratory arrest and other common endoscopic complications.

8.3.4 Diagnosis of ERCP in pancreatic and gallbladder carcinoma

(1) Pancreatic cancer

Pancreatic cancer remains one of the deadliest cancer worldwide. Approximately 75% of the pancreatic cancers occur within the head of the pancreas. ERCP can simultaneously display the pancreatic duct, bile duct, and ampulla, which is valuable for the identification of obstructive jaundice of unknown origin. Therefore, compared to pancreatic angiography, ultrasonography, computed tomography, ERCP is the essential method with the highest diagnostic accuracy rate. In ERCP, the pancreatic duct is irregularly stenotic and obstructed, the end of the pancreatic duct is cut off, the collateral of the main pancreatic duct is destroyed, ruptured, sparse or displaced, the contrast agent spills into the tumor area, and the common bile duct may have stenosis and obstruction. However, the early lesions with no expansion of the main pancreatic duct was difficult to be diagnosed.

（2）Gallbladder Carcinoma

The conventional imaging diagnosis of gallbladder cancer with ERCP is not very significantwith a diagnosis rate about 50%. In the displayed gallbladder cancer, the cystic wall was unclear, the shadow of J-shaped meat-like defects, and the common hepatic duct and common bile duct shift. The advantage of ERCP examination is to collect bile at the same time for cytological examination, and diagnose localized malignant obstructive jaundicequalitatively.

8.4   Lower gastrointestinal endoscopy

Lower gastrointestinal endoscopy includes sigmoidoscopy, colonoscopy, and enteroscopy. Colonoscopy is used more often than others. It can reach the ileocecal regionor even the terminal ileum. Only colonoscopy is discussed here.

8.4.1   Indications

1）Unexplained blood in the stool, bowel habits change, abdominal pain, abdominal mass, weight loss, anemia and other signs, suspected intestinal knot or rectum and distal ileum lesions.

2）Colon stenosis, ulcers, polyps, cancer, diverticulum and other diseases detected by barium enema or sigmoidoscopy need to be further confirmed.

3）Diagnosis and follow-up of inflammatory bowel disease.

4）Primary lesions seeking when CEA, and CA19-9 were elevated.

5）The metastatic adenocarcinomaseeking.

6）Preoperative diagnosis of colon cancer, postoperative follow-up, polypectomy follow-up.

7）Hemostasis, polypectomy, total intussusception, torsion of the intestine, expansion of the intestinal stenosis, placement of stents and other treatment to relieve intestinal obstruction.

8.4.2   Contraindications

1）The anus and rectum are severely narrowed.

2）Acute severe colitis, such as acute bacterial dysentery, acute severe ulcerative colitis, and diverticulitis.

3）Acute diffuse peritonitis, perforation of abdominal organs, multiple abdominal operations, extensive intra-abdominal adhesions and massive ascites.

4）Pregnancy women.

5）Severely heart and lung failure, mental disorders and coma patients.

8.4.3   Complications

（1）Perforation

Perforation of the intestines can cause severe abdominal pain, bloating, signs of acute diffuse peritonitis, and free gas under the armpit under X-ray abdominal fluoroscopy. Once diagnosed, surgery should be performed immediately.

（2）Hemorrhage

Intestinal hemorrhage is mainly caused by endoscopy insertion, excessive biopsy, insufficient electrocoagulation and hemostasis.

(3) Mesenteric laceration

Mesenteric laceration is rare. Intra-abdominal adhesion can easily cause mesenteric laceration. Small amount of bleeding can be treated conservatively. Large amount of bleeding caused blood pressure dropping should be treated by laparotomy.

(4) Cardiovascular and cerebral accidents

Excessive traction of the vagus nerve causes reflex arrhythmias, or even cardiac arrest during examinations. Emotional stress in hypertensive patients can increase the blood pressure and cause cerebrovascular accidents. The operation of endoscopy should be stopped immediately and emergency rescue should be performed.

(5) Gas Explosions

It's rare but can result in colonic perforation to have serious consequences. The risk factors include the oral administration of 20% mannitol for bowel preparation. Mannitol should be avoided or use 6.7% low-concentration mannitol (i. e. ,20% mannitol 500 ml plus 5% glucose saline 1,000 ml) for bowel preparation instead. Inhalation of carbon dioxide during colonoscopy is also recommended as a preventive measure

8.4.4 Endoscopic diagnosis of common intestinal diseases

The basic diseases of intestinal include inflammation, ulcers and tumors. The inflammation of the colon mucosa is caused by various causes. Therefore, it is necessary to combine the changes of the mucosa with the etiology and clinical manifestations to make a comprehensive diagnosis. In patients with ulcerative colitis, extensive mucosal hyperemia, edema, erosion, superficial ulceration, pus and exudates on the surface, or inflammatory polyps were observed under the microscope. In patients with Crohn's disease, a longitudinally distributed or vertical deep ulcer is seen (Figure 8-6).

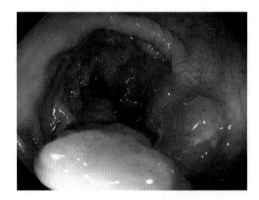

Figure 8-6　Endoscopic image of early colon cancer

8.4.5 Endoscopic diagnosis of colon tumor

Colonoscopy is the major method of diagnosis and follow-up of colon cancer. Adenomas and polyps are more common in benign colon tumors. Their size, shape and presence or absence of pedicles isimportant for the diagnosis and prognosis. Most of the malignant colon cancer is polypoid carcinoma in uplift type, pedicle or semi-pedicle with red, uneven surface, accompanied with erosions or ulcers.

8.5   Fiberoptic bronchoscopy

At the beginning of the 20th century Chevalier Jackson used metal rigid bronchoscopy to check bronchial and pulmonary diseases. In 1964, Ikeda Mao developed a flexible optical fiber bronchoscope (referred to as fiber bronchoscope), which was officially used in clinical practice in 1967. It is one of the important methods for diagnosis and treatment of respiratory diseases. The bronchoscope is thin, flexible, and easy to insert into the bronchi and subsegmental bronchi. At the same time, biopsy or brushing can be performed under direct vision. Bronchial lavage (BL) and broncho-alveolar lavage (BAL) can also be performed. Cytology or liquid components can be examined and photographed.

8.5.1   Indications

1) Unexplained hemoptysis, localization of bleeding site and finding cause of hemoptysis, or localization of lesion when medical treatment is inefficient, hemoptysis repeatedly occur and emergency surgery can't performed.

2) Block shadow, atelectasis, obstructive pneumonia or suspected lung cancer detected by X-ray.

3) "Negative lung cancer" which is negative on the X-ray but has positive sputum cytology.

4) Pathological sections or cytology using forceps or needle-suction required for diffuse lesions, solitary nodules, or masses of unknown in lung tissue.

5) Unexplained atelectasis or pleural effusion.

6) Unexplained recurrent laryngeal nerve paralysis and radial nerve palsy.

7) Unexplained dry cough or local wheezes.

8) Slowly resolving pneumonia or recurrent pneumonia.

9) Draw or brush deep bronchioles secretions of the lungs directly for etiological culture in order to avoid oral contamination.

10) Treatment: bronchial exogenous object, purulent sputum sucking, local drug delivery, sucking sputum after surgery, lung cancer local radiotherapy and chemotherapy and so on. In addition, airway stenosis can be treated with balloon dilation or stent placement such as Nickel titanium memory alloy stents.

8.5.2   Contraindications

1) Those who are allergic to anesthesia and those who cannot cooperate with the examination.

2) Serious cardiopulmonary insufficiency, severe arrhythmia, frequent angina.

3) The general condition is extremely weak and cannot withstand the examiner.

4) Patients with severe blood coagulation disorders that have uncontrollable hemorrhage qualities.

5) Aortic aneurysms are at risk of rupture.

6) Upper respiratory tract infection or hyperthermia, asthma attack, and hemoptysis should be considered carefully.

8.5.3   Clinical application assist in the diagnosis of diseases

Diagnosis of lung cancer: fibrobronchoscopy can greatly increase the diagnosis rate of lung cancer, especially for in-tube proliferative and infiltrating type. At this point can be obtained through the clamp technique for diagnosis, but in the clamp should pay special attention to the first biopsy clamp, require accurate position, clamp the base of the tumor, if the surface with necrosis-like substances need to repeatedly attract or clamp out Then take the tumor tissue. A variety of sampling methods can be used to increase diagnostic positive rates, such as needle aspiration, forceps, brushing, and irrigation.

8.5.4 Complications

Fiberoptic bronchoscopy has been widely used in clinical practice. According to the literature, the incidence of general complications was 0.3%, the incidence of serious complications was 0.1%, and the mortality was 0.04%. The incidence of complications depends on the case and the skill level of the operator. The main complications are bleeding, pneumothorax, fever, throat, anesthetic reactions, occasional cardiac arrest, etc.

(1) Laryngospasm

It is the mostly serious complication caused by anesthetic drugs. It can also occur when patients have bronchial asthma or chronic obstructive pulmonary disease. In addition to the throat, convulsions, respiratory depression, and even cardiac arrest can occur. It is necessary to ask in detail about the history of drug allergy and basic disease before surgery to prevent laryngospasm. It is best to give oxygen inhalation to people with underlying diseases.

(2) Hypoxemia

About 80% of patients have a decrease in PaO_2 when after lens inserted during endoscopy procedure. The decrease is about 10 mmHg. Hypoxemia can induce arrhythmias, myocardial infarction, and even cardiac arrest.

(3) Bleeding

Biopsy specimens collection can cause intraoperative and postoperative bleeding. Lens intubation or coughing can cause local brush bleeding. A small amount of bleeding can stop spontaneously or treated by local injection of hemostatic drugs. Massive hemorrhage should be treated by timely suction under the bronchoscope and local injection of diluted epinephrine or thrombin.

(4) Pneumothorax

It is mainly caused by lung biopsy with incidence about 1%-6%. A few occurs in the tracheal cavity under direct vision biopsy. Death due to pneumothorax rarely occur. About 50% of pneumothorax patient need closed thoracic drainage.

(5) Fever

The incidence of postoperative fever is about 6%. Subsequent bacterial infections, bacteremia, and even postoperative fatal sepsis occur occasionally.

Zhang Tengfei

Chapter 9

Clinical Diagnosis and Evaluation of Tumor

9.1 Clinical diagnosis of tumor

Clinical diagnosis of tumor requires physicians asking patients about their symptoms and medical history, the process of which also includes analysing patients medical tests, and pathological results and radiographer's advice. Based on these results, physicians can provide patients with a suitable treatment plan. Clinical diagnosis is the prerequisite of an effective treatment plan.

9.1.1 Clinical data collection

9.1.1.1 Symptoms and medical history

(1) Patient's systematic symptoms

1) Fever

The fever of cancer patients is mostly caused by the release of fabricant substances from tumor cells into the bloodstream after necrosis of these tumor cells. The type of fever due to this reason is often intermittent fever or irregular fever. In addition, concurrent tumor infection or some antineoplastic drugs can also cause fever.

2) Fatigue

The mechanism of tumor-induced fatigue is not clear. Contributors to fatigue include anemia, hypothyroidism, depression, and antineoplastic drugs.

3) Weight loss

Most cancer patients are accompanied by weight loss. The causes of weight loss include lack of appetite, gastrointestinal diseases, energy consumed by rapid tumor growth, increased catabolism, and increased ineffectiveness of ATP consuming. For patients with significant weight loss, the extent of weight loss should be documented in detail.

4) Jaundice

It is due to lesions getting blocked by the common bile duct.

5) Lack of appetite

Toxins produced by tumors can cause changes in a patient's central intake area in the nervous system and the delay of gastric emptying. In addition, psychological factors can also affect appetite.

(2) Patient's regional symptoms

1) Mass

Mass is the most common local lesion for cancer patients. Superficial mass can be touched. For example, the mass includes enlarged lymph nodes caused by lymphatic metastasis of the tumor, thyroid cancer, parotid cancer, breast cancer subcutaneous mass.

2) Compression

Mediastinal mass compression of the superior vena cava could cause superior vena cava syndrome. The masspressuring the recurrent laryngeal nerve could cause hoarseness. Thyroid cancer could cause breathing and swallowing difficulties.

3) Obstruction

The growth of cancer tissue can cause complete or incomplete lumen obstruction. The types of obstruction include progressive dysphagia due to esophageal cancer, intestinal obstruction, and constipation caused by colon cancer, and dysuria caused by prostate cancer.

4) Ulcers

Some superficial tumor tissues could grow rapidly and therefore lack nutrition supply, resulting in tissue necrosis. Ulcers are the main symptoms of skin cancer, oral cancer, lip cancer. Deep organ tumors, such as gastric and colon cancer, may also be accompanied by ulcers, but they need gastroscopy and colonoscopy to be seen.

5) Pain

Pain occurs when a tumor presses or infringes the related tissue nerves. In the early stage of cancer, the tumor is small in size and generally non-metastatic, so the incidence rate of pain is low. With the enlargement of the lesion, the tumor infiltrates the surrounding tissues and even metastases as well as destroys the bone tissues, so the incidence rate of pain gets higher. The pain caused by a tumor is mostly continuous and partly local, and the position of pain is clear. Some of them are widespread pain, and patients often fail to pinpoint specific areas of pain.

6) Hemorrhage

When cancer tissues invade blood vessels or small blood vessels of cancer tissues, it can result in bleeding. If lung cancer encroaches on the bronchi and blood vessels, it can cause hemoptysis or blood-stained sputum; patients with gastric cancer can have hematopoiesis; colorectal cancer patients often have bloody stool; cervical and vaginal cancers can cause irregular vaginal bleeding.

7) Abnormal secretions

Patients with middle ear tumors can sometimes have hemorrhagic secretions of the external auditory canal; some gynecologic tumor patients have bloody or rice-like leucorrhea in vagina accompanied by stink; nipple discharge may occur in breast cancer patients.

(3) The process of diagnosis and treatment

It should include the occurrence of disease, the whole process of the diagnosis and treatment, the results of the examination, the treatment methods used, the medication regimen and dosage, as well as the evaluation of efficacy. For patients with re-treatment, the last treatment time and the adverse reactions, as well as the occurrence degree of the previous treatment, should be recorded. This information is critical to the diagnosis and treatment of diseases.

(4) Complications

Some cancer patients especially the elderly ones are often accompanied by other chronic diseases such as diabetes, hypertension as well as cardiovascular and cerebrovascular diseases. The complication, medication regimen, and dosage, as well as disease control of patients, should be understood. In the treatment process of a tumor, the interaction between tumor and complications should be taken into account.

(5) Family history

Some tumors have familial heritability, such as retinoblastoma caused by mutation of Rb gene; Li-Fraumeni syndrome caused by mutation of *p*53 gene; familial adenomatous polyposis caused by mutation of APC gene.

(6) Lifestyle

Some bad living habits are closely related to the occurrence of cancer, such as smoking and lung cancer, hot mildew food and esophageal cancer, high-fat diet and colon cancer.

(7) Female reproductive history

Pregnancy abortion has an important reference value for the diagnosis of gynecological tumors such as choriocarcinoma. Early marriage and early pregnancy are risk factors for cervical cancer while late marriage and late childbirth or even infertility are risk factors for breast and ovarian cancer.

(8) Occupational environment

Long-term exposure to ledhs to a significant increase of the risk of some cancers. For example, the incidence of pleural mesothelioma and lung cancer in asbestos workers is significantly increased. The incidence of bladder cancer is significantly increased in chemical workers who engage in the production of benzidine and naphtha mines, as well as manufacturing workers who are exposed to naphthalene and benzidine which are the raw materials of rubber additives and pigments. Workers exposed to coal tar or arsenic compounds are at increased risk of skin cancer.

9.1.1.2　Physical examination

The physical examination of the comprehensive system is an important method to find the positive signs which are of great value for the diagnosis and treatment of the patients.

(1) Systemic examination

Observing the patient's facial features, nutritional status, and mental state. Tumor patients may appear to be thin, anaemic appearance and poor mental state. Patients with liver diseases often have "hepatic facies" with color darkening and poor elastic facial skin. Yellowing of skin or whites of the eyes can occur in patients with jaundice.

Palpation of superficial lymph nodes is one of the key points of physical examination in tumor patients because lymph node metastasis is the most common way of malignant tumor metastasis. Superficial lymph node enlargement occurs in many cancer patients and is the main performance of lymphoma. Lymph nodes have important reference value in determining the nature of the disease and clinical staging of a tumor. Therefore, it is not only necessary to carefully palpate the superficial lymph nodes of the body but also to know the size, texture, mobility as well as whether there exists tenderness or adhesion or not of the lymph nodes.

(2) Local examination

1) Head and neck

Pay attention to whether there is hair loss; whether the eye movement is normal; whether there is abnormal secretion in the ear and nose; whether there is leukoplakia in the mouth; whether there is thyroid enlargement or tracheal displacement. Patients with nasopharyngeal carcinoma or NKT cell lymphoma may have nasal obstruction, nasal bleeding or abnormal secretions from noses. In patients with advanced nasopharyngeal carcinoma, there can be one side of fixation of the eyeball or external abduction of the eyeball accompanied with an upper cervical tubercle. Thyroid neoplasms can cause enlargement of the thyroid gland.

2) Chest

Notice whether there are lumps or varicose veins in the chest wall, whether there is a lump in the breast, or whether the nipple is festering, sag or overflow. The percussion is clear sound, and the auscultation is alveolar breath sound in normal lung. When the tumor patient appears superior vena cava syndrome, there can be facial edema as well as neck and chest blood vessel rage. When the pleural effusion is developed, the percussion of the affected side of chest is dull sound, the speech fibrillation disappears, and the auscultation of the alveolar breath sound is obviously weakened or even disappeared. When the pericardial effusion is complicated, the border of cardiac dullness is enlarged, and the auscultation of the heart gets distant and deep. Some breast cancer patients can have nipple retract, erosion, spillage, or typical orange peel changes. When palpating breast mass, pay attention to the size, boundary, texture, and mobility of the mass, as well as whether there is adhesion to the skin chest wall.

3) Abdomen

Pay attention to observe whether there is abnormal uplift in the abdomen, whether there are flatulence and peritoneal effusion in percussion. Whether there is masses or enlargement of liver and spleen when palpating, whether there is a blood vessel murmur, or whether the bowel sounds are hyperactive in auscultation. Patients with liver cancer can have progressive enlargement of the liver which can be palpated under the right costal margin, the liver is hard and has unsmooth surface or nodules. Portal hypertension can cause varicose veins of the abdominal wall; the patients with lymphoma and chronic myeloid leukemia can develop splenomegaly, and the severe splenomegaly can be below the umbilicus level. Patients with a large number of peritoneal effusion may have a positive transactive sonogram. Ovarian cancer can be palpated on the abdomen when the tumor is large.

4) Spinal and extremities

Osteosarcoma frequently occurs in the lower extremities. Swelling, phyma and increased skin temperature can occur in the diseased regions.

5) External genitalia and anus

Rectal examination is of great significance for patients with suspected prostate cancer and rectal cancer; vaginal touch and bimanual examination are important to understanding the location, range, hardness and activity of the lesions in cervical cancer patients.

9.1.1.3 Auxiliary examination

(1) Imaging examination

Imaging examination methods such as X-ray, CT, MRI, ultrasound, PET-CT and nuclide scan can find the lesions and their location, size, and scope.

(2) Endoscopy examination

Endoscopy examination such as gastroscopy, bronchoscopy, hysteroscopy, and cystoscope can observe the size, shape, location and the relationship with adjacent organs of the lesions, and tissue biopsy can be completed under the guidance of endoscopy.

(3) Pathology examination

Definite diagnosis of most tumors needs histopathological evidence. Pathological classification and type are of great significance to guide clinical treatment.

(4) Laboratory examination

General routine examination is of important reference value for understanding the state of the patient's body, and deciding whether there is any therapeutic contraindication; some tumor markers such as cancer embryo antigen, alpha-fetoprotein, and PSA have important reference value for the diagnosis and disease assessment of tumor.

9.1.2　Define the clinical stages of the tumor

The significance of tumor clinical stages: clinical staging is a comprehensive assessment of the range and degree of the lesions which can provide the basis for the correct clinical treatment plan. Clinical staging is also an important indicator of prognosis in patients. The unified clinical stage is also conducive to the communication between hospitals and the development of clinical research. In general, clinical staging should be determined before anti-tumor treatment, which is very important for the selection of a treatment plan and evaluation of efficacy.

(1) TNM classification

Currently, the TNM staging system is widely used in the world. The system was first put forward by a Frenchman called Pierre Denoix, and was revised by American Joint Committee on Cancer (AJCC) and Union for International Cancer Control (UICC) for many times, it was gradually improved and established as the standard for the International stage.

T (tumor) in TNM stage represents the primary lesion of the tumor which is divided in T_1-T_4 according to the size of the lesion and its invasion range of surrounding tissues; N (lymph node) represents the lymph nodes involvement; M (metastasis) represents the distant metastasis of the tumor. The clinical stages of the tumor are determined according to the comprehensive conditions of T, N, and M indicators (Table 9-1).

Different tumors have different levels of T and N, and the TNM combinations are different in clinical stages of different tumors. Therefore, each tumor has a specific TNM staging.

Table 9-1　TNM staging of the tumor

Staging indicator	Clinical significance
T	The situation of a primary tumor
T_x	Primary tumor cannot be evaluated
T_0	No evidence of primary tumor is found
Tis	Carcinoma in situ
T_1-T_4	The size and scope of the primary tumor (increasing in severity)
N	The situation of affected lymph nodes
N_x	The situation of affected lymph nodes cannot be evaluated
N_0	No lymph node metastasis
N_1-N_3	The extent of the affected lymph nodes (increasing by severity)
M	The situation of distant metastasis
M_x	The situation of distant metastasis cannot be evaluated
M_0	No distant metastasis
M_1	There is distant metastasis

(2) Other staging system

There are also some tumors based on the need for clinical treatment that use other staging systems. For example, small cell lung cancer is often divided into limited and extensive stage in clinical practice. Because of the particularity of its biological behavior, malignant lymphoma often adopts Ann Abor staging which is according to the number and location of affected lymph nodes as well as the infringement of the spleen, bone marrow, and distant metastasis to evaluate the condition of lymphoma. Osteosarcoma often adopts USES Enneking staging system. In this system, histologic grade, location depth, lymph node metastasis and distant metastasis of tumor are combined to evaluate the condition. The MTS staging of soft tissue tumors should also focus on histological grading, location and distant metastasis of tumor.

(3) Molecular staging of the tumor

One of the defects of TNM staging is that it cannot predict the effect of anti-tumor treatment. In the clinical practice, there is a recurrent phenomenon that the curative effect and prognosis are different in the tumors of the same stage, pathological type, and treatment, Therefore, the molecular staging which is more detailed and can guide the prognosis in tumor from the molecular level becomes the new development direction of the clinical tumor staging.

Although many scholars devote to the molecular staging of the tumor and detect many markers associated with prognosis as well as put forward some specific solutions such as the molecular staging of lung cancer. However, due to the diversity of the cell and molecular biology research methods and their own shortcomings, there is no standardized detection method at present, and the stage study requires the joint participation of large sample and multi-center, so there is no mature tumor molecular staging that can be widely used in the clinical practice.

9.1.3 Establish clinical diagnosis

Clinical doctors should comprehensively analyze the patient's clinical data and signs combined with the examination results to make the correct diagnosis. The complete clinical diagnosis should include the primary site of the tumor, the pathological type and clinical stages, and the extent of the lesion at sometimes.

9.2 Evaluation of tumor

9.2.1 Functional status evaluation of tumor patients

In the functional status evaluation of cancer patients, we should take the bear ability to various treatment methods such as surgery, chemotherapy, and radiotherapy of patients into comprehensive consideration which is the necessary step before formulating specific treatment regimen. Currently, there are several methods for evaluating the functional status of tumor patients.

(1) Karnofsky performance status (KPS) score

In 1948, Karnofsky presented a method for evaluating the self-care ability of daily living and physical activity ability of tumor patients, known as kps score. The evaluation system is divided into 10 grades. The higher the score, the better the function status of the patient. See Table 9-2.

Table 9-2   KPS score for functional status evaluation of tumor patients

Score	Status
100	Normal, no symptoms and signs
90	The patient can do activity normally with mild symptoms and signs
80	The patient can manage with an effort to do activity normally with symptoms and signs
70	The patient is able to take care of themselves in daily life, but cannot maintain normal activities
60	The patient can take care of himself/herself in daily life of most of the time, but sometimes they need help
50	The patient often need other's help
40	Patients can't live on their own and need special care
30	Patients can't live on their own seriously
20	The patient is seriously ill and requires hospitalization
10	The patient is critically ill and approaching death
0	Death

(2) Eastern cooperative oncology group score

This is the functional status assessment method specified by the Eastern Cooperative Oncology Group Score(ECOG). The ECOG score is divided into 0–5 points from a normal state to death, and the higher the score, the worse the function of the patients.

(3) QLQ-C30 score system

The 30 indicators of QLQC30 which is established by the European Organization for Research and Treatment of Cancer (EORTC) are evaluated by patients themselves. The evaluation system consisted of five functional scales including body, role, cognition, mood and social function as well as four symptom scales including fatigue, pain, nausea, and vomiting. The QLQ-C30 score system is more systematic than the KPS and Zubrod Performance Status(ZPS) scoring system, but it is more complicated, and the clinical application is not convenient (Table 9-3).

Table 9-3   ZPS score of functional status in tumor patients

Score	Status
0	Normal activity
1	There are symptoms, but almost completely free activity
2	Sometimes bedridden, but the bedtime in day is <50%
3	Need to stay in bed, and the bedtime in day is >50%
4	Completely bedridden
5	Death

9.2.2   Evaluation of the efficacy of tumor therapy

In 1979, WHO developed the evaluation criteria for the objective efficacy of anti-tumor therapy, which was then widely used in the evaluation of solid tumors. With the extensive application of CT and MRI and the progress of clinical research, some problems of the primary WHO standards appeared gradually, for example, there is no unified regulation of the lesions that need to be measured and the lesions that need to be evaluated, there is no minimum size for measurable lesions and there is no specific requirement for the number of lesions to be measured for multiple lesions of the same organ or multiple organs.

In 1999, European Organization for Research and Treatment of Cancer, National Cancer Institute of the United States and National Cancer Institute of the Canada together made the Response Evaluation Criteria in Solid Tumors(RECIST) draft which is standard of evaluating the effect of solid tumor based on the review of common used effect evaluation standard of the WHO. After modified and supplemented, the curative effect evaluation standard named RECIST was formally promulgated in 2000.

One of the major differences between the RECIST standard and the WHO standard is that measuring method of measurable tumor lesions is different. The WHO standard evaluates the size of the tumor by the product of the maximum long diameter and maximum vertical diameter of the tumor, while the RECIST standard evaluates its size only with the maximum long length of the tumor. This is because the study shows that compared with the product of two diameters in a tumor, it is the tumor diameter that more closely related to the number of tumor cells, and the single diameter measurement is more accurate and better in repeatability. Hereinafter, we focus on the RECIST efficacy evaluation criteria.

9.2.2.1　Measurement of tumor lesions

According to whether the tumor lesions can be accurately measured, the lesion can be divided into measurable lesions and non-measurable lesions.

(1) Measurable lesions

The length diameter of the tumor can be measured at least in one direction, and the diameter of the lesion ≥20 mm measured by a conventional method or ≥10 mm measured by spiral CT. The superficial mass or superficial lymph node (the diameter of lesion ≥20 mm) can be measured directly with the ruler, and the chest X-ray can be used as the basis for measuring the lesion if it can clearly show the lung lesions. CT and MRI are recommended methods for measuring the lesion in vivo due to good repeatability. Because of the differences in each scanning plane, the long diameter of measured lesion changes all the time in ultrasound examination which has poor repeatability. What's more, the scan of a deep lesion is affected by gastrointestinal gas and can't be avoided every time. therefore, the measurement of a deep lesion is generally not examined by ultrasound.

(2) Non-measurable lesions

The long diameter of small lesions ≤20 mm measured by the conventional method or ≤10 mm measured by spiral CT. The following conditions are all belonged to the non-measurable lesions: bone lesions, meningeal lesions, pleural effusion, pericardial effusion, peritoneal effusion, inflammatory breast cancer, skin or lungs lymphangitis, the abdominal mass that cannot be determined by imaging and cystic lesions.

9.2.2.2　Efficacy evaluation of tumor

(1) Target lesion and non-target lesion

1) Target lesion

When there are multiple measurable lesions, according to the size of the lesion and the principle of repeatable measurement, there are up to 5 lesions and no more than 10 lesions in total in each organ as target lesions.

2) Non-target lesion

All lesions other than the target lesions are non-target lesions, including other measurable lesions and non-measurable lesions. Non-target lesions do not need to be measured in size, but they should be noted the presence or absence during follow-up.

(2)Standard evaluation of the curative effect

1)Evaluation of target lesions

• Complete response(CR): all target lesions disappear.

• Partial response(PR): the total long diameter of target lesions decreases by more than 30%.

• Progressive disease(PD): the total long diameter of target lesions increases by more than 20%, or there are new lesions.

• Stable disease(SD): the lesion decreases but not reach PR or increases but not reach PD.

2)Evaluation of non-target lesions

• Complete response: all non-target lesions disappear, and tumor markers are restored to normal levels.

• Incomplete response/Stable disease: there is one and/or multiple target lesion(s) or tumor marker (s) that above the normal level.

• Progressive disease: the presence of one or more new lesions and/or already existing non-target lesions has progressed significantly.

3)Overall efficacy evaluation

Correct and timely measurement and recording are the basis for the correct evaluation of the tumor. Overall efficacy is evaluated by the comprehensive condition of target lesions, non-target lesions and the presence of new lesions. Table 9-4 lists the possible combinations of target lesions, non-target lesions, and new lesions.

Table 9-4   Overall efficacy evaluation of solid tumor

Target lesion	Non-target lesion	New lesion	Overall efficacy
CR	CR	Without	CR
CR	Incomplete response/ Stable disease	Without	PR
PR	Not PD	Without	PR
SD	Not PD	Without	SD
PD	Under any circumstances	With or without	PD
Under any circumstances	Progressive disease	With or without	PD
Under any circumstances	Under any circumstances	With	PD

4)Progression-free survival

In addition to the four recent evaluation indexes of CR, PR, SD and PD in the RECIST standard, the concept of progression-free survival (PFS) have been increased. PFS is the time from randomization to the progression time of the tumor or death of the patient. To a certain extent, PFS represents the duration of mitigation, which can better reflect the curative effect of tumor therapy on the basis of excluding the influence of subsequent therapy.

9.2.2.3   Outlook of standard efficacy evaluation

With the development of imaging technology and the clinical application of 3D imaging technology, many hospitals can perform the three-dimensional measurement of lesions. This will provide new requirements for tumor measurement in RECIST standard.

Ma Wang, Du Yabing

Chapter 10

Surgical Treatment for Tumor

10.1　Concept of surgical oncology

According to the difference of management, clinical oncology is divided into medical oncology, surgical oncology, and radiation oncology. Surgical oncology is the branch of surgery applied to oncology; it focuses on the surgical management of tumors, especially malignant tumors. It was generally thought that pharmacotherapy was the only treatment of cancer with a chance of success. Now surgery takes an indispensable role in treatment of solid tumor. Usually, surgery is feasible only when there are indications that the tumor can be removed entirely. When there are metastases elsewhere, curative surgery is often impossible. However, the survival rate of patients improves after surgery, even if part of tumor tissue remains. Also, it is used for the palliative treatment for some cancers, which will be introduced in detail in 1.3. Surgical oncology has significance not only in the treatment of tumors, but in precaution, diagnosis, staging, reestablishment and recovery.

Surgeons who specialize in treating cancer patients regard themselves as surgical oncologists. Mostly, surgical oncologist refers to the general surgical oncologist, but those surgeons who are anatomical site specific and retain the remit to treat patients relating to their organ of interest can all be considered as surgical oncologists, like thoracic surgical oncologists, gynecologic oncologists and so forth. As surgical oncologists, our obligation is not only to the patient who is sitting before us in the office, but the progression of patients who will follow. The improved success and decreased morbidity of the treatments that we offer today are only possible because of the involvement of surgeons and their patients in clinical trials of the past. As the newest discoveries in all fields of oncology will have a direct impact on the surgical therapy, it is imperative that surgeons continue to play prominent roles as both leaders and participants in multidisciplinary cooperative group trials. All surgical oncologists should not only incorporate clinical trials into their practice but strongly encourage the participation of the general surgical community.

10.2　History and evolution of surgical oncology

Dating back to 1600 B. C. , ancient Egyptians treated tumor patients with simple excision or cautery to destroy tumors, limited to the tumor of limbs, breast, and superficial tumor. The concept of breast was known to the ancient Egyptians, as shown by the papyri of Ebers and Smith. It was 7th century that operations for breast cancer were described by Aetius of Amida, the first surgeon to emphasize the significance of the resection margin that the knife should cut around the tumor, remaining in the healthy tissue. As the development of anatomy and physiology in mid-18th century, John Hunter, the father of scientific surgery, described principles of surgical oncology including cancer as local disease and lymphatic spread, based on the writings of Jean-Louis Petit, who firstly described the spread of breast cancer to the regional axillary lymph nodes. In 1809, the first modern elective surgery for abdominal cancer is performed: the removal of a 22-lb ovarian tumor by Ephraim McDowell. The advent of general anesthesia and antisepsis pushed the further development of surgery, as the first major cancer operation performed under general anesthesia: the excision of the submaxillay gland and part of the tongue by John Collins Warren, and Lister's description of the antisepsis principles and introduction of carbolic acid, greatly reducing the morbidity of surgery.

In the last half of the 19th century, surgical oncology was flourishing. Billroth in vienna, the founding father of modern abdominal surgery, was the first surgeon to excise a rectal cancer and by 1867, he had performed 33 such operations. But he is famous for accomplishment of the first successful gastrectomy of cancer. On January 29, 1881, Billroth performed the first successful resection for antral carcinoma on Therese Heller, who lived for almost 4 months and died of liver metastases. He accomplished this operation by closing the great curvature side of the stomach and anatomizing the lesser curvature to the duodenum, in an operation that is still know as the Billroth I to this day. It should also be remembered that Pean performed a partial gastrectomy in 1879 in Paris and Rydigier performed a similar procedure in 1880. W. S. Halsted held the belief that cancers spread through the bloodstream, which led him to think that the sufficient local removal of the tumor would cure cancer and he performed the first radical mastectomy in 1882, thus ushering in the modern era of surgical treatment for breast cancer. The en bloc removal of breast tissue became known as the Halsted mastectomy before adopting the title "the complement operation" and eventually, "the radical mastectomy" as it is known today (Figure 10-1).

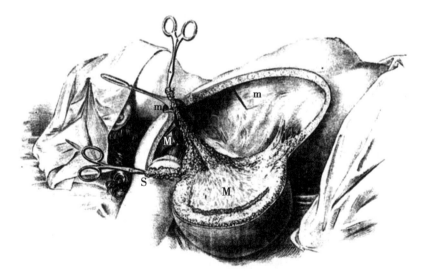

Figure 10-1 Original drawing of the radical mastectomy reported by William S. Halsted in 1894. Introduction of this operation led to improved local control in the treatment of breast cancer.

(From Halsted, by permission of *Annals of Surgery*)

Hugh H Young, credited with conceiving of the of radical perineal prostatectomy to treat prostate cancer, performed the first operation of that kind on April 7, 1904. He learned the procedure from Dr. George Googfellow, who first performed the operation in 1891. In 1909, Kocher became the first surgeon to win the Nobel Prize in Pyhsiology or Medicine for his work in the physiology, pathology and surgery of the thyroid. During the first half of the 20th century, more surgeons applied surgery to can-cer patients. Other milestones in cancer surgery include that Ernest Miles described the first abdominal-perineal resection for rectal cancer in 1908, Franz Torek performed the first successful transthoracic resection for carcinoma of the esophagus in 1913, and Evarts Graham performed the first pneumonectomy for primary bronchogenic carcinoma in 1933, following the first successful resection of a lung metastasis by Davis in 1927.

In retrospect, there is no doubt that these pioneers explored blind alleys in surgery to conquer cancer. Recent years, standing on the shoulders of giants, surgical oncology has been developing rapidly. It becomes more easier for lots of patients to diagnosis cancer at a early stage in their disease progress, due to the improving awareness of symptoms and the advanced modern screening programs. Kinds of examinations in pre-operation can specify the stage of cancer, which helps to estimate the surgical resection. And there appears more and more new treatments, such as laser, endoscopic surgery, cryotheropy and so on. As the vigorous development of microsurgery, the complications of surgery decrease obviously and patients achieve better therapeutic effects. There is reason to expect a brighter future in surgical oncology (Table 10-1).

Table 10-1　Important milestones in surgical oncology

Time	Events
1700 B. C. –1600 B. C.	Egyptians use cautery to destroy breast cancer
400 B. C.	Hippocrates describes the clinical symptoms of cancer and coins the terms "carcinoma" and "sarcoma"
1st and 2nd century A. D.	Roman physicians use surgery to treat breast cancer
5th century A. D.	The Greek physician Lenoidas first describes a mastectomy as a treatment of breast cancer
1760s	John Hunter, the "Father of Scientific Surgery," describes principles of surgical oncology including cancer as local disease and lymphatic spread
1775	Percival Pott describes scrotal cancer in chimney sweeps, first identifying a specific etiology of cancer
1809	The first modern elective surgery for an abdominal cancer is performed: the removal of a 22-lb ovarian tumor by Ephraim MacDowell
1829	Joseph Recamier first describes the principles of tumor metastasis
1846	The first major cancer operation is performed under general anesthesia: the excision of the submaxillary gland and part of the tongue by John Collins Warren
1867	Lister describes the principles of antisepsis and introduces carbolic acid, greatly reducing the morbidity of surgery
1873	First total laryngectomy for laryngeal cancer by Theodore Billroth
1881	First partial gastrectomy for cancer by Theodore Billroth
1885	First colectomy for colon cancer by Robert Weir
1887	New York Cancer Hospital becomes the first hospital in the United States specifically for cancer treatment

Continue to Table 10-1

Time	Events
1891	First hemipelvectomy by Theodore Billroth; first radical mastectomy for breast cancer by William Halsted
1896	Roentgen discovers X-rays, ultimately leading to radiation oncology; G. T. Beason performs the first oophorectomy as hormonal treatment for breast cancer
1906	First abdominoperineal resection for rectal cancer by W. Ernest Miles
1909	Theodore Kocher first describes thyroid surgery
1913	Both the American Association for the Advancement of Cancer (which would become the American Cancer Society) and the American College of Surgeons are established
1919	James Ewing publishes *Neoplastic Diseases*, promoting the concept of the multidisciplinary treatment of cancer
1927	First resection of pulmonary metastases by George Divis
1935	First pancreaticoduodenectomy for pancreatic cancer by Allen O. Whipple
1940	The James Ewing Society is established to "further our knowledge of cancer"
1940s	Chemotherapy begins with the discovery of nitrogen mustards and folic acid antagonists
1957	The initiation of the National Surgical Adjuvant Breast Project (NSABP)
1960s	Dr. Walter Lawrence establishes a division of surgical oncology at the Medical College of Virginia
1975	The Society of Surgical Oncology (SSO) is established
1978	The term *surgical oncologist* is defined by the SSO and NCI, and the SSO formulates guidelines for postresidency surgical oncology training
1998	The American Board of Surgery establishes the Advisory Council for Surgical Oncology The American College of Surgeons Oncology Group (ACOSOG) is established

10.3   Principles of surgical therapy in oncology

The principles of surgical oncology involve screening and TNM staging, pathological biopsy, assessment of patient, and the principles of surgical therapy in oncology. It is a big challenge for surgeons to choose the proper operation for the correct patient in the tumor type and staging, physically and psychologically.

Same as all surgical intervention, in modern surgical oncology, there are open surgery, laparoscopic surgery, robotic surgery, ablative interventions and other technical interventions. According to the purpose of operation, usually, it is divided as prophylactic surgery, diagnostic surgery, radical surgery, palliative surgery, rehabilitative surgery, and so forth. Among these, the most common surgeries are the radical surgery and the palliative surgery.

Radical surgery, also called curative surgery, is only performed when a total excision of all the tumor is possible, including the primary tumor and associated lymph node drainage fields in continuity. One of the major principles of surgical therapy of the primary tumor is to obtain adequate *negative margins* around the primary tumor, which could mean different operative approaches depending on the tumor type and its local involvement with adjacent structures. For example, the removal of a primary colon cancer that involves an adjacent loop of small bowel or bladder requires the en bloc resection of the primary tumor along with removal of the involved segment of small bowel and bladder wall. This approach avoids violation of the primary tumor margins that could lead to tumor spillage and possible implantation of malignant cells in the surrounding normal tissues. Aside from biopsies of the primary tumor, the lesion should not be entered during a definitive resection. In fact, any biopsy tract or incision that was performed before the tumor resection should be included in the procedure to reduce the risk of local recurrence. The regional lymph nodes represent the most prevalent site of metastasis for solid tumors. Because of this, the involvement of the regional lymph nodes represents an important prognostic factor in the staging of the cancer patient. For this reason, the removal of the regional lymph nodes is often performed at the time of resection of the primary cancer. Besides staging information, a regional lymphadenectomy provides regional control of the cancer. Examples of this are patients with melanoma who have tumor metastatic to lymph nodes. It is well documented that the removal of these regional lymph nodes can result in long-term survival benefit in approximately 20% –40% of individuals depending upon the extent of nodal involvement. Hence, the removal of regional lymph nodes can be therapeutic.

Palliative surgery is aimed at overcoming any symptom-producing consequences of the tumor. Surgical intervention is sometimes required in the patient with unresectable advanced cancer for palliative indications. The common indications for palliation in this setting are pain, bleeding, obstruction, malnutrition, or infection. There are examples as follow: to alleviate gastric haemorrhage or block disease that endangers life. Subtotal gastrectomy is of great importance in terminal gastric cancer patients. Ovariectomy is applied for terminal mastocarcinoma female patient before menopause, especially with estrogen receptor positive. The surgeon needs to consider several factors regarding each situation as to whether the surgical intervention will significantly to the quality of life of the patient. Factors include the expected survival of the individual, the potential morbidity of the procedure, the likelihood that the procedure will palliate the patient, and whether there are alternative nonsurgical methods of palliation. Probably the most common oncologic emergency that the surgeon confronts is the obstruction of a hollow viscus, which can give rise to an acute abdomen, perforation of the viscus, and possibly bleeding. Malnutrition is a common problem in the cancer patient, especially one with advanced, unresectable disease. Nutrition can be supplemented or replaced by intravenous hyperalimentation or enteral feedings via a gastrostomy or jejunostomy tube. Occasionally, the surgeon is involved in palliating pain caused by a metastatic lesion compressing an organ or adjacent nerves.

There are special considerations when planning operative procedures on cancer patients beyond the normal planning done for the same operation on a nononcologic patient (Table 10-2).

Table 10-2   Special considerations in the cancer patient

Oncologic factors	Potential associated problems
Tumor-specific factors	
Gastrointestinal	Obstruction and aspiration risk, gastrointestinal bleeding, bowel perforation
Head and neck/mediastinal	Reduced oral intake, superior vena cava obstruction, airway compromise, difficulty with ventilation or intubation
Cerebral tumors/brain metastasis	Decreased mental status, syndrome of inappropriate secretion of antidiuretic hormone, increased intracerebral pressures
Paraneoplastic syndromes	Syndrome of inappropriate secretion of antidiuretic hormone, hypercalcemia

Continue to Table 10-2

Oncologic factors	Potential associated problems
Cancer factors	
Cachexia/malnutrion	Increased infection, fluid and electrolyte management, wound healing
Hypercoagulability	Venous thrombosis, superior vena cava syndrome, pulmonary embolism
Bone metastasis	Hypercalcemia, increased fracture risk, potential for cord compression, potential for difficulty with intubation
Treatment-specific factors	
Steroids	Gastritis and gastrointestinal bleeding, diabetes, adrenal insufficiency, difficulties with wound healing
Chemotherapy	Neutropenia and anemia, pulmonary fibrosis, cardiac dysfunction, stomatitis, alteration in mucosal integrity of the gastrointestinal tract, constipation, bowel perforation, nausea, vomiting, diarrhea, hypercoagulability
Radiation therapy	Pulmonary fibrosis, difficulty with wound healing
Tamoxifen	Hypercoagulability

As the management of cancer is altered by new discoveries in genetics, molecular biology, immunology, and improved therapeutics, so too will the functions of the surgical oncologist change. With our increased understanding of the genetic predisposition to cancer, the surgeon is increasingly being asked to remove healthy organs to prevent malignancy. However, as other effective methods of prevention are developed, such as chemoprevention or gene therapy, this role will certainly diminish. Improving imaging technologies may have diminished the need for surgical intervention for staging, but the expanded use of neoadjuvant therapies often requires interventions to accurately assess response to therapy. In addition, harvesting tumors may become increasingly important for molecular staging as well as identifying molecular targets for specific therapies.

However, what should never be ignored is the complications after surgery, especially metastasis led by surgery. Surgical oncologists should comply with not only the general principles of surgery, but the basic principles of surgical oncology, which is aimed at the prevention of tumor cell implant and transvascular metastasis in operation. There are three basic principles of operation of tumor as follow, no-cut, en bloc resection, and no-touch. No-cut requires that surgeon should dissect tumor from sides to centre without directly cutting any tumor tissue. Any operation should be performed in correct tissue away from tumor. En bloc resection is intended to excise the primary tumor with lymph nodes of related irrigation region in successively and totally. No-touch means that surgeon should avoid touching tumor and local metastasis region in operation, designed to prevent the implantation and metastasis led by surgery.

10.4   Principles of quality control in surgical oncology: surgical consequence of abdominal irradiation

Quality can be defined as the totality of features and characteristics of a product or service that meet or exceed the customer requirements and expectations. Usually in medicine only the professional quality is mentioned. However, two other domains can be distinguished: logistic and relational quality. The first reflects the quality of the organization of cancer care and the second the way of addressing the patient.

Quality control is the way to achieve optimal treatment results in all domains that meet a certain set standard. It is the operational process of techniques and activities to fulfill these requirements. This standard of outcome can be set by the community or by the professionals themselves. The result of a certain diagnostic or treatment procedure can be expressed in outcome or process indicators.

The potential benefit of treatment has to be carefully balanced against radiotherapy-induced side-effects prior to administration of adjuvant radiotherapy. Radiotherapy-induced side-effects can be broadly classified as early (acute) or late, based on the time-frame of their manifestation. Early toxicities (Table 10–3) from radiation tend to arise during radiotherapy and can last from 6 weeks to 3 months after conclusion of radiotherapy. These are usually due to direct damage to the parenchymal tissue cells that are sensitive to irradiation. Late toxicities are usually apparent from 3 months after completion of radiotherapy (Table 10–4) and are attributed to damage to microvasculature and mesenchymal cells. However, the exact etiology is unknown and given the differences of th extent of toxicities observed between patients, inheren radiosensitivity of patients is also likely to contribute to the development of late effects.

Table 10–3   Summary of early side-effects with radiotherapy

Site	Side effects
Skin	Erythema, pruritus, dry desquamation, moist desquamation
Oral mucosa	Mucositis
Esophagus	Esophagitis-dysphagia
Lung	Radiation pneumonitis-cough, shortness of breath
Liver	Radiation hepatitis-nausea, vomiting, raised hepatic transaminases
Stomach	Gastritis-indigestion, heartburn, excess wind
Small bowel	Enteritis-abdominal cramps, nausea, vomiting, diarrhea
Rectum	Proctitis-tenesmus, diarrhea
Bladder	Cystitis-frequency, urgency, dysuria
Systemic	Lethargy
Hemopoietic	Anemia, leucopenia, thrombocytopenia

Table 10–4   Summary of late side-effects with radiotherapy

Site	Side effects
Skin	Fibrosis, pigmentation, telangiectasia, late ulceration
Mucosa	Fibrosis, stricture, fistula
Salivary glands	Xerostomia [permanent in 80% after 40–60 Gy (2Gy/fraction)]
Kidney	Chronic radiation nephritis (inability to concentrate urine, nocturia), benign hypertension, proteinuria, malignant hypertension
Bone/cartilage	Growth retardation in young children (limb shortening, scoliosis), radionecrosis (mandible/femoral head), external ear cartilage necrosis
Lung	Radiation pneumonitis
Marrow	Myelofibrosis
Gonads	Sterility, genetic mutations
Tumorigenesis	Induction of second malignancies

Radiation to the abdomen or pelvis administered in therapeutic doses for neoplastic disease can adversely affect the structure and function of any organ system or viscus in the path of the radiation beam. The gastrointestinal tract is by far the organ system most vulnerable to abdominal irradiation. Injury other structures may incur such as liver, pancreas, kidneys, ureter, and bladder. The surgical consequences of injuries to these structures are much less prevalent and are discussed briefly after injuries to various portions of the gastrointestinal tract.

There are several maxims in the management of radiation enteropathy.

1) Operation should always be a measure of last resort.

2) Optimal nutritional status should be achieved preoperatively.

3) Incision into heavily irradiated areas of skin should be avoided. Dilated bowel should be decompressed preoperatively, by long tube if possible.

4) Antibiotic bowel preparation should be done preoperatively and broad-spectrum parenteral antibiotics should be given postoperatively.

5) Resection of severely damaged bowel ismore definitive than bypass, but judgment at the time of operation should determine this decision.

6) Excessive adhesiolysis should be avoided. It rarely is definitive treatment for obstructive enteropathy; it may aggravate it and risks fistula formation.

7) Hand-sewn, stapled, end-to-end, or side-to-side anastomoses are equally effective, but each requires meticulous fashioning. Anastomoses in radiation-damaged bowel are precarious.

8) Anastomosis should be identifiable either by staple lines in stapled anastomoses or by hemoclips in hand-sewn anastomoses.

9) Oral feeding should be delayed until effective peristalsis returns and the anastomosis is functional. A minimum 5-day delay is recommended.

10) Low rectal anastomoses in irradiated bowel should be protected against leaks with a proximal colostomy for maximum safety.

11) Intestinal stomasmadewith irradiated bowel or in irradiated skin are prone to complications. An ample segment should be exteriorized.

12) Radiation-induced fistulas rarely respond to nonoperative therapy or simple closure. Resection or tissue transfer is usually necessary. Bypass exclusion is an option, although it is less desirable.

10.5   Progress on surgical oncology

10.5.1   Organ transplantation and malignancy

The first successful orthotopic liver transplantation was performed for a 19-month-old girl with hepatocellular carcinoma(HCC) on 1967, by Thomas E. Starzl. Although it had been over 50 years ago and the evolution has been remarkable, generally, the application of organ transplantation for the treatment of malignancy is extremely limited, especially in kidney, pancreas, small bowel, heart, and lung. The most important exception is that of liver transplantation for a primary hepatic malignancy, only of HCC, under circumstances in which all disease will be removed with the explanted organ. Achievements of better outcomes relies heavily on key components of peritranslpant care: ①accurate radiographic delineation of disease extent; ②early listing for patients with disease extent within the Milan criteria; ③effective locoregional therapy prior to transplantation; ④ en bloc resection of all intrahepatic disease. Preoperative imaging is of great significance in documenting the tumor location, size, number and association with adjacent important organ or tissue, as well as ruling out some absolute contraindications to liver transplantation including extrahepatic disease spread, tumor-related portal vein thrombosis, and encasement of the hepatoduodenal ligament. The Model for End-Stage Liver Disease (MELD) scoring system introduced in 2002 now offers priority for patients with HCC within conventional Milan criteria. The Milan Criteria, as they came to be known, were adopted by UNOS for directing organ allocation in the United States. The details of the Milan Criteria and the UNOS staging system are shown in Table 10-5 and Table 10-6. In 2003, priority scoring for HCC was reduced from 20 to 24 for stage I tumors (one tumor ≤ 1.9 cm) and from 24 to 29 for stage II tumors (single tumor 2 to 5 cm or three or less tumors, none larger than 3 cm). Despite these improvements, overall outcomes remain significantly lower for patients transplanted for HCC compared with those with end-stage liver disease but free of hepatic malignancy.

Table 10-5　Hepatocellular carcinoma: eligibility criteria for liver transplantation

Milan criteria	UNOS criteria
1 tumor ≤ 5 cm	1 tumor ≤ 6.5 cm
or	or
up to 3 tumors, none >3 cm	Multiple tumors, none >4.5 cm and total tumor diameter ≤ 8 cm

Table 10-6　UNOS-modified TNM staging system

Installment	Content	
T(primary tumor)	T_1	one nodule ≤ 1.9 cm
	T_2	One nodule 2.0-5.0 cm; two or three nodules, all< 3.0 cm
	T_3	One nodule >5.0 cm; two or three nodules, at least one >3.0 cm
	T_{4a}	Four or more nodules, any size
	T_{4b}	T_2, T_3, or T_{4a} with gross intrahepatic portal or hepatic vein involvement
N(regional lymph nodes)	N_1	Regional lymph node(s) involvement
M(distant metastasis)	M_1	Any extrahepatic metastatic disease beyond regional nodes
Stage	I	T_1
	II	T_2
	III	T_3
	IV A1	T_{4a}
	IV A2	T_{4b}
	IV B	Any N_1, any M_1

For the surgical oncologist, there are additional issues and concerns, as well as some fascinating and instructive aspects in the simultaneous consideration of immunosuppression and malignancy. Indeed, surgical oncology and transplantation overlap in a number of areas, obligating physicians in each discipline to maintain an understanding of the problems common to both. The two areas of greatest interest include the treatment of malignancy with organ transplantation and the consequences of immunosuppression on the development of malignancy. The true magnitude of the relationship between immune system and malignancy was dramatically illustrated when an early organ recipient succumbed to a donor's malignancy, establishing that immunosuppression can facilitate transplantation of more than just organ. Over time, immunosuppression was found to be a risk for both incidence and aggression of certain de novo tumors, as well as affecting outcomes of common sporadic cancers (Table 10-7).

Table 10-7   De novo malignancy after transplantation: relative incidence of some specific tumors

	General transplant	Population recipients
Lymphoma	5%	24%
Lip cancer	0.2%	6%
Kaposi's sarcoma	Negligible	6%
Anogenital	0.4%	3.5%
Hepatobiliary	1.5%	2.4%
Other Sarcomas	0.5%	1.8%

Immunosuppression related malignancy: ①direct carcinogenic effects of immunosuppressants; ②facilitation of oncogenic viral mechanisms; ③sensitization to environmental carcinogens; ④diminished immune surveillance; ⑤chronic antigenic stimulation: hyperplasia to neoplasia; ⑥impaired immunoregulation/unrestrained lymphoid proliferation; ⑦decreased interferons/altered cytokine milieu.

Although undeniable evidence implicates immunosuppressive drugs in the development of tumors following transplantation, the exact mechanisms by which they facilitate malignancies remain unclear. Possibilities include diminished immunosurveillance, facilitation of viral oncogenesis, increased sensitivity to environmental carcinogens, chronic antigenic stimulation with hyperplasia, or a host of effects at the cellular level. It seems likely that none are mutually exclusive, but rather the overall effect is multifactorial. The candidate with a history of malignancy presents one of the most difficult aspects of transplantation. The risks of a recurrent neoplasm in the immunosuppressed environment must be weighed against the alternatives without a transplant. A number of early reports documented the disastrous potential to transmit malignancy with a transplanted organ. Failure to elicit a prior history of a malignancy or an unrecognized lesion in a deceased donor has led to the transmission of a broad variety of tumors. Treatment options always include immunosuppression dose reduction but, if feasible as with kidney or pancreas transplants, these drugs can be completely discontinued with removal of the organs. Even diffuse metastases have been reported to resolve in the absence of ongoing immunosuppression. Given the increasing shortage of organs, further assessment of the risks may allow expansion of the donor pool into this previously avoided area. Malignancy among transplant candidates, recipients, and donors continues to be an area of major significance. Continued experience and research in the areas common to both surgical oncology and transplantation will, without doubt, provide the foundations for future successes in the treatment of malignancy.

10.5.2   Minimally invasive surgery for cancer

As surgery has been developing maturely, we pay more attention to the psychology, physiology and social demands of patients, thus minimally invasive surgery emerges as a new concept with the goal of small trauma, mild pain and rapid recovery to improve life quality and rehabilitation. Minimally invasive surgery refers to the use of laparoscopy, thoracoscopy and other modern medical devices and related equipment. Mouret, a French surgery, accidentally and successfully performed the first laparosopic surgery in 1987, which was marked as a milestone of new medicine. It has been resent decade that minimally invasive surgery is wildly applied to surgery and plays a more and more important role in surgery.

Although, it has achieved established success in the treatment of several benign diseases, mature data on the safety of these procedures is keenly awaited, as to date they are mostly restricted to the field of colon cancer. The application of this concept to surgical oncology is already common practice in certain fields such as the rectum, while it still needs to be thoroughly investigated in many others. Natural orifice transluminal endoscopic surgery (NOTES) is currently of major research interest as it may offer significant clinical potential for endoscopic procedures in the future, although many further issues are still unresolved.

Endoscopic mucosal resection (EMR) and endoscopic submucosal dissection (ESD) are advanced techniques and may be considered the ultimate "minimally" invasive treatments for early stage cancers. Therefore, NOTES may initially have a role in furthering the application of such endeavors to slightly more advanced stages. NOTES could supplement ESD by providing for direct sampling of sentinel nodes from the perigastric lymph basin. And NOTES may provide a complement for endoscopic sentinel node biopsy and an oncological supplement to current EMR/ESD techniques.

Transanal endoscopic microsurgery (TEM), pioneered and disseminated by Gerhard Buess, is considered as the direct ancestor in the lineage to NOTES in the field of general surgery. TEM was firstly applied to excision of benign rectal neoplasms, and then to curative surgery of "low risk" pT1 rectal adenocarcinomas and palliative surgery of invasive rectal adenocarcinomas. However, TEM instruments are currently designed for intraluminal tasks low in the pelvis, with 5–10 mm port sizes. For this reason Gerhard Buess is now working to a newly designed instrumentarium derived from the original TEM device, consisting of specially designed instruments and a single-port technique, to allow abdominal surgery with rigid instruments under the principles of NOTES.

10.5.3 Radioguided surgery in oncological surgery

Radioguided surgery refers to the use of radionuclides to locate lymph nodes or other tissues to excise during an operation. The use of gamma detection probe technology in radioguided surgery has expanded tremendously and has evolved into what is now considered an established discipline within the practice of surgery, revolutionizing the surgical management of many malignancies, including breast cancer, melanoma and colorectal cancer. The two main functions of radioguided surgery in oncological surgery are the localization of tumors and biopsy of the sentinel lymph nodes.

About two decades ago, radioguided occult localization was used to localize non-palpable breast lesions, which marked a natural evolution from earlier studies on radioguided sentinel node biopsy for breast carcinoma. And it shows great advantages, compared with wire localization, that it can provide specimen with better centering of the lesion and less healthy tissue, as well as a quicker and more simple way to locate and excise the lesion during operation. However, there are amount of difficulties in technique. For instance, the injection needle is not always insert to the correct depth or the centering of lesion, especially for superficial lesions or lesions in the central quanrant of the breast. Patient selection should never be of ignorance. For example, it can be deemed as contraindication in patients with diffuse microcalcifications and multifocal or multicentric lesions.

It is now generally acknowledged that high-quality scintigraphy with ^{99m}Tc-sestamibi can accurately localize parathyroid adenomas in 85% –95% of patients with primary hyperparathyroidism. ^{99m}Tc-sestamibi scintigraphy is used as a preoperative localization technique for unilateral neck exploration and minimally invasive radioguided parathyroidectomy, in which the use of a gamma probe helps finding the overproducing parathyroid gland and the volume of hormone produced by any individual parathyroid gland, based on metabolic activity as mirrored by the uptake of ^{99m}Tc-sestamibi.

Although pancreatic endocrine tumors are difficult to localize, endosonography is highly accurate in localizing the gastric and pancreatic neuroendocrine tumors. Up to 20% of insulinomas are not palpable at the time of surgery, whereas gastrinomas are not found during surgery in up to 40% of cases. Concerning the intraoperative tumor localization rate, the combination of intraoperative ultrasound and surgical palpation leads to 97% cure rate in patients with benign insulinomas. Furthermore, intraoperative ultrasound does not allow accurate detection of small lymph node metastases because of their normal size. Therefore, the intraoperative use of gamma probes makes it possible to identify recurrent tumor tissue when the normal anatomy has been altered or primary tumors in unusual anatomic locations.

Sentinel lymph node biopsy is accepted worldwide as the method of choice to stage regional lymph nodes in patients with melanoma. Radioguided surgery is particularly useful in patients with melanomas that are located in the perineum, since lymph drainage is clinically ambiguous. These lesions may drain to nodes in the groin, iliac, and obturator regions, as demonstrated by lymphoscintigraphy. Regional lymph node metastases (N_1 to N_3) define stage III disease and are cardinal prognostic variables for patients with cutaneous melanoma. Sentinel node staging can be considered for prognostic purposes, and to evaluate eligibility for clinical trials and the need for adjuvant therapy. Accurate staging can identify patients whose risk of recurrence is sufficiently high to justify adjuvant systemic treatment.

10.5.4　Prosthetic materials in surgical oncology

Protheses are wildly used in surgery, though there has been a heated discussion on whether these protheses have the potential carcinogenicity. The mechanism of this effect was suggested in 1975 by Brand et al. who asserted that the reaction of a foreign body creates the conditions required for the neoplastic development and maturation of cells with a neoplastic determination

already present in the body, although without inducing their mutation in itself. Some cases have been reported in the literature of angiosarcomas and sarcomas of other origin associated with stimulation by a foreign body as referred by Jennings et al. In contrast, more recently in 2002 Ghadimi et al. showed in a molecular study that although millions of hernia repairs are performed in the world with prostheses, no patient has subsequently reported the development of a soft tissue tumor.

The oncological surgery fields where prostheses are now largely used can be singled out as: oncological surgery in the true sense, surgery for wall defects and surgery for inguinal hernia.

Gray et al. suggested in 1996 that obtaining correct and sufficient resection of soft tissue tumors of the anterior abdominal wall required the removal of the tumor en bloc from the wall, and that this was enabled by the possibility of reconstructing the wall with the use of polypropylene mesh, which was also used by Puppo et al. in 2005 to reconstruct pelvic floor integrity following radical cystectomy for a stage T_2 bladder tumor with associated vaginal prolapse after subtotal hysterectomy, associated with an ileal reservoir for the urethra. It has been proposed the use of prothesis in pure Marlex or combined with methylmetacrylate or with a prothesis in stainless steel, while they are not usable in all cases and present contraindications being placed in contact with the intestine or used in a potentially or actually infected field. Modern technology has produced a solution for these situations, with the introduction of new biological prostheses derived from porcine or bovine collagen, with various products that differ in some of their details that might be important in particular situations. The use of a biological prosthesis to create a pelvic neo-diaphragm with the aim of isolating the zone to be radiated from the overlying intestinal loops and rendering it immune to infections and adherences might reveal itself to be the ideal solution for enabling the application of multimodal treatment for the rectal tumor, which certainly offers greater advantages than surgery alone. The incidence of incisional hernias following laparotomy varies from 2% −11% up to 16% in some case series. Chronic obstructive pulmonary disease, wound infections and diabetes are significantly correlated with the incidence of postoperative incisional hernias, while tumor disease seems not to be concluded as the predisposing factor. In the case of an already present hernia and the need to treat a tumor with a potentially contaminated operation (colon tumors, abscessualized, perforated), up to some time ago a prosthesis could not be used given the risk of infection and failure of the wall reconstruction. The positioning of a retromuscular mesh might be attempted in the case of low contamination of the surgical field, though bearing clearly in mind the risks run of infection in these cases. The realization of new biological prostheses offers an optimal solution for these cases. The new concept of mesh in low cost material (polypropylene) and low weight provides excellent materials for treating post-laparotomy hernias with traditional techniques (Rives) and with satisfactory results in terms of success and patient compliance. The use of human fibrin-based glues for fixing them also reduces the discomfort created when stitches are used, adding a relatively small cost to the operation in the face of decidedly favorable results.

The implementation of an operation that is "not clean" would make a simultaneous hernioplasty inadvisable, forbidding "tailoring" with the usual prosthetic meshes for reasons that can been imagined connected with a possible infection. Nevertheless, even if plausible, all this is only partially true due to the evolution that the materials used have undergone in recent years. New composition prostheses, other fully biological prostheses made up of bovine collagen, light meshes or meshes which are resorbable by the body after implantation, or combined with non-stick substances, and lastly the use of aids like adhesives able to secure the prostheses without suture are all innovations able to disprove past statements questioning the ability of the prosthesis to be held safely in place and the risk of complications in the field of sepsis, and able to achieve a high percentage of success.

10.5.5   New technologies in oncological endocrine surgery

Endocrine surgery involves kinds of organs, such as thyroid, parathyroid, adrenal gland and even digestive organs, and variant theraputic approaches, especially in the oncological fields. and the emergence of new technologies pushes the rapid development of oncological endocrine surgery.

In the last ten years, the adoption in selected cases of a mini-invasive surgical approach to neoplastic thyroid disease has made it possible to perform the procedure with greater respect for the esthetic elements of a zone, i. e. the front of the neck, which is so important for relational life. In the third millennium we are trying to establish diagnostic potential with methods alternative to the surgical procedure and with less impact for the patient. With the intention of making this aspect tolerable, the indication of mini-invasive (MIVAT) techniques has been extended in the oncological field (Table 10−8), an appreciably different approach throughout the world produced by dissimilar habits and the multiple skills of individual operators. Nevertheless, over the course of the years there has been a convergence in the area of video-assisted techniques without pneumo-neck, with a direct approach in the anterior region. Manageable systems of coagulation and section have reduced the use of metal clips or laces, which has made dissection and obliteration of vascular pedicles just as safe, rapid and efficacious, almost determining potentially "sutureless" thyroidectomy, and has been coupled with optical devices of ever smaller dimensions so as to allow reassuring control of the operative field through an incision of around 2 cm. The ultrasound and the radiofrequency dissector compete in the operating theatre to produce maximum hemostatic safety, optimization of operating times and stability of results.

Table 10-8 Current indications and contraindications for MIVAT

Indications	Contraindications
Thyroid nodules with diameter less than 3–3.5 cm	History of thyroiditis (positive antibodies)
Indeterminate cytology	Previous neck irradiation
Follicular lesions	Previous thyroid or parathyroid surgery
"Low risk" papillary carcinoma	
Basedow's disease with gland not exceeding 20 ml	
Prophylactic thyroidectomy in patients who are carriers of RET gene mutation	

Radiofrequency ablation is a treatment already in use to manage many neoplasms, as carcinoma of the liver, hepatic metastasis, bone metastasis and renal tumor; recently its efficacy and safety were also assessed in the treatment of nodular thyroid disease, in subjects not referable to surgery due to a high operative risk or who expressly refused surgical treatment. Laser ablation of nodular thyroid formations through the skin has been applied both in the oncological field and for the treatment of hyperfunctioning adenomas. In the oncological field ablation with the laser technique seems efficacious in obtaining a rapid reduction in tumor mass before chemotherapy and/or radiotherapy of a thyroid carcinoma not susceptible to surgical resection or radiometabolic ablation with iodine.

High-energy shock waves have been used since the beginning of the 1980s in lithotripsy. More recently, applications of this technology have been tested which appear able to open up new perspectives in the oncological field. In particular, some research projects have taken on the aim of verifying a method of antitumor therapy that will enable a greater cytostatic effect to be obtained with notably reduced doses of chemotherapy drugs compared with those adopted in common treatment plans. Another innovative technique proposed for the treatment of differentiated thyroid carcinomas aims at recovering the efficacy of radiometabolic therapy with iodine in tumors.

As in bilateral exploration of parathyroids, it is possible to single out three parathyroids in 87%, while four glands are visualized only in 45% of cases, the glands may quiet frequently be localized in atypical sites, and thus the pathological gland may be more difficult to be localized. In 1996, Norman proposed to use an isotopic tracer, sestamibi, pre-operatively and intra-operatively with the purpose of localizing the site of the adenoma and then carry out a mini-invasive radio-guided parathyroidectomy. With the aim of performing an extremely efficient, targeted maneuver, rigid inclusion and exclusion criteria are needed (Table 10-9). The procedure may also be carried out under local anesthesia, as widely published by Lo Gerfo, with different types of cervical plexus block and recently proposed again by Miccoli for his personal minimally invasive parathyroidectomy technique.

Table 10-9　Inclusion and exclusion criteria for radio-guided parathyroidectomy

Inclusion criteria	Exclusion criteria
Parathyroid scintigraphy with sestamibi documenting uptake of a single gland	Lack of visualization of parathyroids in preoperative imaging
	Demonstration of 2 or more enlarged glands at scintigraphy and/or ECT
	Concomitant presence of thyroid nodule disease

At the beginning of the 1990s, the laparoscopic adrenalectomy technique was first described by Ganger, and then it has systematically become established as the alternative to conventional surgery for the treatment of surgical disease of the adrenal gland, even becoming the theraputic standard for some indications, such as functioning benign tumors of small dimensions, aldosteronomas and so forth (Table 10-10). The laparoscopic approach has significantly reduced some of the complications or consequences of conventional surgery, such as paralytic ileum, respiratory problems, infections and wound complications. Among the complications of laparoscopic adrenalectomy, intra-or postoperative hemorrhage is certainly the most frequent and the accidental lesion of large vessels is the main cause of laparotomic conversion. The most feared complication for oncological aims is undoubtedly adrenal capsule lesion with dispersion of glandular tissue, a situation which proves decisive in the choice of surgical approach in particular in suspected adrenal carcinoma, pheochromocytoma and the case of extremely large myelolipoma. Robotic surgery is the new technological challenge and has been coupled with imaging fusion techniques with intraoperative video-laparoscopic visualization aimed at improving surgical orientation.

Table 10-10　Indications and contraindications for adrenal laparoscopic surgery

Project	Content
Indications	Functioning benign tumors of small dimensions; aldosteronomas; Cushing's Syndrome induced by cortisol producing adrenal adenoma or bilateral hyperplasia; non-functioning incidentalomas of small dimensions (however >3. 5-4 cm); primitive tumors including suspected malignancy without signs of infiltration
Relative contraindications (connected with the tumor)	Tumors of large dimensions (>12-14 cm); pheochromocytoma (due to risk of bleeding or anesthesiological problems); malignant tumors (risk of capsular breakage or "spillage"); rapidly growing myelolipomas, large dimensions, compressing neighboring organs
Relative contraindications (connected with the patient)	Obesity; previous surgery for nephrectomy or duodenopancreatectomy
Absolute contraindications	Contraindications for pneumoperitoneum, coagulopathy, serious cardiopulmonary disease; malignant tumors with signs of infiltration

Except from the laparoscopic approach, radiolocalization of the forms expressing receptors for somatostatin, with the help of nuclear medical imaging, is the only innovative event in the field of surgery for neuroendocrine disease of the gasrto-entero-pancreatic zone. Endocrine pancreatic tumors belong to the large group of neuroendocrine tumors of the gastro-entero-pancreatic tract, the cells of which contain enzymatic structures capable of amine precursor storage and decarboxylation, an essential process for the production of monoamine neurotransmitters like serotonin, histamine and dopamine, and often express somatostatin receptors on their surface. Nuclear medical molecular imaging exploits both these characteristics to develop new tracers able to visualize these tumors.

10.5.6   Robots in oncological surgery

The term "robotic surgery" refers to the surgical technology that places a computer-assisted electro-mechanical instrument between the surgeon and the patient. The exact term for the instruments currently used is "remote presence manipulator", since the available technology does not generally work without the explicit and direct control of a human operator. The key elements of this "remote presence" are the implementation of the surgeon's skills and the alteration of the traditional direct contact between surgeon and patient.

Robotic surgery was used for the first time in neurosurgery; it dates back to the first half the 1980s when the Unimate PUMA 2000 was built specifically to be used with neurosurgical instruments in stereotactic biopsies. Subsequently used in orthopedics, robotic systems have been more recently used in general and specialized abdominal surgery. Computer Motion and Intuitive Surgical were the main manufacturers of robotic surgery systems until 2003, when Intuitive Surgical bought out Computer Motion, which was founded in 1989 by Yulun Wang. It marketed AESOP, which became the first surgical robot approved by the FDA (in 1994) and started the concept of solo-surgery. The same happened with the Zeus Robotic Microsurgical System, introduced in 1998 and used in 2001 for the first experience of remote surgery on humans.

It can be divided as three main parts: operating console, surgical cart and vision system. The operating console is a non-sterile workstation that is kept distant from the operating table; it has wheels for easy movement, a power cable for connection to the electricity main and three more cables for connection to the slave (Figure 10-2). The surgical cart is located next to the operating table, partially inside the sterile area; its position changes depending on the surgical procedure (Figure 10-3). The vision system includes several devices that process and optimize the image quality during surgery.

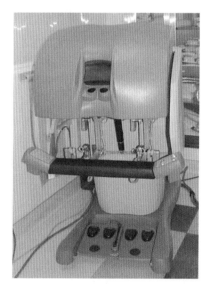

Figure 10-2   **Operator console**
(dimensions 166 cm×97 cm×158 cm, weight 227 kg)

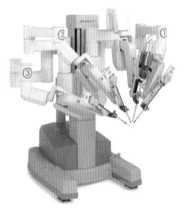

Figure 10-3   **Robotic arms**
(dimensions 198 cm×94 cm× 97 cm, weight 544 kg)

The literature describes two types of approach for the treatment of esophageal pathology with robotic technology: the transthoracic approach and the transhiatal approach. In both cases, the technique is similar to that used in traditional laparoscopic and laparotomic surgery. The robotic technique with longer instruments and with 7 degrees of freedom results in operations performed in a very small space which overcome the limits found both in the laparoscopic and thoracoscopic techniques. The use of the robotic technique in the treatment of stomach cancer has been documented by very few authors, the first being Giulianotti in 2003. In the available literature, the use of robots seems to suggest easier performance of lymphadenectomies. What emerges from the data presented in the literature is that the robotic approach to the surgical treatment of stomach cancer is feasible and its results are comparable to those of the traditional technique; the removal of lymph nodes for D2 lymphadenectomy is easy and safe. Also, robots surgery is applied in other fields, such as in oncological urology for the treatment of parenchymal kidney tumor, blander cancer and radical prostatectomy.

10.5.7 Endoscopy and oncology

Endoscopic therapy has emerged as a highly effective and minimally invasive way to control and cure early neoplasia of the digestive tract. Firstly, it was used to polyectomy. And more recently, ablation and endoscopic mucosal resection(EMR) has been successfully applied to treatment of flat neoplasia of gut mucosa. The emergence of endoscopic ultrasonograph(EUS) improves accuracy for cancer staging, and EUS-guided fine-needle aspiration helps tissue diagnosis outside the gut lumen, by specimen biopsy. On the other hand, in advanced cancer, it plays a key role in palliation with the use of stents to bridge obstruction, ablation and the placement of tubes for drainage and nutrition.

EMR provides a valid alternative to surgical resection for the treatment of early cancer of gastrointestinal tract, which can completely or curatively remove the affected mucosa, by excising the middle or deeper part of the submucosa. Submucosal injection used to facilitate EMR can help in the decision of whether or not to continue with the procedure, by the observation of a bleb formation with elevation of the overlying mucosa indicating the absence of deep submucosal involvement and the feasibility of EMR. Nevertheless, like any invasive procedures, EMR has complications. The most frequent complication of EMR is bleeding, which occurs in 1.5% ~24.0% of cases. And perforation is the most worrisome complication, which occurs when the muscle layer is included in the snare resection, generally, due to a lack of submucosal saline solution injection while performing the procedure. Specially, stenosis is a consequence of EMR in the esophagus with deep thermal injury of the esophageal wall.

Endoscopic submucosal dissection(ESD) is a newly developed technique which require the use of special knives, suitable for en bloc resection of large lesions in the gastrointestinal tract and now being used in other locations. Conventional techniques of EMR are thought to be inadequate for en bloc resection of large colonic lesions. The multiple fragments that result from this piecemeal resection make the histopathological evaluation of the completeness of polyp removal difficult. Therefore, en bloc resection with a satisfactory tumor cell-negative margin is considered a more desirable outcome. The technical limitations in endoscopic treatment of large colonic lesions can sometimes be overcome by a device enabling the performance of en bloc resection, thus allowing the acquisition of a single large specimen for the correct evaluation of the resection margins.

Narrow-band imaging (NBI) is a novel endoscopic technique that may enhance the accuracy of diagnosis by using narrow-bandwidth filters in a red-green-blue (R/G/B) sequential illumination system. Magnifying endoscopy by using NBI has two distinct applications; the analysis of the surface architecture of the epithelium (pit pattern) and the analysis of the vascular network. Magnifying endoscopy by using NBI provides the most effective method of detecting premalignant and malignant precursors of advanced cancer in which the tumor process is restricted to the superficial layers of the gastrointestinal wall. Premalignant lesions often develop against a background of inflammation and diffuse alterations in the mucosa; these are considered to be risk factors for cancer and are called "premalignant conditions". Premalignant conditions of the gastrointestinal tract include intestinal metaplasia of the esophagus and stomach, chronic gastritis associated with H. pylori infection, chronic inflammation in ulcerative colitis, and gastrointestinal adenomas.

EUS has been one of the most important innovations to occur in gastrointestinal endoscopy during the last 25 years. It has extended the range of possibilities for endoscopic diagnosis, supplying the endoscopist with the unequalled opportunity to see not only the mucosal surface but within and beyond the wall of the gastrointestinal tract. Presently, EUS is still the most accurate imaging technique for pre-theraputic clinical staging, both T and N, of early gastrointestinal neoplasia. However, conventional EUS, with dedicated echoendoscope (5, 7.5 and 12 MHz), has not sufficient accuracy in differentiating T_1 from T_{1s} cancers. Small miniaturized echographic probes (miniprobes), which can be passed through the operative channel of a standard endoscope, can achieve better results providing high spatial resolution of the GI wall, depicted as a 9-layered structure instead of a 5-layered one, seen with the lowest frequencies. Miniprobes can assist EMR and increase its safety by reducing the risk of complications, especially perforative ones. Compared with other imaging techniques, such as transabdominal US, CT and MRI, the advantage of EMR is its superior pancreatic parenchymal resolution.

Xiong Li

Chapter 11

Principle of Chemotherapy for Tumor

11.1 Overview of chemotherapy

Medical oncology is a subspecialty of internal medicine that focuses on care and treatments to patients with cancers. Chemotherapy is one of the three main treatment approaches for cancers. It has been an effective tool of medical oncologists since 1940s. With rapid development of pharmaceutical industry and some breakthroughs in molecular targeted therapy, tools of medical oncologists for fighting cancer have been varied from conventional cancer drugs to targeted therapy. In this chapter, conventional chemotherapy agents will be mainly introduced.

11.1.1 History and development of chemotherapy

During both World Wars, the United States developed a secret gas program as chemical weapons, and the astute observation that exposure to mustard gas resulted in bone marrow and lymphoid hypoplasia. This experience led to the first clinical use of nitrogen mustard in a patient with non-Hodgkin's lymphoma in 1942. Subsequent treatment with this alkylating agent resulted in dramatic regressions in advanced lymphomas and thereby generated significant excitement in the field of cancerpharmacology. In the late 1940s, Sidney Farber reported that folic acid had a significant proliferative effect on leukemic cell growth in children with lymphoblastic leukemia. These observations led to the development of folic acid analogs as cancer drugs to inhibit cellular folate metabolism, which initiated the era of cancer chemotherapy. In the latter half of the 20th century, cytotoxic drugs took the predominant position with continuous appearance of new agents.

11.1.2 Curability of cancers with chemotherapy

Some cancers may be cured by chemotherapy agents. These include but are not limited to cancers like acute lymphoid or acute myeloid leukemia, Hodgkin's diseases, lymphoma (certain type), germ cell neoplasms, some pediatric neoplasms, gestational trophoblastic neoplasm. Selections of drugs or regimens for different types of cancers are mainly based on the results of prior clinical trials.

Some advanced diseases such as relapsed lymphoid/myeloid leukemia, relapsed Hodgkin's/non-Hodgkin's lymphomas, multiple myeloma are still possibly cured by "high-dose" chemotherapy with stem cells support. "High-dose" chemotherapy is mainly based on the observation that higher proportion of cancer cells could be killed and decreased incidence of drug resistance while dose increased. However, life-threatening complications that require intensive supportive care should be noticed, but it still worth because there are definite curative potentials in some diseases. "High-dose" chemotherapy with stem cell transplantation is usually indicated in hematological diseases, such as lymphoma, leukemia, and myeloma.

Chemotherapy can be administered after radical surgery or eradication by radiotherapy, which is also known as adjuvant chemotherapy. Adjuvant chemotherapy can reduce relapse rate, increase the survival rate and improve the curability of some certain types of solid tumors. Cancers like breast cancer, colorectal cancer, osteogenic sarcoma, non-small cell lung cancer and so on are likely to benefit from adjuvant chemotherapy. Standard regimens and dose with evidences should be chosen with intent of adjuvant chemotherapy.

When the tumor is too large or clinical stage is relatively advanced but there is no evidence of distant metastasis, chemotherapy can be employed before radical surgery or radiotherapy in order to decrease the size and down staging of tumors, in order to get chances of radical treatment. This type of chemotherapy is also known as neo-adjuvant chemotherapy. Neo-adjuvant chemotherapy can kill micrometastic foci and decrease chances of tumor cell spread during surgery. It also helps conserve more normal tissue and avoid impairment of normal organ functions.

Palliative chemotherapy is usually applied in advanced, metastatic cancer which has little chance to be cured. Chemotherapy can relieve symptoms caused by cancers progression and improve patient's life of quality, and some agents even prolong survival. Cause the objective of this type of therapy is not curing the cancer but just to improve the life of quality mostly, medical oncologists always have to balance the efficacy and side effects of the treatments. Individualized therapy based on evidences of prior clinical trials is often applied.

Although chemotherapy agents have gained achievements among different cancers, there are some cancers are not sensitive to conventional chemotherapy agents. Cancers like hepatocellular carcinoma, melanoma, and thyroid carcinoma seldom get benefit from conventional chemotherapy. Nevertheless, thanks to development of targeted therapy and immune therapy, these cancers may benefit from the new treatment approaches.

11.2　Cell cycle and tumor biology

Cell cycle refers to a series of events that take place in a cell leading to its duplication and division of DNA to produce two daughter cells. There are four phases. Gap1 (G1) phase, from the end of previous mitosis phase to DNA synthesis, is when large amount of RNA and proteins are synthesized and prepared for DNA synthesis. In this phase, organelles inside the cell increase in sizes and numbers. A cell in G1 phase can stop cell cycle and enter resting phase (G0 phase) to undergo differentiation or just get arrested in which situation it can re-enter G1 phase, or proceed to synthesis phase (S phase). S phase is the phase when DNA duplicates. Then a cell goes into Gap2 (G2) phase, when protein synthesis and cell growth are prepared to mitotic phase (M phase). In M phase, two identical daughter cells were produced by mitosis which involves sequential events and phases.

The cell cycle is regulated by a series of cyclins, cyclin-dependent kinases (CDK) and cyclin-dependent kinase inhibitors (CDKI). Cell cycle regulatory genes encoding these proteins are usually mutated or deletion in tumor cells, which leads to loss of control in tumor cell cycle and rapid growth of tumor tissues.

Growth fraction (GF) refersto percentage of proliferative cells to total cells. Tumors that have higher GF are more sensitive to chemotherapy. And when proliferative cells are killed, cells in G0 phase will re-enter into cellcycle and be killed by chemotherapy agents. Doubling time (DT) is defined as the time tumor cells need to increase twice of the total amount and volume. Both GF and DT can provide information of tumor's growth speed and sensitivity to chemotherapy. Some agents are more effective to cells in proliferative phases (most are specific to S and Mphases), which also called cell cycle specific agents (CCSA); while some can kill cells not depending on specific phases, which are classified into cell cycle non-specific agents (CCSNA). Most chemotherapy agents are more sensitive to tumors with high growth rates (i. e. Hodgkin's lymphoma) than those with slower growth rates (i. e indolent lymphoma). Phases of tumor cells have influences on sensitivity of a chemotherapy agent. Generally, cells in proliferative phases (G1, S, G2 and M) are more sensitive to chemotherapy than those in quiescent phase (G0).

Chemotherapy agents follow the "first order kinetics" when kill tumor cells, which is killing a proportion, not an exact number of tumor cells each time. If concentration increases in arithmetic, tumor cells will be killed in logarithm way. For example, if we define the tumor cell survival rate is 100% when drug concentration is 0 mg/L; then when theconcentration is added from 0 mg/L to 1 mg/L, the tumor cells survival rate will fall from 10% to 100%. Clinical complete remission does not equal to cure. To cure the can-cer means to eliminate all the cancer cells within the body. Total kill of the cancer refers to not only remove all cancer cells by multiple modalities including surgery, chemotherapy, radiotherapy and biological targeted therapy, but also kill cancer cells by the host immune system. Combination, sequential or synchronized use of CCSA and CCSNA can kill cancer cells more effectively (Figure 11–1).

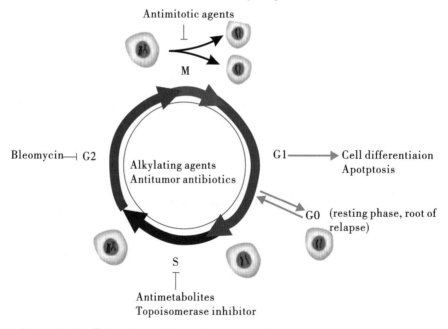

Figure 11–1   Cell cycle and chemotherapy agents

11.3   Chemotherapy agents: overview and mechanisms

According to source and chemical structure of the drugs and their mode of acting mechanisms, conventional chemotherapy agents can be divided into five subtypes. Commonly used agents are seen in Table 11–1.

Table 11-1　Commonly used chemotherapy agents

Drug	Usual dose	Toxicity	Indications	Cautions
Alkylating agents				
Cyclophospha-mide (CTX)	$400 - 2,000$ mg/m^2 IV, 100 mg/m^2 PO, qd	Myelosuppression, common alkylator*, hemorrhagic cystitis	Broad-spectrum, commonly used in lymphoma, myeloma, SCLC, et al.	Not use locally
Ifosfamide (IFO)	$1.0-1.5$ mg/m^2, qd, 5-7 d	Myelosuppression, common alkylator*, hemorrhagic cystitis	Broad-spectrum, soft tissue sarcoma	Simultaneous hydration and mesna
Myleran	2 mg, tid or qid, PO	Myelosuppression, hyperpigmentation, amenorrhea, pulmonary fibrosis,	Chronic myeloid leukemia, MDS	
Melphalan	0.25 mg/kg, qd, PO, 4 d, every 4 - 6 weeks; 2 - 4 mg qd, PO	Myelosuppression, nausea, vomiting	MM, testicular seminoma	
Carmustine (BCNU)	200 mg/m^2 IV; 150 mg/m^2, PO	Delayed myelosuppression, nausea, vomiting	Brain tumors, lymphoma, SCLC	Penetrate BBB; thrombocytopenia
Lomustine (CCNU)	100 mg/m^2 PO, every 4-6 weeks	Delayed myelosuppression, vomiting	Brain tumors, lymphoma, SCLC	Same as above
Semustine (Me-CCNU)	175 mg/m^2 PO, every 4-6 weeks	Delayed myelosuppression, vomiting	Brain tumors, lymphoma, SCLC	Same as above
Dacarbazine (DTIC)	250 mg/m^2 IV, qd, 5 d, every 3 weeks	Myelosuppression, nausea, vomiting	Melanoma, Hodgkin's lym-phoma, soft tissue sarcoma	Protect from light
Temozolomide	$150 - 200$ mg/m^2, qd, 5 d, every 4 weeks	Myelosuppression, nausea, vomiting, headache, fatigue	Brain tumors, melanoma	Penetrate BBB
Procarbazin (PCB)	$100-200$ mg/m^2 qd, 14 d, every 4 weeks	Myelosuppression	Hodgkin's lymphoma, brain tumors	Delayed myelosuppression when high-dose used
Cisplatin (DDP)	20 mg/m^2 qd, 5 d, IV; 100 mg/m^2 IV, every 3-4 weeks	Nephropathy, neuropathy, myelo-suppression, nausea, vomiting	Broad-spectrum head and neck cancer, ovarian cancer, lung cancer, et al.	Hydration and diuresis before, during and after treatment
Carboplatin	$300 - 350$ mg/m^2; or AUC 5-6 IV, every 4 weeks	Myelosuppression, thrombocytopenia, nausea, vomiting, nephropathy,	Broad-spectrum, indications similar to DDP	Nephropathy and vomiting relatively mild
Oxaliplatin	130 mg/m^2 IV, per 3 weeks; 85-100 mg/m^2 IV, every 2 weeks	Neuropathy, nausea, vomiting, myelosuppression, allergy	Colorectal cancer	Avoid cold

Continue to Table 11-1

Drug	Usual dose	Toxicity	Indications	Cautions
Antimetabolites				
Methotrexate (MTX)	15–30 mg PO,qd, 3–5 d;or 30 mg IV, D1, D8; or 1.5–12 g/m² IV with CF	Myelosuppression, mucositis, nephropathy,nausea,vomiting,	Broad-spectrum, acute leukemia, squamous cell carcinoma, lung cancer, breast cancer,et al.	Monitor plasma drug concentration,hydration and alkalization when use in high-dose
6-mercaptopurine(6-MP)	2.5 mg/(kg·d), 5 d,every 4 weeks	Myelosuppression, mucositis, nausea,vomiting,liver toxicity	Acute leukemia	
6-thioguanine (6-TG)	2.5 mg/(kg·d), 5 d,every 4 weeks	Myelosuppression, mucositis, nausea,vomiting,liver toxicity	Acute leukemia	
Hydroxyurea (H.U)	20–40 mg/kg,qd, PO	Myelosuppression,mucositis	Acute leukemia,head and neck cancer	
5-fluorouracil (5-FU)	15 mg/kg IV, per week; or 400–500 mg/(kg·d), 5 d,very 3–4 weeks	Mucositis, diarrhea, myelosuppression, vomiting, alopecia, hyperpigmentation, hand-foot syndrome	Gastrointestinal cancer, breast cancer, head and neck cancer,ovarian cancer,choriocarcinoma	Simultaneous use of CF can increase efficacy and toxicity
Capecitabine	1,250 mg/m²,bid, PO, 2 weeks on/1 off; or 665 mg/m² bid continuous	Hand-foot syndrome,diarrhea, mucositis,fatigue	Breast cancer, gastrointestinal cancer, head and neck caner	
Gimeraciland oteracil porassium capsule (S-1)	40 mg/m², PO, 28 d on/14 d off	Diarrhea, myelosuppression, fatigue,anorexia,nausea	Gastrointestinal cancer, head and neck squamous cell carcinoma	
Cytosine arabinoside (Ara-c)	100–150 mg/m², qd, IVD, 5–7 d, every 3 weeks	Mucositis, myelosuppression, nausea,vomiting	Acute leukemia	Can be used intrathecally
Gemcitabine	1,000–1,250 mg/m², qw, IV, 2–3 d,every 4 weeks	Myelosuppression, nausea, vomiting,fever/flu syndrome	NSCLC,pancreatic cancer,breast cancer,et al.	Notice thrombocytopenia
Pemetrexed	200 mg IV,every 3 weeks	Myelosuppression	NSCLC,pleural mesothelioma	Supplement folate/B_{12}; caution renal failure
Fludarabin L-asparaginase	2.5 mg/(kg·d), 5 d,every 4 weeks	Neutropenia, thrombocytopenia, nausea, vomiting, hypoalbuminemia	Indolent non-Hodgkin's lymphoma	Allergic test before use
Antimitotic agents				
Vincristine (VCR)	0.7–1.0 mg/m², qw, IV (maximal dose of 2 mg)	Neuropathy,constipation	Acute leukemia, lymphoma	Leakage of drug cause vesicles and necrosis of the local tissue
Vinblastine (VLB)	4–6 mg/m², qw, IV	Neutropenia,neuropathy	Hodgkin's lymphoma, testicular cancer	Same as above

Continue to Table 11-1

Drug	Usual dose	Toxicity	Indications	Cautions
Vinorelbine (NVB)	$20-30$ mg/m^2, qw, IV; or $40-80$ mg/m^2, qw, PO	Myelosuppression, phlebitis	NSCLC, breast cancer	Same as above
Paclitaxel	175 mg/m^2 (alone) or 135 mg/m^2 (in combination) IV, every 4 weeks	Myelosuppression, allergy reaction, alopecia, neuropathy	Broad-spectrum, breast cancer, NSCLC, et al.	Premedicate with anti-allergic treatment (dexamethasone, Diphenhydramine, ranitidine)
Docetaxel	$60-100$ mg/m^2 IV, every 3 weeks	Myelosuppression, allergy reaction, alopecia, neuropathy, edema	Breast cancer, NSCLC	Same as above
Nab-paclitaxel	260 mg/m^2 IVD, every 3 weeks	Neuropathy, myelosuppression	Breast cancer, gastric cancer et al.	Caution in hepatic insufficiency
Ixabepilone	40 mg/m^2 IV, every 3 weeks	Neuropathy, myelosuppression	Breast cancer	

Antitumor antibiotics

Drug	Usual dose	Toxicity	Indications	Cautions
Adriamycin (ADM)	$40-50$ mg/m^2 IV, every 3 weeks	Myelosuppression, cardiotoxicity, alopecia, nausea, vomiting	Lymphoma, breast cancer, SCLC, soft tissue sarcoma, myeloma	Cardiotoxicity is cumulative, total dosage should be less than 450 mg/m^2
Liposomal adriamycin	$20-50$ mg/m^2 IV, every 3–4 weeks	Myelosuppression, cardiotoxicity, hand-foot syndrome	Ovarian cancer, breast cancer	Mild cardiotoxity compared to ADM
Epirubicin (EPI)	$60-100$ mg/m^2 IV, every 3 weeks	Myelosuppression, cardiotoxicity, hand-foot syndrome	Same as above	Same as above
Daunorubicin	30–60 mg/m^2, qd, 1–3 d, IV, every 2–3 weeks	Same as ADM	Acute leukemia	Same as ADM
Pirarubicin (THP)	$30-50$ mg/m^2 IV, every 3 weeks	Similar to EPI	Same as ADM	Cumulative dosage 900 mg/m^2
Bleomycin (BLM)	5–10 mg/m^2 IV, qod or qw	Pulmonary fibrosis, skin toxicity, fever, occasional allergic reaction	Lymphoma, testicular cancer, head and neck cancer	Pulmonary fibrosis related to cumulative dosage
Mitomycin-c (MMC)	10 mg/m^2 IV, every 3–4 weeks	Myelosuppression, nausea, vomiting, phlebitis	Breast cancer, gastrointestinal cancer, lung cancer	Caution in leakage of the drug
Mitoxantrone	12 mg/m^2 qd, 3 d; or $12-14$ mg/m^2 IV, every 3 weeks	Myelosuppression, mild cardiotoxicity, phlebitis, change of nails, blue urine	Lymphoma, leukemia, breast cancer, et al.	
Actinomycin D	$250-400$ g/(kg · d), 5 d, every 4 weeks	Myelosuppression, nausea, vomiting, alopecia	Soft tissue sarcoma, testicular cancer, embryonal carcinoma, pediatric tumors	Caution in leakage of the drug

Continue to Table 11-1

Drug	Usual dose	Toxicity	Indications	Cautions
Topoisomerase inhibitors				
Etoposide (VP-16)	50 mg/m², qd, 5 d, IV, every 3 - 4 weeks; or 50 mg, qd, 14-20 d, PO, 2 weeks off	Myelosuppression, alopecia, nausea, vomiting	SCLC, lymphoma, testicular cancer	
Vumon (VM26)	70 mg/m² qd, 3 - 5 d, IV, every 3 weeks	Myelosuppression, alopecia, allergy	Lymphoma, metastatic brain tumors	Penetrate BBB, caution in allergic reaction
Topotecan (TPT)	1. 25 mg/(m² · d), 5 d, every 3 week	Myelosuppression, alopecia, nausea, vomiting	Ovarian cancer, SCLC, gastric cancer	Caution in drug leakage
Irinotecan (CPT-11)	300-350 mg/m² IV, every 3 weeks	Delayed diarrhea, neutropenia, alopecia, nausea, vomiting	Colorectal cancer, gastric cancer, SCLC	Loperamide (2 mg, q2 h) to manage delayed diarrhea

* commonalkylator: alopecia, infertility, and teratogenesis.

Abbreviations: SCLC, small cell lung cancer; MDS, myelodysplastic syndrome; MM, multiple myeloma; AUC, area under curve; NSCLC, non-small cell lung cancer.

11.3.1 Alkylating agents

Alkylating agent has active R-CH2-, which forms a cross linking with DNA molecular or between DNA molecular and protein by foralkylation, then causes destruction of cellular structure and cell death. Nitrogen mustard is a prototypic representative of this subtype, and nowadays, cyclophosphamide, ifosfamide and so on are more often used in clinic. Cyclophosphamide is a derivative of nitrogen mustard, which is inactive unless metabolized by cytochrome P450 in liver and then transform into 4-hydro-cyclophoshpamide. Alkylating agents are frequently used in combination therapy to treat a variety of types of cancer. Because of early successes, many disease states are managed with drug combinations that contain several alkylating agents. Cyclophosphamide is employed to treat a variety of immune-related diseases and to purge bone marrow in autologous marrow transplantation. Dacarbazine (DTIC) is activated in the liver to gain the highly reactive methyl diazonium cation. Temozolomide is structurally related to DTIC and can pass the blood-brain barrier. Platinum drugs can form crossing link between DNA molecules and works like alkylating agents. Since the introduction of cisplatin in the 1970s, three agents have come to constitute the most broadly used class of anticancer agents, the platinum compounds. Cisplatin is still very important in neck and head malignancy and lung cancer. Carboplatin with slighter renal impairment and GI tract reactions is applied in various types of cancers. Oxaliplatin has litter impairment to the kidney functions but cause peripheral neuropathy, is now commonly used in colorectal carcinomas.

11.3.2 Anti-metabolic agents

Anti-metabolic agents interrupt the metabolism of nucleic acids thus to impair synthesis of DNA, RNA and proteins. They usually have similar structure to the normal metabolites, competitively inhibit the main enzymes of nucleic acid metabolismand replace the precursor materials for DNA or RNA synthesis, thus affect DNA synthesis. They interfere with nucleic acid synthesis, and are most effective in Phase S (cell cycle specific agents), little effect on non-proliferatingcells. Methotrexate (MTX) is a dihydrofolate reductase (DHFR) inhibitor, interferes with formation of tetrahydrofolic acid thus to inhibits synthesis of DNA. MTX can be used in high-dose accompanied with calcium folinate (CF) in order to kill cancer cells with greater effect but reduce the damage of normal tissue. 6-Mercaptopurine (6-MP) and 6-Thioguanine (6-TG) can block the conversion from hypoxanthine to adenine. 5-Fluorouracil (5-FU) is metabolized and activated to FdUMP, then inhibits thymidylate synthetase (TS) which prevents dUMP from turning into dTMP. 5-FU is metabolized by dihydropyrimidine dehydrogenase (DPD), deficiency of this enzyme can cause excessive toxicity. The oral anti-metabolic agent capecitabine is also a prodrug of 5-FU. It is firstly metabolized to 5-Deoxy-5-fluorouridine (5-DFCR) by carboxylesterase in gastrointestinal tract, then converts to 5-Fluoro-deoxyuridine (5-DFUR) by cytidine deaminase in the liver and finally to 5-FU in the tumor by thymidine phosphorylase (TP). Capecitabine is convenient and with relatively lower toxicity. Commonly seen side effects include hand-foot syndrome, diarrhea and fatigue. Cytosine arabinoside (ara-C) inhibits DNA polymerase and incorporates into DNA thus inhibit DNA synthesis. Tumor cells can't synthesize asparagines; L-asparaginase can prevent protein synthesis in tumor cells by hydrolyzing asparagines into aspartic acid and ammonia.

11.3.3　Anti-mitotic agents

Microtubules are cellular structure in interphase cells that form mitotic spindle. Mitotic spindle inhibitors are cell-cycle specific. Two major drugs are included in this subtype. One is vinca alkaloids including vincrstine, vinblastine and vinorelbine. they can bind to microtubules and disaggregating them, then blocking the growing cells in M phase. The other is taxanes including paclitaxel and docetaxel. These agents stabilize microtubules against depolymerizaiton. So the growing cells cannot form the mitotic spindle and complete the cell cycle.

11.3.4　Antitumor antibiotics

Antitumor antibiotics include actinoycin D, idarubicin, mitoantrone and antracyclines. They interfere with transcription of DNA and synthesis of RNA by inserting into the base pair near the DNA double strands and dissociating the DNA double strands. Bleomycin directly break DNA single strand, while mitomycin for crossing link with DNA molecules, which is similar to alkylating agents.

11.3.5　Topoisomerase inhibitors

Topoisomerase iinhibitors such as irinotecan (CPT-11) and topotecan, stabilize the enzyme linked to DNA against re-connection of the DNA, and break the DNA single strand and interfere DNA replication. CPT-11 causes acetylcholine syndrome, delayed diarrhea, nausea, vomiting and bone marrow suppression. Topoisomerase Ⅱ inhibitors including etoposide and teniposide, break the double strands of DNA and interfere with DNA replication. The main toxicity of topoisomerase Ⅱ inhibitors are bone marrow suppression, transient hypotension may occur during rapid infusion.

11.4 Side effects of chemotherapy

11.4.1 Bone marrow suppression

Bone marrow suppression is the major obstacle in chemotherapy of clinical application. Most chemotherapy drugs except hormonal agents, bleomycin, L-asparaginase, can cause neutropenia, anemia or thrombocytopenia in different extents. Severe bone marrow suppression leads to greater chance of severe infection, even septicemia and visceral hemorrhage. Appropriate use of granulocytecolony stimulating factors (G-CSF) can prevent and reduce risk of infection due to neutropenia. Prophylactic use of G-CSF should be given if risk of febrile neutropenia is over 20% according to NCCN guideline. Anemia is also a common complication of chemotherapy, but use of erythropoiesis stimulating agents (ESAs) is limited use in clinic due to some evidences have shownincreased risk of thromboembolism and even potentially decreased survival due to cancerrelateddeaths. Red blood cell transfusion may be an alternative option to manage symptomatic anemia, especially when intent of chemotherapy is cure. Chemotherapy-induced-thrombocytopenia can be managed with interleukin-11 and platelet transfusion. Dose escalation should be made ifsevere bone marrow suppression is very likely to occur again even prophylactic approaches applied.

11.4.2 Gastrointestinal toxicity

Chemotherapy induced nausea and vomiting is the most stressful side effect to most patients. Most chemotherapy agents can cause both symptoms. Nausea and vomiting can be acute, which occur minutes or hours after chemotherapy, and delayed which can last for 7 days. Combination of 5-hydroxytryptamine subtype 3 (5HT3) antagonists, neurokininsubtype 1 (NK1) antagonists and dexamethasone can prevent and relieve the symptoms in great extent. Mucositis can be induced by 5-FU, MTX, bleomycin and adriamycin. Oral hygiene is essential to prevent mucositis. Pretreatment dentist examination and caries treatment can reduce risk of occurrence of mucositis. 5-FU and CPT-11 can cause severe diarrhea, and loperamide can be used to manage delayed diarrhea caused by CPT-11. Dehydration and electrolyte imbalances caused by severe diarrhea should be managed immediately in hospital because it can be life-threatening.

11.4.3 Liver function impairment

Chemotherapy agents like MTX, 6-MP, 5-FU, VP-16 and so on cause liver function impairment. Regimens containing oxaliplatin (i. e. FOLFOX) may induce damage and hemorrhage of hepatic sinusoids. Regimens with CPT-11, FOLFIRI as an example, may cause steotohepatitis. Abnormal bilirubin level influences metabolism of antracyclins and vinca alkaloids. Dose modification should be adjusted for patients with impaired liver function. Patients with chronic hepatitis, like chronic hepatitis B which is common in China, should receive antiviral therapy before administration of chemotherapy because acute fulminate hepatitis may be induced due to low immunity.

11.4.4 Renal function impairment

Active metabolic product of CTX and IFO, acrolein, excreting in the urine can cause hemorrhagic cystitis. Mesna prevent generation of acrolein and thus prevent hemorrhagic cystitis. High dose application of MTX can cause damage of renal tubules and thus induce oliguria and uremia. Simultaneous hydration, alkalization, use of CF and serum concentration monitoringcan help to manage toxicity of MTX. cisplatin (DDP) can cause renal damage directly, vigorous hydration and diuresis must be applied with high dose DDP, and renal function and electrolytes must be monitored. Some chemo-sensitive cancer can cause acute tumor lysis syndrome (TLS) which manifested as metabolic abnormalities due to massive tumor cell rapture. TLS is characterized as hyperuremia, hyperkalemia and hyperphosphatemia and cause renal function impairment. The best treatment is preventive approaches, for example, pretreatment hydration, alkalization of the urine, and administration of allopurinol.

11.4.5　Cardiotoxicity

The representative of chemotherapy agents that can cause cardiotoxicity is antracyclines antibiotics. The most severe complication is congestive heart failure. So it's important to monitor heart function before and during administration of antracyclines. Besides, cardiac toxicity caused by antracyclines is cumulative and dose-related. The maximum total dose of adriamycin is less than 550 mg/m^2 when adiministered alone and less than 450 mg/m^2 in combination with other chemotherapy agents or targeted agents such as trastuzumab. Dose should be lower if prior chest radiotherapy has been applied. Cardiotoxicity of epirubicin and liposomal doxorubicin are relatively mild, which allows expand the dose of clinical use.

11.4.6　Pulmonary toxicity

Long term use of bleomycin and busulfan can cause chronic pulmonary fibrosis. Cautious control of total dosage should be taken to avoid fatal situations. The drugs are discontinued and high-dose corticosteroids along with antibiotics are instituted if nonproductive cough, dyspnea and pulmonary infiltrates develop.

11.4.7　Neuropathy

Peripheral neuropathy caused by vincristine and taxanes is usually described as numbness of the fingers and feet. Intensive pain and hypersensitivity to cold, which initially begin on hands and feet, is the typical kind of neuropathy caused by oxaliplatin. The total dose of this drug should be limited strictly because the neuropathy caused by oxaliplatin is irreversible and progressive.

11.4.8　Allergy reaction

Taxanes such as paclitaxel and docetaxel can cause chilling, fever, edema and evenanaphylactic shock; thus prophylactic use of dexamethasone, diphenhydramine, ranitidine is necessary. The novel formulated agent Nab-paclitaxel has low potential of allergy reaction, so no prophylactic treatment is needed. Allergic test should be done when first time use of L-Asparaginase. A number of agents such as bleomycin, Ara-C, gemcitabine, oxaliplatin, may cause different extents of allergy reactions; similar treatment can prevent the occurrence.

11.4.9　Skin toxicity

Alopecia is a concerning side effect for most patients which can be caused by a lot of chemotherapy agents. But this symptom istemporary rather thanpermanent. Hair usually re-grow after discontinue of chemotherapy agents in nearly all patients. Severe hair loss occurs often with doxorubicin, MTX, IFO, VP-16 and so on. Palmar plantar erythroderma also called hand-foot syndrome is commonly seen when continuous infusion of 5-FU or oral use of capcitabine. It's characterized as hyperpigmentation, nail changes, pain, erytherma, swelling, desquamation, even ulcers in the palm of the hand and soles of the feet. Dose escalation or temporary discontinuation of the drug can palliative the symptoms greatly in most patients. Some studies have shown preventive use of oral pyridoxine, NAIDS, or cold packs to the extremities may help relieve the symptoms.

11.4.10　Infertility and teratogenecity

Most chemotherapy agents have influence on gonadal functions and lower ability of fertility. Fertility preservation including cryopreservation of semen, ovarian tissue, oocytes, embryos, or use of LHRHa in some studies should be chosen prior to chemotherapy in patients with child-bearing intention. Most chemotherapy agents are teratogenic during pregnancy, especially the first trimester. It may increase risk of complications in pregnancy and fetal myelosuppression.

11.4.11　Carcinogenesis

Some alkylating agents such as HN2, melphalan, procarbazine can increase risk of secondary neoplasm in months or years. The most commonly seen secondary neoplasm is secondary acute myeloid leukemia, which develop safter treatment with alkylating agents or topoisomerase inhibitors.

11.5　Principles of clinical application of chemotherapy

11.5.1　Basic principles

Patients who are going toreceive chemotherapy must have pathologic or cytological diagnosis of a cancer. And chemotherapy agents should be administered by experienced medical oncologists. The medical oncologist should make rational regimen under fully consideration of patients' medical history, general condition, performance status and personal will. Standard regimens with evidences should be chosen as first choice. Consent should be signed after fully informing the treatment intent, efficacy, cost, toxicity and potential risks to the patients and their family members. In the situation combination therapy is used, there are some notifications as follow: ①each drug should be effective; ②drugs in combination should act in different mechanisms; ③drugs in combination should have different, non-overlapping toxicities; ④regimens are proven to be effective in clinical applications.

11.5.2　Ensure intents of chemotherapy

Intents of chemotherapy include curative, adjuvant, neo-adjuvant, palliative and investigative chemotherapy. Curative, adjuvant and neo-adjuvant chemotherapy are likely to cure cancer and improve survival, so standard dosage and regimens should be applied. Every attempt should be made to schedule chemotherapy on time at full dose. Palliative chemotherapy applies for patients with advanced, metastatic disease. Balance of toxicity and efficacy should be notified. Investigative chemotherapy refers to clinical investigations of new drugs or new regimens. It should comply with medical ethics and good clinical practice (GCP).

11.5.3　Manage the toxicities

Chemotherapy-induced toxicities are inevitable and it's always the main obstacle for cancer chemotherapy. Rational use of antiemetic drugs, G-CSF and other symptomatic treatments can help ensure next cycle of chemotherapy on time and improve compliance of patients. Sometimes, intensive supportive care is needed when severe infection occurs. Prophylactic approaches are necessary in patients with weak immunity or elder patients with complications.

11.5.4   Overcome drug resistance

Drug resistance can exist before chemotherapy agents are applied (primary drug resistance) or acquired after chemotherapy (secondary resistance). Multiple drug resistance refers to resistance of multiple natural drugs that are completely different in structures and acting mechanisms. Changes in targeted receptors or transduction signaling, for example, increased numbers of receptors or enzymes, change of affinity, blockage of apoptosis pathway, improvement of DNA repairmen and establishment of alternative pathways, lead to failure of drug cytotoxicity effect. Besides, increased efflux, decreased uptake or impaired metabolism of drug lower concentration inside the cell thus weakens the drug lethality. Tumor stem cells refer to a group of cells in tumor that haveability of self-regeneration and infinite differentiated potential. These cells have strong repair ability and are highly expressed multidrug resistance associated protein (MRP) and P-glycoprotein (P-gp). They areusually in quiescent phase and born to be resistant to chemotherapy and radiotherapy. Existenceof TSCs is the major reason of failure of treatment and relapse or recurrence of the tumor.

Strategies to overcome drug resistance are as fllows:

1) Combine effective chemotherapy agents in fully dose when tumor burden is low, total kill of tumor cells in different phases and prevent generation of predominant colony of drug resistant cells.

2) Rational application of multiple modalities to decrease cells in G0 phase.

3) Rational use of regimens containing drugs with different targets or pathways.

4) Develop novel targeted drugs to overcome drug resistance.

11.5.5   Individualized and multidisciplinary therapy

Multidisciplinary therapy refers to taking full advantage of different modalities to achieve greatest treatment effect and lowest toxicity, improve patients' quality of life in greatest extent with appropriate economic cost in cancer treatment. According to intent of treatment, tumor heterogeneity, patient's tolerance, patients' will, life expectancy and psychologicalstatus, individualized therapy should be made to balance advantages and disadvantages of chemotherapy. Pain is a common symptom in patients with advanced disease, supportive care and management of pain are essential. Rational application of antiemetic drugs (Table 11-2), G-CSFs, painkillers, antidepressants and Chinese medicine is necessary to improve quality of life, patients' compliances and reduce toxicities.

Table 11-2   Commonly used antiemetic drugs

Drugs	Usage and dosage
Steroids	
Dexamethasone	12 mg PO or Ⅳ, day 1; 8 mg PO, qd, days 2-4 12 mg PO or Ⅳ, day 1; 8 mg PO, days 2; 8 mg PO, bid, days 3 and 4
Serotonin (5-HT3) antagonists	
Dolasetron	100 mg PO
Palonosetron	0. 25 mg Ⅳ, day 1
Ondansetron	16-24 mg PO or 8-24 mg (max 32 mg/d) Ⅳ, day 1
Granisetron	2 mg PO or 1 mg PO, bid, day 1, mg/kg (max 1 mg) Ⅳ, day 1

Continue to Table 11-2

Drugs	Usage and dosage
Neurokinin 1 antagonists	
Aprepitant	125 mg PO, day 1; 80 mg PO, qd; days 2-3
Fosaprepitant	150 mg IV, day 1; 115 mg IV, day 1
Others	
Lorazepam	0.5-20 mg PO or IV or sublingual, q4 h or q6 h, days 1-4
Mirtazapine	15-45 mg PO, qd
Metoclopramide	5-10 mg PO, tid; 10-20 mg IM
Metoclopramide	

Wang Shusen

Chapter 12

Basics of Radiation Oncology

12.1 Introduction

Radiation Oncology, also known as radiotherapy, is an interdisciplinary science that includes gradiology and oncology. It is one of the three established clinical cancer treatments for most types of tumors and some hematologic malignancies. It is basic purpose is to fundamentally eliminate the tumor, while at the same time maximizing the preservation of normal tissue structure and function, improving the patient's survival rate and long-term quality of life. Radiotherapy is routinely combined with surgery, chemotherapy, or both to improve therapeutic outcomes. It is often used with surgery to destroy the microscopic regions of tumor extension and together with chemotherapy to more effectively destroy the primary tumor.

12.2 Brife history of radiation oncology

X-rays were first discovered emanating from an energized Crooke's tube by Wilhelm Roentgen in 1895. In 1896, Henri Becquerel discovered that some naturally occurring elements emitted ionizing radiation. The radioactive elementsradium and polonium were isolatedand characterized by the Curies in 1898. With the discovery of radium, the biological effects of radiation were revealed, and within a year or so, ionizingradiation was in use worldwide formedical imaging and radiationtherapy. The first patient was cured in 1898. In 1906, Bergorine and Tribondeau proposed the B-T law about the radiation sensitivity of cells and tissues in their study of the radiation effect on testicular cells. Due to the constraints of scientific developmentat the time, radiobiology progress lagged behind itsclinical application. With over 20 years of painstaking work, in 1922 Coutard and Hautant used X-ray to successfully cure apatient of advanced laryngeal cancer without complications, which formally established the clinical status of the radiotherapy.

At the 2nd International Conference on Radiology, the radiation dosage unit, Roentgen, was approved, which moved the field of radiotherapy to be more scientific and standardized. In 1930, Paterson and Parker established the Manchester system, which formalised the dosage-distribution law of inter-organizational planting, and prompted the development of after-loading branchy therapy. In 1934, Coutard reported the use of fractionation external beam radiation therapy. Clinical practices were upgraded to such an extent that fractionated radiation therapy, i. e. using small dose with prescribed increments over several weeks, became the standard of care and has largely remained so to the present day.

In 1953, Gray described the effects of oxygen, which demonstrated the role of hypoxia in increasing cell radiation resistance. In the early 1950s, John successfully established the ^{60}Co therapy unit, which marked the end of the "KV era" and the beginning of the "MV era". In 1955, Kaplan installed a linear accelerator at Stanford University, which consequently became the mainstream of radiation devices. Compared with the ^{60}Co therapy machine, the linear accelerator greatly reduced the adverse reaction of radiation therapy even though it couldn't significantly improve the curing effect.

In 1975, Withers HR published a seminal book chapter entitled "The Four R's of Radiotherapy". The chapter was an attempt to explain the biological basics or foundation of fractionation. This publication described in simple terms the key radio biological processes thought to affect the outcome of fractionated radiotherapy: Repair, Repopulation, Reoxygenation, and Redistribution. The theory of the Four R's formed the guidance for the practice of clinical radiotherapy, which remained the basis of radiation biology research despite some new conceptual development. Although the term "radiosurgery" was coined in 1951, the first radiosurgical approaches were not designed until 1968 for treatment of intracranial lesions by the Swedish neurosurgeon Leksell. The head gamma knife approach was the first widely used technique, using a large number of 60Co radiation sources for the treatment of intracranial lesions. In 1980, the application of the multi-leaf collimator laid the foundation for modern precision radiotherapy, based on which new radiotherapy techniques such as intensity-modulated radiation therapy (IMRT), image-guided radiation therapy (IGRT), was designed to further improve the effectiveness of radiotherapy. Stereotactic body radiotherapy (SBRT) is a hypofractionated treatment applied to extracranial targets, such as in the abdominal, pelvic, and spinal areas. First reported in 1995, the SBRT has a much shorter history than Stereotactic Radiosurgery (SRS), Early SBRT studies focused on the treatment of lung and liver lesions, while more recent efforts have included studies of the spine, prostate, kidney, pancreas, and gynecologic cancers. Most recently, with progresses made in molecular biology, computer and electronic technology, radiation oncology has entered the new era of precision radiotherapy.

A comprehensive understanding of the therapeutic use of ionizing radiation requires a basic knowledge of both the physics of radiation therapy delivery and the biological effects of the interaction of radiation with other matters.

12.3   Overview of radiation physics

The toxic biological effects of ionizing radiation, although complex, varied, and incompletely understood, form the basis for the use of radiation therapy as a cancer treatment. These biological effects are initiated when packets of energy are deposited in a volume of tissue to remove electrons from constituent atoms through a process called ionization. Accordingly, the physics of radiation oncology is focused on the details of how, where, and how much energy can be deposited on the unhealthy tissue to eradicate it, while at the same time minimizing the energy released on the healthy tissues nearby. This process requires an understanding of the nature of the radiation and the matter through which it passes and how that matter is changed as a result of the energy deposition.

Several types of ionizing radiation are used to treat patients; most are of the low linear energy transferal, and lessbiologically potent varieties. To be effectivein radiation therapy, radiation must be generated in a manner in which it can be directed at thetarget tissues. Radiation for cancer therapy is predominantly generated through two means; linear accelerators (linacs) and radioactive sources.

Therapeutic X-rays (photons) and electrons are generated from linear accelerators. They can also be produced by nuclear isotopes undergoing radioactive decay. These in turn form the basis of external-beam radiotherapy and brachytherapy, respectively.

Ionizing radiation interacts with other matters via several processes, of which Compton scattering is the most important for clinical radiation therapy.

Megavoltage photons from linear accelerators have the desirable property of delivering, you will need to link this paragraph together, it is jumpling from one thought to another maximum dose at depth within the patient, thereby sparing the skin and, tosome extent, other normal tissues.

12.4　The radiobiology of radiation therapy

Radiation biology is the study of the biological effects of ionizing radiation in individuals, tissues, cells and molecules. The main research objects are electromagnetic radiation, such as ultraviolet ray, X-ray and gamma ray. Particle rays include electron rays, proton rays, heavy hydrogen rays, alpha rays, and the role of neutron radiation.

Ionization of biomolecules from the deposition of energy by photons orparticles can occur directly andindirectly. The most important cellular target for radiation is DNA, with irreparable or "misrepaired" double-stranded breaks believed tobe the lesions most responsible for cell killing.

Irradiation elicits diverse cellular responses that include the sensing of DNA damage, mobilization of DNA repair proteins, repair (or attempted repair) of DNA damage, triggering of cell cycle checkpoints, and, forirreparable or mis-rejoined damage, cell death by one of several mechanisms (e. g. , mitotic catastrophe, apoptosis, and senescence).

Cell survival is essential for the success of radio therapy. Therefore, the calculation of cell survival is most important. The most commonly applied model of cell survival probability is the linear quadratic (α/β) model, with the surviving fraction of irradiated cells calculated by the equation $S = e^{-(\alpha d + \beta d2)}$. The α/β ratio is a convenient metric for describing cellular radio sensitivity and has been adopted to model the response ofirradiated tissues based on a function oftime, dosage, and fractionation.

DNA damage and repair were initially inferred by monitoring increases incell survival or tissue tolerance with fractionation. These phenomena were termed sublethal and potentially lethal damage repair orrecovery.

Cells in different cell cycle phases possess different radio sensitivity; cells are most radiosensitive in the G2 and M phases of the cell cycle, and most resistant in the S phase, particularly the late S phase(Figure 12-1). Cells in the G1 phase are of intermediate need a graph of the phases, to illustrate.

Well-oxygenated cells are as much as three times more sensitive to radiation-induced cells killing than (severely) oxygen-deprived cells. Viable hypoxic cells that exist inmany human tumors but aremostly absent in normal tissues maybe an impediment to tumor control. The elimination of such cells has been a long-termclinical goal. Hypoxia may present a potential path for therapeutic success through the use of hypoxia-directed therapies.

Radiation sensitizers, particularly cytotoxic chemotherapy and, to alesser extent, radiation protectors, aim to improve the therapeutic ratio.

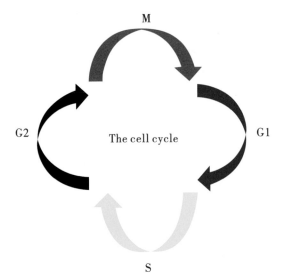

G1 (cell grows phase) , S (DNA replication phase) , G2 (cell prepares to divide phase) , M (mitosis phase).

Figure 12−1 **Cell cycle**

12.5　Clinical radiation oncology

12.5.1　Indications and contraindications of radiotherapy

With theprogress of radiation physics , radiobiology and related disciplines , the radiation oncologyis also becoming more and more important in cancer therapy. Radiation therapy is used in more than half of all patients with cancer , either as an adjuvant or neoadjuvant treatment in combination with surgery ; as a destinctive treatment alone or in combination with chemotherapy ; as an organ-sparing therapy ; or to palliate symptoms. Radiation therapy has the substantial benefit of being able toprovide organ preservation in many clinical situations and to be ableto sterilize microscopic disease when used in conjunction with surgery.

12.5.2　The use of radiation therapy can be categorized as the following

（1）Radiation therapy alone

Radiation therapy is often used for small tumors for which surgery would be excessive either because of the precise location of the tumor or the limitations of surgical resection. Radiation therapy can also beused in this manner when a patient is too frail for a surgical procedureor when a patient refuses surgical intervention. Radiation therapy alone is used much less commonly for locally advanced disease , for which it is now often combined with concurrent chemotherapy , and surgical procedures. Examples of this categoryinclude treatment of early stage cancers of the head and neck , prostate cancer of all stages , early-stage cervical cancer , and selected basal cell carcinomas of the skin.

（2）Preoperative or postoperative radiation therapy

For sometumors , surgical therapy is required , but surgery alone is likely to leave residual disease either in the tumor bed or in regional lymphatics that are not completely resected. In this situation , Radiation therapy will often be performed/applied with concurrent chemotherapy for the radiation-sensitizing effects of the chemotherapy. Examples include soft tissue sarcomas, certain cancers of the head and neck, intermediate and high-grade gliomas, and early-stage breast cancers.

(3) Primary radiation therapy with concurrent chemotherapy

For many tumors, surgical resection is not an option because of the inability to perform a grossly complete surgical resection. As such, radiation therapy becomes the primary local therapy. Chemotherapy can be added either concurrently as a radiation sensitizer to enhance local control or before or after radiation therapy for the control of systemic disease. Examples include all anal cancers and locally advanced tumors of the uterine cervix, esophagus, pancreas, and head and neck.

(4) Tri-modality therapy

Often all three primary therapeutic modalities—surgery, radiation therapy, and chemotherapy—are needed for the control of local, regional, and systemic disease. The timing of the therapies is dependent on the individual clinical situation. Tri-modality therapy is perhaps the most common approach at the present time. Examples include a large group of tumors, including esophageal, glioblastoma, head and neck, esophagus, pancreas, breast, and rectum tumors.

(5) Palliative radiotherapy

Palliative radiotherapy is aimed at pain relief, trying to prolong the survival time of cancer patients. It is mainly used for terminal cancer patients to stop bleeding, pain, to relieve obstruction, and to inhibit tumor growth. The technology of palliative radiotherapy is relatively simple. Although it is difficult to accurately determine the survival rate of terminal patients, Palliative radiotherapy should still be taken seriously, in case of complications.

(6) Side effects and contraindications of radiotherapy

Radiation's immediate effects may include mucositis, skin erythema, or desquamation, while long term effects may include fibrosis and carcinogenesis.

There are also a few contraindications to radiotherapy, which are mainly organ perforation, cachexia, myelosuppression, etc.

12.6   Delivery techniques for radiation therapy

There are multiple tools a radiation oncologist can sue for the delivery of radiation therapy, depending on the specific circumstances.

12.6.1   Brachytherapy

The brachytherapy is also known as internal irradiation. This technique is most commonly used in gynecologic tumors and in the treatment of prostate cancer. For gynecologic malignancies such as cervical cancer, external radiation therapy is initially used to treat the pelvic primary tumor and for draining lymphatics. Then an implant is used to give an even higher dose of radiation to the primary tumor through the use of tubes placed in the uterus and vagina which contains radioactive sources.

Temporary implants are also used for the treatment of selective head and neck squamous cell carcinomas, melanomas of the choroid in the eye, and occasionally for tumors of other anatomic sites where it is difficult to deliver the desired radiation dose otherwise. Prostate brachytherapy is delivered by the placement of permanent radio active seeds into the prostate. Depending on the radioisotope, the treatment will be delivered over the course of months, with the implanted radiation sources continuously delivering therapy until the sources have decayed to the point that they are barely radioactive. Reassuringly, the energy of the radiation deposited by these isotopes is low, thus there is minimal risk to the public health or to family members. This approach is probably the most cost-effective way to treat early-stage prostate cancer and is very effective due to the high dose of radiation delivered to the prostate.

12.6.2 External beam fractionated radiation therapy

(1) Overview of external beam fractionated radiation therapy

External beam fractionated radiation therapy (EBRT) is by far the most common technique used clinically. Radiation beams are usually delivered through multiple angles to reach the lesion, with each of the beams shaped and altered in intensity to maximize the delivery of dosage to the tumor, while minimizing the dosage to normal tissues.

External beam therapy can be delivered with conformal radiationtherapy techniques (i. e. , shaping the beams based on the 3D reconstructions of the tumor size, shape and the location of nearby normal tissues). Intensity-modulated radiation therapy changes the intensity of each small segment ("beamlet") of an individual beam to obtain even more precise dose localization and avoidance of normal tissue irradiation. Image-guided radiation therapy usesreal-time and/or daily imaging toensure that the tumor is located/targetedsothat the radiation beams are precisely delivered to the appropriate location inside the patient.

Generally these treatments are given using either low (6 MV) or high (≈ 10 to 15 MV) energy X-rays, but they can also be delivered with electrons of various energies, with the higher energy beams having agreater depth of penetration into tissues. The radiation oncologistdecides the most appropriate treatment based on experience and literature estimates of tolerance doses for normal tissue complications and curative doses for tumors for different fractionation schedules. This decision is a balancing effort, in an attempt to give the highest probability of tumor control with the lowest reasonable level of clinically significant normal tissue injury. Often, depending on the individual anatomy and stages of tumor development, radiation doses will need to be modified.

The radiation used by external beam radiation therapy often targets areas of presumed subclinical disease (such as nodaldrainage regions), as well as the clinically apparent tumor. As a result, it is critical for the radiation oncologist to have an excellent understanding of the nature and history of each disease and its specific spreading pattern.

Radiation treatments are usually given daily, i. e. 5 days a week, and can extend in duration from 1 week (or less) for certain types of palliative therapy to courses over 6-7 weeks of daily therapy.

Fractionation of radiation and altered fractionation schedules, such as accelerated hyperfractionatedradiation therapy, make use of differences in the responses of normal and malignant tissues toirradiation to achieve higher rates of treatment.

(2) Simulation, treatment planning, and deliveryof ebrt

After diagnosis, the first step in designing and delivering radiation therapy is called "simulation". Simulation is a process for determining the proper selection andorientation of beams so that they covera target properly. Invirtual simulation, the patient is placed in the orientation and position that is the best for treatment delivery. A CT scan is required. When the patient is positioned on the scanning table, the physician uses the superior soft tissue contrast of the CT scan to select a location asisocenter within the target area. Next, an integrated lasersystem moves to indicate the position of the physician-selectedisocenter on the patient surface, allowing the external markers ortattoos to be placed for future alignment with the linear acceleratorvault laser systems. The superior soft tissue contrast on CT images allows improved tumor localization and better beam selection compared with fluoroscopy-based conventional simulators.

After simulation, the CT scan and other images are sent to a computer-based planning workstation, where the teamof physicians, dosimetrists, and physicists can begin the treatment planning process. Treatment planning includes the identification of target volumes and normal structures required for dose tracking, and the selection and modification of beams to achieve specified dosimetricgoals. The contouring process of identifying the boundaries of all treatment and avoidance structures happens on the CT scan from the previous simulation stage, and it maybe supplemented by other imaging modalities, such as magnetic resonance imaging, positron emission tomography, or ultra sound. Normal structures are typically defined by their anatomic boundaries. The volume to be treated, named as the target volume by the International Commission on Radiation Units & Measurements Report 60 (ICRU 60), is created by combining three structures: the gross tumor volume (GTV), the clinical tumor volume (CTV), and the planning target volume (PTV) (Figure 12-2). The GTV includes all detectable disease areas on each imagingmodality, including visible primary tumor and involved lymph nodes. The CTV is an expansion of the GTV that includes regions of possibleor potential microscopic disease, including both adjacent tissues and draining lymph nodes. The PTV is a further expansion of the CTV to include the anatomic motion and the expected variations of a patient's daily setup. Expansions from GTV to CTV and to PTV vary with disease types, techniques applied, and patient's history, but typical expansion numbers from CTV to PTV are usually on the border of 1 cm or less. Expansion from GTV to CTV is entirely dependent on the biology of the clinical situation. At times, no GTV is present (for example in the treatment in the postoperative setting), in which case the CTV is based entirely on the assumed high-risk areas for residual disease.

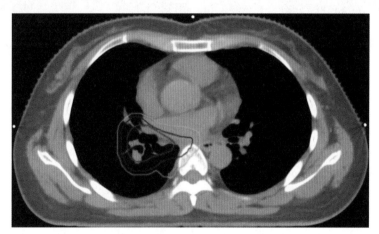

GTV (the red isodose line), CTV (the blue isodose line), PTV (the green isodose line).

Figure 12-2   Treatment plan for a thoracic lesion

Once the target and avoidance structures are identified and defined on the patient images, a specific strategy for dose delivery can be developed by the physicians, physicists, and dosimetrists involved. The essential task of treatment planning is to select, arrange, and characterize a group of radiation beams to deliver a high dose to the tumor while keeping the dose delivered to normal structures under acceptablelimit. The treatment plan must be specified in terms of the total dosage and the number of fractions in which the dose will be delivered. Individual beam is customized by specifying the beam energy, orientation, and shape. Beams are typically shaped to match the cross section of the PTV plus asmall margin to maximize coverage of the tumor while limiting the amount of normal tissue directly exposed to the radiation beam. This goal can be accomplished by designing a customized block made from an easily castmetal alloy such as Cerrobend, but on modern machines it is typically performed with the use of automated beam-shaping devices such as amultileaf collimator (Figure 12-3). Use of multiple beams overlapping on the tumor site can maximize the dose received by the tumor. The appropriate number, orientation, and relative weighting of beams in a treatment plan will depend on geometric factors, such as tumor location and the proximity of normal structures, as well as clinicalfactors, such as prior or planned surgery, overall patient health, history of prior irradiation, likelihood of future irradiation, and the effects of concurrent chemotherapy.

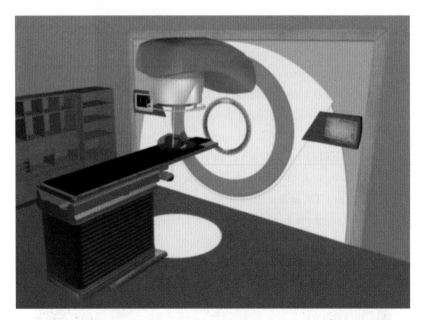

The individual collimator leaves can be adjusted to form arbitrarily shaped fields.

Figure 12-3　Sample intensity-modulated radiation therapy beams for treatment of a patient with lung cancer

The dosimetry of a sample treatment plan must be evaluated for likely treatment efficacy of the tumor and the possibility of toxicity to normal structures. Dosimetry can be evaluated by examining isodose lines and dose-volume histograms. Isodose lines are a 3D representation of dose levels superimposed on the patient's image toindicate regions of high and low dose on any user-selected plane. Isodose lines correlate dose with anatomiclocation and specify regions of insufficient or excessive dose and suggest beam arrangements and weightings that can better meet the dosimetric goals for the plan. Aggregate dose to contoured structures are illustratedas dose-volume histograms, which display the percentage or absolute volume of the structure receiving a specified dose orlower (Figure 12-4). Most of the dose constraints applied to treatment planning are expressed in terms of dose-volume histograms.

12.6.3　Stereotactic radiosurgery and stereotactic body radiotherapy

Stereotactic radiosurgery (SRS) and stereotactic body radiotherapy(SBRT) combine a high dose perfraction with highly conformal treatment delivery to increase the therapeutic ratio while reducing treatment time.

Stereotactic radiosurgery refers to a single-fraction delivery of a high dose to a target. Depending on the precise location, if the volume irradiated to high dose is small, the likelihood of clinically significant injury is low, similar to what would be the case with surgical excision. This technique is entirely dependent on very precise dose localization and the use of many radiation beams so that only the tumor and immediately adjacent tissues receive a high dose.

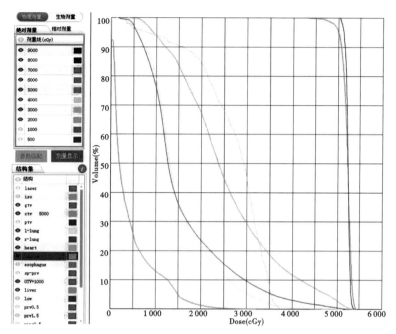

Figure 12-4 A dose-volume histogram expressed in terms of what percentage of the structure volume receives at least what percentage of the total dose

The first radiosurgical approach was designed for treatment of intracranial lesions, but the same technique is now used for multiple anatomic sites. The ability to deliver radiation in this manner is heavily dependent on the development of radiation therapy hardware and computer software to design a large number of radiation beams that intersect at the tumor. The Gamma Knife approach was the first widely used technique, using a large number of ^{60}Co radiation sources for the treatment of intracranial lesions. However, a number of different approaches exist now which use linac techniques for delivering X-rays stereotactically.

Stereotactic body radiotherapy is a hypofractionated treatmentapplied to extracranial targets, such as in the abdominal, pelvic, and spinal regions. SBRT has a much shorter history compared to the SRS, with the first clinical outcomes for SBRT reported in 1995. Early SBRT studies focused on the treatment of lung and liver lesions, but more recent efforts have included studies of spine, prostate, kidney, pancreas, and gynecologic cancers.

12.7 Specialized radiotherapy techniques and facilities

Investigators have great interest in the use of specialized radiation modalities that require different machines to produce protons, neutrons, or other high-energy particles.

12.7.1 Protons

Protons are charged particles that can be accelerated and directed into tissue, where they deposit their dose. Protons can first deliver a lower dose to superficial tissues, then a higher radiation dose at depth where the tumor is, while leaving virtually no damage to normal tissues beyond the tumor. This provides a clear advantage compared with conventional X-rays, which deliver the highest doses (from a single beam) to more superficial tissues. Thus protons can allow for more precise delivery of the radiation dose to the tumor in comparison with normal tissues. The RBE for protons is approximately 1.1, and thus they are only slightly more biologically effective than X-rays or electrons. The primary advantage of proton therapy, therefore, is improved dose distributions.

Proton therapy is the most common type of heavy particle therapy. Proton beams are produced by accelerating ionized hydrogen in acyclotron or synchrotron to energies in excess of 100 MeV. The required devices are conside rably larger and more expensive than conventional clinical accelerators, therefore, they tend to be built as stand-alone facilities, although research into smaller scale proton devices isongoing. Unlike electrons that lose energy roughly evenly across therange of therapeutic energy spectrum, protons lose their energy at an increasing rate as the beams loses energy with depth. This effect culminatesin a region of rapid dose deposition near the depth of maximum penetration, called the Bragg peak. The depth of the Bragg peak increases with beam energy, allowing careful energy selection to ensure that the highest dose is delivered to the tumor volume, with lower dose at the upstream of the target and negligible dose downstream of the target. The width of the Bragg peak is virtually alwaysnarrower than the region to be targeted, requiring a range of protonenergies to "paint" high, uniform doses across the target.

This widened dose distribution, known as a spread out Bragg peak, can be created either by varying the proton beam energy in a synchrotron or by using a spinning modulator of varying thickness to selectively vary the beam energy. The principal clinical application with the use of proton radiotherapyhas been for the treatment of prostate cancer. However, although their use in this site has a theoretical advantage, this advantage has never been demonstrated in clinical trials. Protons are very appealing for the treatment of certain pediatric tumors, because the effects of unwanted irradiation of normal tissues can be severe in children. In this context, protons have been used extensively in the treatment of pediatric central nervous system tumors. Studies on the use of protonsfor therapy of lung cancer and tumors at other anatomic sites areongoing. Because the cost of a proton irradiator (and its specialized facility) is far greater than traditional X-ray and electron linacs, it is obligatory upon staffusing protons for radiotherapy to demonstrate that the extra expense translates into better tumor controlrates and/or fewer normal tissue complications. The lack of satisfactory evidence to date has hindered the rapid proliferation of proton facilities.

12.7.2 Neutrons

Neutrons are heavy particles that are not charged, and they are also generated by specialized machines. Neutrons interact with matters through different mechanisms than thephotons and particles previously discussed; these interactions can cause low-energy protons and heavier ions to be ejected during collisions between neutrons and target nuclei. These ejected particles cause biological damage in line with their LET. Neutron beams therefore have an energy dependent average RBE that can vary between 5 and 20. Neutrons have no advantage in dose distribution over X-rays and infact have a disadvantage in dose delivery. However, they are more potent biologically due to their higher RBE and therefore have the potential to destroy certain tumors more effectively, such as those that are relatively radio-resistant, including melanomas, sarcomas, and salivarygland tumors. Although there have been many clinical studies involving neutron therapy, it remains difficult to identifya clear advantage of this approach over conventional treatment methods.

12.7.3 Heavy ions

Till now, investigators have been interested in using other heavily charged particles, such as accelerated carbon or neon ions, for therapeutic purposes. These particles have the potential to combine both the biological advantage of neutrons and the dose distribution advantage of protons. The machines to generate these particles and the associated operating costs are veryhigh, which has substantially limited their development and application to only a handful of facilities worldwide.

12.8   Future directions

Over the past two decades, great achievements have been made in radiation therapy, enabling it to localize tumors more accurately and to deliver radiation more precisely, while minimizing impact on normal tissue. Most of these advances have been technological, and it is highly likely that further advances will follow. Some areas of interesting development is the increasing merge of biology and therapy to improve the biological definition of the tumor location with functional imaging. In addition, better illumination of tumor subtypes will allow us to identify more precisely which type of patients are at higher risk of local recurrence and therefore require additional local therapy, or which group of patients will benefit from combination of treatments. It is also likely that combining radiation therapy and biologics (as well as new cytotoxics) will have substantially greater benefits in clinical practice in the near future, which will enhance the rate of selective killing of tumor cells.

Wen Juyi

Chapter 13

Endocrine Therapy of Cancer

The functioning of endocrine system is an important mechanism for multicellular animals, integrating activities across different cell populations to maintain environmental stability in the body to adapt to environmental changes. Steroid molecules are conservative throughout evolution and can be traced back to single-cell organisms. In insects, steroid hormones have played an important role. The secretion of ecdysone in the anterior thymus is related to growth, development and metamorphosis. In vertebrates, steroid hormones are important endocrine signals that not only play an important role in sugar, protein, fat metabolism and water-electrolytes metabolism, but also a major regulator of reproductive activity. In addition, steroid hormones are involved in physiological activities closely related to individual survival, such as stress response and immune homeostasis. The physiological effects of steroids are very broad, targeting at almost all tissues. Mammary gland and prostate are important target organs of steroid hormones, and cancer tissues derived from breast ductal epithelium and prostate epithelium often retain reactivity against steroid hormones. The steroid hormone signal pathway in the internal environment can promote the proliferation and metastasis of endocrine-dependent cancer cells. A specific targeted therapy that plays an important role in the treatment of endocrine-dependent cancers through blocking steroid hormone signal pathways is known as Endocrine therapy.

Some other cancers, such as endometrial cancer, breast cancer and prostate cancer, share the characteristic of rich steroid receptors in cancer cells, and therefore can be stimulated by host physiological steroids . Hormones associated with cancer endocrine therapy also include other type of steroid hormones, such asglucocorticoids, which can treat lymphoid-derived tumors. Some non-steroidal hormones, such as thyroxine, can act as a negative feedback to thyrotropin to treat thyroid cancer. Somatostatin Analogue (SSA) can be used to treat gastrointestinal neuroendocrine tumors. Briefly speaking, this article mainly focus on estrogen and breast cancer, androgen and prostate cancer, in which endocrine therapy plays an important role in the treatment strategies, as examples to show the basic principles of cancer endocrine therapy.

13.1 Brief history of endocrine therapy

The origin of cancer endocrine therapy is based on the observation and analysis of certain clinical events and animal reproductive phenomena, and later promoted by chemistry and molecular biology. After more than 100 years of development, doctors achieved certain understanding of the molecular mechanisms of cancer endocrine therapy, enabling release of new effective drugs constantly.

13.1.1 Brief history of endocrine therapy research of cancer

The relationship between cancer growth and endocrine has been noticed for a long time. The fact that gonadal activity affects the development of specific organs has led to attempts to open the door to endocrine therapy with surgical techniques. At the end of the 19th century, the efficacy of oophorectomy for breast cancer was assured. At the beginning of the 20th century, chemistry promoted medical progress, and soon molecular biology emerged, promoting the understanding of the microscopic mechanism of cancer endocrine therapy. The industrialization of drug research and development has promoted the entry of a number of effective endocrine drugs into the clinic application. These drugs have basically replaced surgery in cancer endocrine therapy.

13.1.1.1 Scientific observation gave birth to the first cancer endocrine therapy practice

In 1836, Astley Cooper, the British surgeon, noticed the relationship between tumor growth and the menstrual cycle, and found that breast cell proliferation was related to reproductive activity.

In 1895, Georage Thomas Beatson, a surgeon at the Glasgow Cancer Hospital in Scotland, performed oophorectomy on a case of advanced young breast cancer and achieved tumor regression. Subsequently, in 1896, he reported the efficacy of bilateral oophorectomy in local recurrence and advanced breast cancer on the Transactions of the Medico-Chirurgical Society of Edinburgh, opening the door to endocrine therapy.

In 1941, Huggins et al. reported that orchiectomy had a significant therapeutic effect on advanced prostate cancer based on animal experiments.

13.1.1.2 Exploration of microscopic mechanism of cancer endocrine therapy

With the development of chemistry in the early 20th century, the main hormones secreted by the gonads were identified, and the main mechanism of action of sex hormones was also understood. The nuclear receptor family was discovered. Research on sex hormone receptors has promoted the development of new drugs, switching endocrine therapy to the era of drug therapy.

In 1929, German biochemist Adolf Butenandt extracted estrone from the urine of pregnant women and speculated on its chemical structure. Soon, Croatian-born Swiss scientist Leopold Ruzicka artificially synthesized estrogen analogues and experimentally confirmed the estrogen-like effects of the chemical and derived the general structure of steroid hormones. American scientist Edward Adelbert Doisy and Adolf Butenandt, each separated and identified the chemical structure of estrogen independently.

In 1958, based on isotope-labeled estrogen tracer in animal experiments, Elwood Jensen proposed existence of pro-estrogen-producing proteins in tissues such as breast uterus. It is believed that this receptor-like protein is present in the cell, not on the cell membrane. He subsequently sequestered the estrogen receptor and elucidated the predictive effect of the ER receptor on the effectiveness of endocrine therapy.

In 1986, French scientist Pierre Shambon cloned the ER gene. With the continued efforts of other scientists, humans eventually discovered the nuclear receptor superfamily.

Studies of sex hormones and their receptors explain the mechanisms of endocrine therapy and also help predict endocrine efficacy, and these studies have greatly facilitated the development of related drugs.

13.1.1.3 Discovery of the regulation mechanism of gonadal function

In 1945, British physiologist Geoffrey Harris proposed the neurohumoral regulation hypothesis that the hypothalamus contains chemicals that regulate pituitary function.

In 1955, Geoffrey Harris published the book *Neural Control of the Pituitary Gland*, which promoted research in this field.

In 1971, American scientist Andrew Schally isolated the hypothalamic hormone LHRH and identified its chemical structure. Several LHRH analogues have been developed since, such as leuprolide, goserelin, and triptorelin.

13.1.2 Brief history of endocrine drug development for cancer

The advances in chemistry and molecular biology in the 20th century have promoted the understanding of the molecular mechanism of cancer endocrine, which greatly promoted the development of related drugs.

13.1.2.1 Drugs acting on estrogen receptors

Tamoxifen is the first anti-cancer drug targeting at ER and the first molecular target drug to some extent.

In 1962, Tamoxifen was developed by Arthur Walpole, the reproductive endocrinologist and Dora Richardson, the chemist of ICI Pharmaceuticals in the United Kingdom. In 1971, the first clinical trial at Christie Hospital proved the efficacy of tamoxifen in the treatment of advanced breast cancer. In 1973, it was used in advanced breast cancer, and later approved by FDA in 1977.

In 2002, Fulvestrant developed by AstraZeneca was approved by FDA in US.

13.1.2.2 Aromatase inhibitor

In 1969, the first report of Aminoglutethimide in the treatment of breast cancer was published.

In 1973, Schwarsel first proposed the aromatase inhibitors which can specifically cause target enzyme inactivation, block aromatization, inhibit estrogen production, and lower estrogen levels in the blood to achieve breast cancer treatment.

In 1981, the first generation of AI, Aminoglutethimide was launched in the US.

In 1992, Lentaron, the second generation of AI, was approved.

In 1995, the third generation AI, Anastrozole was approved for medical use, which was patented in 1987.

In 1999, the third-generation AI, Exemestane was approved for marketing. It was researched and developed by Pharmaela & Upjoin of Italy in 1988.

In 2001, the third generation of AI, Letrozole was approved for listing.

13.1.2.3 Androgen receptor antagonist

In 1983, Flutamide was launched in Europe.

In 1995, Bicalutamide was listed in the UK.

In 2012, Enzalutamide was launched in the US.

13.1.2.4 Androgen synthase inhibitor

In 2010, Johnson& Johnson developed abiraterone, which was approved in US.

13.1.2.5 LHRH analogues

LHRH, also known as GnRH, of which precursors is synthesized in hypothalamic neurons and is transported through the axons to the pituitary gland in the form of decapeptides. LHRH analogue refers to a peptide similar in structure to LHRH. The peptide bond is weak between amino acids 6/7 and 9/10, which is easily cleaved by lyase to inactivate LHRH. An agonist can be obtained by modification and substitution with the amino acid at position 6 and 9, while an antagonist can be obtained by modifying or replacing the amino acid at position 2 and amino acids at positions 3 and 6.

In 1971, shortly after the chemical structure of LHRH was identified, LHRH was synthesized.

In 1972, antagonists of LHRH receptors were synthesized, but they were not used in clinical practice due to allergic reactions.

In 1973, leuprolide was synthesized.

In 1985, the daily dosage form of leuprolide was marketed in the US.

In 1989, monthly dosage of leuprolide developed by Takeda Pharmaceutics in Japan was launched in the US and Europe.

In 1996, three-month dosage of leuprolide developed by Takeda Pharmaceutics in Japan was launched in the US and Europe.

In 1989, Goserelin developed by AstraZeneca was approved for the treatment of prostate cancer in the United States.

In 1999, Cetrorelix (trade name Cetrotide), developed by Asta Medica in Germany, was approved in Germany. It was the first LHRH antagonist approved for market, as well as the first third generation drug approved.

13.2   Biological basis of cancer endocrine therapy

The proliferation-driven mechanism of about 50% of breast cancers and more than 80% of prostate cancer cells is related to the steroid hormone signaling pathway. Blocking this signaling pathway can lead to apoptosis of cancer cells and inhibition of tumor development.

13.2.1   Synthesis and metabolism of steroid hormones

Steroid hormones are converted from cholesterol. Cholesterol is also an important cell membrane structural component and is important for maintaining the stability of cell membranes. Human cholesterol is mainly synthesized and secreted by the liver cells into the blood, and only a small amount comes from the absorption of food components. In the blood, cholesterol and carrier proteins are combined and transported throughout the body.

95% of the sex hormones in the human body are from the gonads. The estrogens are synthesized by the combination of ovarian follicular cells and granulosa cells, and androgen is synthesized by Leydig cells. 5% of the sex hormones come from the adrenal cortex reticular cells, and the androgen can also be produced in the breast tissue and prostate tissue. In addition, aromatase is widely existed in various peripheral tissues such as fat, muscle, liver, bone, etc., which can convert androgens into estrogens.

The route of steroid synthesis is complicated, and the synthetic pathway of sex hormones can be simplified as a three-step process: production of progesterone, androgen and estrogen (Figure 13-1).

The first step is the conversion from cholesterol into progesterone by the cholesterol side-chain lyase in the mitochondria, and the subsequent steps are performed on the endoplasmic reticulum of the cytoplasm. The rate-limiting enzyme for the conversion of progesterone to androgen is CYP17, and the rate-limiting enzyme for the conversion of androgen to estrogen is CYP19, also known as aromatase.

Human 5α-reductase has two isoforms, type I isoenzymes are mainly distributed in the skin, and type II isoenzymes are mainly distributed in the prostate. In the prostate, 5α-reductase converts testosterone to dihydrotestosterone, which increases activity by 5-10 times.

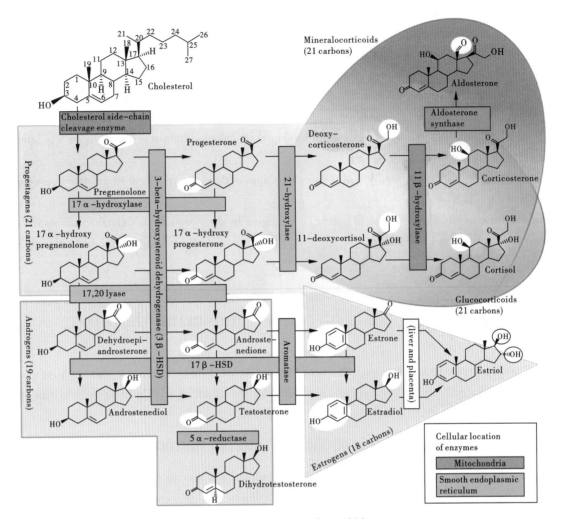

Figure 13-1　The synthesis of steroid hormone

13.2.2　Regulation mechanism of steroid hormone synthesis

The hypothalamic-pituitary-peripheral endocrine gland axis controls the endocrine activity of the peripheral gland. The pituitary gland plays the central role in integration and has a dominant position in the peripheral gland(Figure 13-2).

The hypothalamus connects endocrine and central nervous system, which synthesizes and secretes gonadotropin-releasing hormone, and reaches the endocrine cells of the pituitary gland through the pituitary portal system, stimulating or inhibiting the secretion of pituitary hormones.

The pituitary gland releases gonadotropin and adrenocorticotropic hormone under the action of hypothalamic regulatory peptides, and controls the secretion levels of sex hormones such as ovary, testis and adrenal cortex.

The gonads and adrenal glands synthesize and secrete progesterone, androgen, estrogen, etc. , under the regulation of peptide hormones secreted by the pituitary gland, and act on various parts of the body to achieve physiological function regulation.

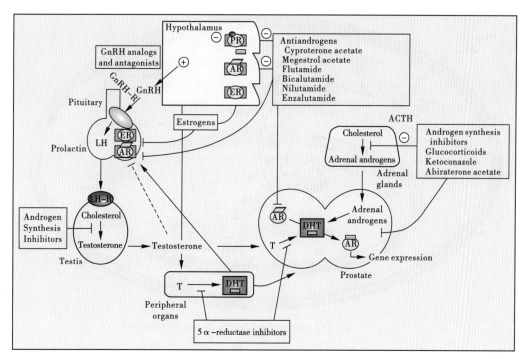

Sites of action of different treatments that affect androgen action. ACTH, adrenocorticotropic hormone; AR, androgen receptor; DHT, 5α-dihydrotestosterone; ER, estrogen receptor; GnRH, gonadotropin-releasing hormone; LH, luteinizing hormone; PR, progesterone receptor; T, testosterone.

Figure 13-2   **Target of endocrine therapy**

13.2.3   Sex hormone receptor

Sex hormones can exert a wide range of physiological effects when combined with sex hormone receptors. The sex hormone receptor belongs to the superfamily of transcription factors and the nuclear receptor superfamily, which is widely distributed in various tissues of the human body.

The sex hormone receptor is synthesized in the rough endoplasmic reticulum. It is distributed in the cytoplasm when it is inactive, and binds to heat shock protein 90. After activation, dimerization occurs and then enters the nucleus(Figure 13-3). In the nucleus, the sex hormone receptor complex binds to a region of the DNA called hormone-responsive element that activates or inhibits the expression of a variety of gene. The action mechanism of sex hormone receptors is extremely complicated. It recruits some helper regulatory complexes to enhance or inhibit transcriptional activity before transcription. Most of these helper regulatory molecules belong to enzymes, which modify hormone receptor complexes by acetylation, methylation, phosphorylation, and ubiquitin. Over hundreds accessory molecules provide regulatory functions for chaperones, transcriptional machinery recruiters, and RNA splices.

Receptors of androgens, estrogens, progestins, etc, belong to steroid receptors, and their structures are generally similar. It consists of four distinct functional regions, including an active regulatory region, a DNA binding region, a hinge region, and a ligand binding region(Figure 13-4).

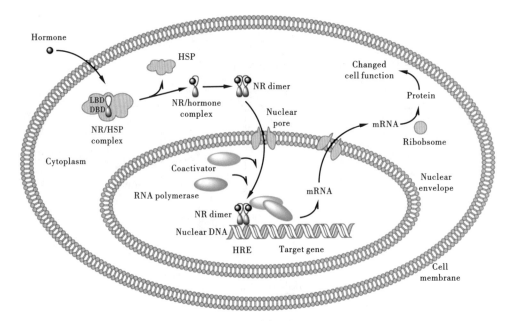

Figure 13-3　The action mechanism of nulear receptor

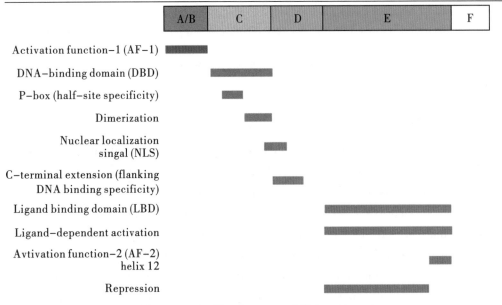

Figure 13-4　The Structure of Nulear Receptor

13.2.4　Main target organs of steroid hormones

Sex hormone receptors are widely distributed, and the hormone, endometrium and prostate are rich in sex hormone receptors; sex hormone receptors are also distributed in the parenchyma of many organs such as bone, muscle, fat, liver and cardiovascular. Estrogen receptors are predominant in breast ductal epithelial cells, and progesterone receptors are predominant in lobular epithelial cells. Androgen receptors are distributed in prostate epithelial cells.

The level of estradiol in breast cancer tissue is 4-6 times higher than that in plasma because of the high expression of enzymes involved in estrogen synthesis in breast tissue. For example, aromatase, 17β-estradiol hydroxysteroid dehydrogenase, estrone sulfatase. Prostate cancer tissue itself can synthesize androgens, or convert testosterone into more active dihydrotestosterone.

13.3 Endocrine therapy strategy for cancer

There are two basic treatment strategies for blocking the endocrine signaling pathway: lowering sex hormone levels and blocking sex hormone receptors.

In the early stages of cancer endocrine therapy, since effective drugs were lacking, castration surgery was the main treatment. Castration surgery could reduce sex hormones level within 12 hours. It once played an important role in endocrine therapy for breast and prostate cancer. At that time, adrenalectomy and pituitary resection were developed to reduce hormone production. In the past, attempts have been made to destroy these organs by radiotherapy to inhibit hormone synthesis. At present, except for the application of the potential surgery, other surgical endocrine treatment methods have been abolished for the treatment of complications. Nowadays, low-toxic and effective drugs have become the main strategy for cancer endocrine therapy.

13.3.1 Reducing sex hormone level

The gonad steroid hormone requires at least two conditions. Firstly, the Leydig cells or the ovarian cells/granulosa cells should be activated by the pituitary gonadotropin LH/FSH and secondly, the various steroid hormone synthesis-related enzymes should have sufficient activity. Hence, the goal of reducing sex hormone levels can be achieved both by reducing the release of the pituitary LH/FSH and inhibiting the activity of steroid synthesis-related enzymes.

13.3.1.1 Luteinizing hormone releasing hormone analogue and luteinizing hormone releasing hormone antagonist

Luteinizing hormone releasing hormone analogue (LHRHa) and luteinizing hormone releasing hormone antagonist (LHRHA) can compete with pituitary receptors for gonadotropin releasing hormone (GNRH, also known as LHRH, which is the two acronyms of the same hormone), reduce the secretion of LH / FSH, thereby reducing the levels of estrogen, progesterone and androgen, which is also known as drug castration.

LHRHa is one of the most commonly used castration drugs in endocrine therapy for breast cancer and prostate cancer. It has the advantages of reversible and small adverse reactions.

LHRH antagonists (LHRHA/LHRH-ant) are currently only used for endocrine therapy of advanced prostate cancer, and their clinical use is limited for the adverse reactions.

13.3.1.2 Inhibition of sex hormone synthase

(1) CYP17 inhibitor: abiraterone

Abiraterone acetate is an oral CYP17 inhibitor that is metabolized in vivo and function as abiraterone, which reduces androgen synthesis by inhibiting the activity of C17/C20-lyase and 17α-hydroxylase.

(2) CYP19 inhibitor: aromatase inhibitor

According to the AI structure and mechanism of action, it can be divided into two types.

Steroidal aromatase inhibitors compete with androgen for occupying the active site of aromatase and can irreversibly bind to the enzyme by covalent bond, causing permanent enzyme inactivation. The representative drug is exemestane.

Non-steroidal aromatase inhibitors compete with androgen for aromatase active site, and reversibly binds to the enzyme by ionic bond, thereby reversibly inhibiting enzyme activity. The representative drugs are letrozole and anastrozole.

13.3.2　Receptor modulator

Commonly used sex hormone receptor regulating drugs include three kinds of drugs.

13.3.2.1　Androgen receptor antagonists

Androgen receptor antagonists competitively bind to endogenous AR, which inhibit androgen from entring into the nucleus, and blocks the stimulation of androgen on prostate cancer. The drug can accelerate the formation of LH and FSH, and increase the levels of testosterone and estradiol in plasma, so it is often used in combination with LHRH analogues, thus it becomes the basic treatment for prostate cancer.

Androgenreceptor antagonists can be divided into steroid antagonists and nonsteroid antagonists. Steroid antagonists have steroid structure; for instance, cycloproterone and megestrol. Cycloproterone is rarely used because of its obvious cardiovascular toxicity. Nonsteroid antagonists have no steroid structure; for instance, the first generation of drugs flutamide, bicalutamide, the second generation of drugs enzalutamine.

13.3.2.2　Selective estrogen receptor modulators

Selective estrogen receptor modulators (SERMs) are drugs that have an agonistic effect on one of the estrogen receptor subtypes ERα or ERβ and no effect or antagonism on the other subtype. Its representative drug, Tamoxifen, competes with estrogen for binding to ER, blocks the expression of estrogen target genes, arrests cancer cells in G1 phase, and slows cell division and growth. Tamoxifen can be used in premenopausal and postmenopausal patients. It is more effective after menopause and is widely used in endocrine therapy of breast cancer. Tamoxifen has a partial estrogen agonistic effect, exhibits an antagonistic effect in the breast and reproductive system, and exhibits an agonistic effect in bone tissue, which is beneficial for osteoporosis. From the point of the lesion, tamoxifen are effective for skin, lymph nodes and soft tissues involvement but has poor effects on bone and visceral metastasis.

13.3.2.3　Selective estrogen receptor down-regulator

Unlike Tamoxifen, which only blocks AF2 site of the estrogen receptor, Fulvestrant blocks both AF2/AF1 sites and therefore has no agonistic effects and is known as a pure estrogen receptor blocker(Figure 13-5). In addition, Fulvestrant binds to the estrogen receptor and induces estrogen receptor degradation. However, the drug can only exert its therapeutic effect in the post-menopausal population. If the blocking effect is reached in the pre-menopausal state, the toxicity at the required dose is intolerable.

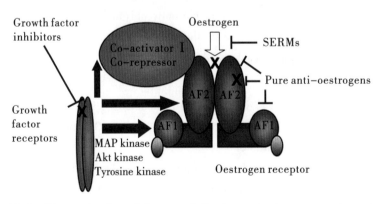

Figure 13-5　The mechanism of the pure Anti-estrogen(estrogen receptor antagonist)

13.4　Toxicity management of endocrine therapy

In addition to the dense distribution of reproductive related organs, sex hormone receptors are also widely distributed in almost all human tissues and have complex physiological functions. While cancer endocrine therapy attempts to produce an inhibitory effect on cancer cells, it also has a significant effect on the physiological function of the host cells, most of which are adverse effects. The down regulation of-sex hormone during cancer endocrine therapy leads to endocrine disorders, and even complicated steroid hormone disorders, which are the main side effects of treatment. In a few cases, treatment brings additional benefits, such as the activation effect of selective estrogen receptors which can enhance osteoporosis.

13.4.1　Hyperlipidemia and cardiac events

Estrogen can lower LDL levels, increase HDL levels, and have a protective effect on cardiovascular disease. According to one epidemiological survey in America, cardiovascular disease was the first cause of death for women older than 66 years, accounted for 15.9%, while breast cancer-related deaths accounted for 15.1%. Postmenopausal women will experience further decline in estrogen after AI treatment, which may have adverse effects on hyperlipidemia and cardiovascular events. TAM also has an effect on hyperlipidemia, and the incidence of fatty liver in long-term users reaches to 43.2%.

13.4.2　Osteoporosis

Bone density is regulated by sex hormones. AI causes bone loss due to a decrease in estrogen levels. Low androgen levels are associated with osteoporosis. The steroidal AI, exemestane, has an androgen-like effect and causes relatively less bone mineral loss than non-steroidal AI. The protective effect of tamoxifen on bone is proved.

13.4.3　Musculoskeletal joint pain

The incidence of this symptom is 15% –35%. Generally, it is heavier in the morning and improves after the activity. The symptoms are heavier within 6 months after onset of treatment, and the symptoms gradually decrease after 6 months. Tamoxifen has a lower incidence than AI.

13.4.4　Embolization

Endocrine therapy can lead to venous thrombosis, thromboembolism, and tamoxifen has a higher incidence than AI.

13.4.5　Endometrial thickening and endometrial cancer

Tamoxifen has estrogen stimulating effect, can mildly (1%) increase the risk of endometrial cancer mainly in the elderly. While AI reduces estrogen levels, 50% of patients with endometrium thickening (>10 mm) may return to normal (endometrial thickness <5 mm).

13.4.6　Hot flashes

30% –40% of patients with postmenopausal breast cancer may experience hot flashes during AI or tamoxifen treatment. The mechanism of hot flash is due to the decrease of 5-HT3 in the central nervous system, leading to narrow the sensory range of temperature changes. Patients are more sensitive to feel-like temperature. Auxiliary clinical trial data showed that the incidence of hot flashes during AI treatment was slightly lower than during tamoxifen. Glycine max can reduce the symptoms of hot flashes.

13.4.7 Decreased libido

Complete androgen blockage leads to decline in the quality of life of patients, such as libido reduction, erectile dysfunction, fatigue, mental decline, depression, decreased muscle strength, accumulation of fat, and decreased mobility. Female endocrine therapy can also cause adverse reactions such as vaginal dryness, painful intercourse, decreased libido, and hot flashes.

13.4.8 Adrenal steroid hormone secretion disorder

Abiraterone blocks the conversion of progesterone to androgen by acting on a specific enzyme system, and also prevents the conversion of progesterone to the glucocorticoid precursor, but does not prevent the conversion of progesterone to mineralocorticoid. Thus, after treatment with abiraterone, patients may present adrenocortical hormone disorder, manifested as increase of mineralocorticoids and decrease of glucocorticoids. Increasing level of mineralocorticoids cause hypokalemia, high blood pressure, and fluid retention (edema), while glucocorticoid deficiency leads to intolerance of infection or stress. Glucocorticoids must be added when using abiraterone. Glucocorticoid may also present therapeutic effect on prostate cancer, which may relate to negative feedback on inhibition of ACTH release and reduction of androgen synthesis.

13.4.9 Others

The lower the level of testosterone in men, the greater risk for metabolic syndrome, which leads to diabetes, heart disease, cardiovascular disease, and even vasogenic erectile dysfunction in turn. Some patients may have cataracts and retinal changes.

13.5 Mechanism of endocrine therapy resistance

The presence of sex hormone receptors in cancer cells indicates the sensitivity of blockade treatment on hormone signaling pathway. More than one third of ER-positive breast cancer patients are not sensitive to endocrine therapy, and about 20% of prostate cancer patients are ineffective for androgen removal therapy. Even if the initial treatment is effective, most of the drugs are resistant to hormones finally.

The occurrence of drug resistance is related to the heterogeneity of tumor cells. Based on the sensitivity to hormone blockade, there are at least two cell subpopulations in cancer tissue. After treatment, sensitive cells are inhibited whereas insensitive cells are allowed to grow, and thus resistance occurs for a long time. In terms of specific mechanisms, endocrine therapy resistance is associated with drug metabolism, tumor endocrine microenvironment, hormone synthase or receptor polymorphisms, and abnormal activation of non-receptor-associated bypass or downstream pathways (Figure 13-6).

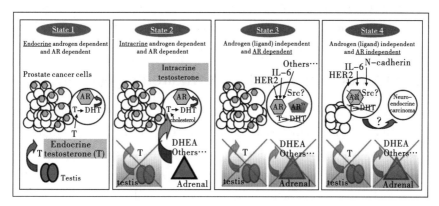

Figure 13-6   Drug resistance mechanism of cancer endocrine therapy (prostate cancer as an example)

13.5.1   Drug metabolism

Some drugs need to be degraded by drug-metabolizing enzymes to produce effective activity. Tamoxifen exerts pharmacological effects mainly by metabolizing to its active form, 4-OH-TAM and valsoxifen. The difference in the treatment outcome of tamoxifen is often related to the activity variation of metabolic enzymes. The main mechanism is the decline of metabolism activity of the enzyme CYP2D6.

13.5.2   Tumor endocrine microenvironment

Both breast cancer and prostate cancer cells are able to synthesize sex hormones, and some mesenchymal cells in cancer foci can also synthase sex hormone. Some mesenchymal cells even have the ability to secrete cell growth factors.

Some enzymes in cancer cells can reactivate hormone metabolites or convert sex hormones into active forms. For example, type II 5α-reductase can catalyze the conversion of testosterone to dihydrotestosterone, which is approximately 5 times more active than the former.

13.5.3   Polymorphisms of hormone synthase and nuclear receptor

Whether the drug is effective is related to the expected structure and function of the target. If the target is mutated, the drug will be ineffective, not as expected. Recently, some target abnormalities closely related to endocrine therapy drug resistance are identified, including hormone synthetase polymorphism, nuclear receptor loss, down-regulation, hypersensitivity and or reverse activation (Antagonists change into agonists due to receptor changes, which is also the reason of prostate cancer drug withdrawal effect.), ligand-independent nuclear receptor activation.

Studies have confirmed that the mechanism of ER action and target genes is very complex, which is regulated by a variety of different transcriptional regulators at different stages. Dysfunction of regulatory factors are also important causes of resistance to nuclear receptor inhibitors.

13.5.4   Hormone bypass activation

Mutations in the PI3K/AKT/mTOR signaling pathway occur in up to 70% of breast cancers, leading to abnormal activation. Signals transmitted by PI3K/AKT/mTOR activate non-estrogen-dependent ER transcriptional activity, allowing cells to proliferate without estrogen.

Growth factor receptors associated with endocrine resistance also include human epidermal growth factor receptor 2 (HER2), epidermal growth factor receptor (EGFR), insulin-like growth factor-1 receptor (IGF-1R), and estrogen receptors. The crosstalk of signaling pathways between the ER and other growth factor receptors is one of the mechanisms of drug resistance.

13.5.5   Abnormal activation of the downstream pathway of the receptor

Cell cycle abnormality is a common phenomenon in breast cancer cells. About 20% of ER-positive breast cancers have cyclin D1 gene amplification, and about 50% of cyclin D1 is overexpressed. Abnormal cell cycle is also considered an early event in breast cancer, with cyclin D1 overexpression observed in 72% of ductal carcinoma in situ. Cyclin is an important component involved in the cell cycle, which binds to cyclin-dependent kinase (CDK) to form a heterodimer promotes the cell cycle from G1 to S phase.

In ER-positive breast cancer patients, mitotic signals such as estrogen signal activate promoter of cyclin D1 encoding gene (CCND1), driving the expression of Cyclin D1 and binding to CDK4/6, phosphorylating RB as well as activating transcription factor E2F, which initiates downstream gene transcription and promotes G1-S phase transformation, leading to initiation of cycle progression.

Interaction between cyclin D1 and ER promotes transcriptional activity of ER, which leads to a higher dependence of ER-positive breast cancer on Cyclin D1.

13.6   Strategy for endocrine therapy resistance

The endocrine therapy of survivors with tumors is effective at the beginning. But if cure cannot be achieved, endocrine therapy would turn into the palliative therapy. As long as the life expectancy extends, almost all patients will eventually become resistant. About 50% of breast cancers and 80% of prostate cancers respond to initial endocrine therapy. The median effective time for first-line treatment of breast cancer is about 12 months, while the second line is about 5 months, and the third line is only 3 months. The effective period of prostate cancer treatment is longer than that of breast cancer, and the median effective time for first-line treatment is between 18 and 24 months.

13.6.1   General principles

The presence of sex hormone receptors is an effective marker for endocrine therapy. The detection of ER/PR receptors can be used as an effective marker for endocrine therapy in breast cancer. For example, if ER/PRis negative, the effective rate of endocrine therapy is less than 10%. ER is also a marker for predicting the effectiveness of CDK4/6 inhibitors. In almost all patients with prostate cancer, AR is positive, and the initial endocrine therapy response rate is over 80%, so there is no need to detect AR receptors.

When resistance occurs, an alternative endocrine drug with a different mechanism of action is generally used. Chemotherapy or other different types of anticancer drugs should be considered when the disease progresses rapidly or if appropriate endocrine drugs are unavailable.

13.6.2   Combination strategy

The polyclonal evolutionary pattern of cancer cells makes it highly adaptable. Under the pressure of endocrine therapy, clonal selection ultimately leads to the tolerance of a certain therapy. An important reason is the networking and diversity of molecular driving mechanisms in cancer cells, including cross-channel, bypass, and downstream path activation. Designing a more effective endocrine-resistance strategy requires further understanding of the molecular drive systems for cancer cell survival. Some combination regimens have been proved for their efficacy.

13.6.2.1 CDK4/6 inhibitor

The key regulatory site of the cell cycle from the G1 phase (pre-DNA synthesis) to the S phase (DNAsynthesis phase) is called the "R" point which is the key rate-limiting mechanism for cell proliferation. The "R" point is controlled by the CDK4/6 and Cyclin D complex. The abnormal activation of the complex activity has been officially established in ER-positive breast cancer cells. CDK4/6 inhibitors inhibit the binding of CDK4/6 and cyclin D1, thereby inhibiting the phosphorylation of Rb protein, arresting the cell cycle in the G1 phase, making it unable to transform to S phase.

Clinical trials have shown that the CDK4/6 inhibitor, Palbociclib, in combination with letrozole, extends PFS as long as 24 months, which prolongs PFS on letrozole treatment alone for more than one fold.

13.6.2.2 Inhibitor of the mTOR signaling pathway

The PI3K/AKT/mTOR signaling pathway is one of the important pathways in cells and is closely related to cell growth, proliferation and apoptosis. About 70% of breast cancers show activation of this signaling pathway. Major genetic mutations include loss of PTEN activity, PIK3CA activation point mutations, and AKT mutations, and can cross the downstream pathway of endocrine signaling, leading to drug resistance.

The mTOR inhibitor Everolimus is an analog of rapamycin, the natural mTOR inhibitor. Clinical trials have confirmed that Everolimus combined with tamoxifen, exemestane or fulvestrant significantly prolonged PFS compared with single-agent endocrine therapy for hormone receptor-positive HER2-negative breast cancer.

13.6.2.3 Receptor tyrosine kinase inhibitor

Lapatinib is a small molecule receptor tyrosine kinase inhibitor that blocks the epidermal growth factor receptor (ErbB1) and human epidermal factor receptor 2 (ErbB2). For patients with advanced breast cancer who are positive for hormone receptors and human epidermal factor receptor 2, letrozole combined with lapatinib, shows approximately three fold longer PFS (3.0-8.2 months), and almost doubled efficiency (15%-28%) compared to letrozole alone.

Although the tumor endocrine therapy functions slowly, it presents similar efficacy compared to molecular targeted therapy. It has the advantages of low toxicity, good tolerance and long remission period, and can be used as the first choice for patients with slow disease progression. Endocrine therapy is not isolated, and the best efficacy depends on the right time and the combination or conversion of other treatments if needed. The main problem of current endocrine therapy remains on drug resistance. Perhaps drug resistance is an inherent character of cancer cells. Conquering cancer is still a challenge that modern medicine has to face.

Qin Jianyong, Shi Yanxia, Chen Meiting, Yang Wei

Chapter 14

Immunotherapy of Cancer

The evolution of immune mechanisms can be traced back to a molecular system called CRISPR/Cas in single-celled organisms, which recognizes exogenous DNA and cuts it to silence the expression of exogenous genes. In the evolutionary history of multicellular animals, innate immunity is the basis of immune function, which first appeared. Adaptive immunity did not evolve until the advanced stages of multicellular animals. cellular immunity appeared early, and humoral immunity appeared late. Immunity as a structure that is ancient and scattered in its phylogeny and is closely related to every organ in the whole body. It achieves continuous monitoring and steady-state maintenance of the whole-body tissue through the circulatory system.

14.1　Brief history of tumor immunotherapy

The exploration of tumor immune mechanisms by humans has been more than 100 years, there are still many unknown areas.

14.1.1　Early immunotherapy practice

The earliest documented immunotherapy for tumors was in 1868. Dr. Wilhelm Busch of Germany used an erysipelas pathogenic bacteria (Group A Beta Hemolytic Streptococcus) to infect a patient with inoperable facial sarcoma, it was observed that the tumor showed a significant shrink.

In 1891, William Coley, an orthopaedic surgeon at Memorial Hospital in New York, United States, treated cancer by injecting bacteria into the tumor. Initially, the efficacy of this method was not stable, and the patient might die of infection; after many improvements being made, heated inactivated bacterial fluid became safe. This method has indeed enabled many cancer patients to be relieved or even relieved in the long term without medical treatment.

14.1.2　The origin and development of immunoediting theory

Immune editing is the main theory of tumor immunotherapy. Its appearance has experienced three historical development stages.

In 1909, German scientist Paul Ehrlich proposed the theory of immunosurveillance, in which human cells would develop abnormal proliferation (generating tumors) at a certain frequency under natural conditions. If not under the surveillance of the immune system, these abnormal proliferations would eventually become fatal(Paul Ehrlich's original words: if not kept in check by immune system, there was a high frequency of "aberrant germ", which would overwhelm us). He thought that the immune system could suppress the occurrence of tumors, and abnormal immune function was the basic factor of tumorigenesis.

In 1959, Australian scientist Frank Macfarlane Burnet and American medical scientist Lewis Thomas proposed the hypothesis of "tumor immune surveillance" that the immune system could recognize and eliminate malignant tumors, thereby inhibiting the occurrence and development of tumors.

In 2002, the American medical scientists Gavin Dunn and Robert Schreiber first proposed the theory of tumor immunoediting, systematically expounding the three-stage relationship between cancer and the immune system: early elimination, mid-term equilibrium, and late escape.

14.1.3   Adoptive cellular immunotherapy

The historical origins of CART-T cells—today's mainstream adoptive cellular immunotherapy can be traced back to 1984. In that year, the Steve Rosenberg team of the National Cancer Institute of the United Statesused large doses of IL-2 and LAK cells to treat 25 patients with renal cell carcinoma, melanoma, lung cancer, colon cancer, and other tumors. In 11 cases, tumor shrinkage exceeded 50%. A 33-year-old patient with metastatic melanoma had a complete regression of tumors, which brought a glimmer of hope to tumor immunotherapy. This is the first report of the success of Adoptive cell transfer, and the remarkable efficacy has made tumor immunotherapy gain attention once again after William Coley.

Israeli scientist Professor Zelig Eshhar is known as the father of CAR-T. In 1989, he first came up with the design of the first generation of CAR-T therapy, an adoptive T cell therapy based on Single Chain Antibody Fragment that corresponded to tumor antigens. ScFv antibodies were expressed on T cells by gene editing techniques to replace MHC-restricted TCR to target antigens of cancer cells. In the United States, Carl June and Michel Sadelain further developed the therapy by adding 4−1BB or CD28 costimulatory signals to develop the second-generation CAR-T therapies, and later developed the third and the fourth generation CAR-T therapies. In 2017, the United States approved the first CAR-T product to go public.

14.1.4   Brief history of the development of immune checkpoint inhibitors

In 1987, American scientist James Allison discovered CTLA-4. In 1996, James Allison reported the results of an animal experiment with CTLA-4 antibody in the journal of Science, tumors in mice disappeared after treatment. In 2011, the CTLA-4 antibody (trade name Ipilimumab) was approved for marketing in the United States to treat malignant melanoma tumors.

In 1992, Japanese scholar Tasuku Honjo discovered PD-1. In 1999, the Chinese-American scholar Lieping Chen discovered PD-L1 (it was also called B7-H1). In 2000, Tasuku Honjo demonstrated the negative regulation of T cells by the PD-1/PD-L1 pathway. In 2003, Lieping Chen used PD-L1 antibody to cure 60% of head and neck cancers in mice. In 2014, PD-1 antibody (trade name Keytruda/Opdivo) was approved for marketing in the United States; in 2016, PD-L1 antibody (trade name Tecentriq) was approved for marketing in the United States.

14.2 The biological basis of tumor immunotherapy

The reason why cancer cell clones can reach the clinical stage lies in immune escape. Cancer cell clones shape the tumor microenvironment in an immunosuppressed state, and the cytokines secreted by cancer cells also have a certain immunosuppressive effect on the whole host. Understanding the immunosuppressive mechanisms in TME(tumor microenvironment) and systemic immune status are the basis of immunotherapy. The current immunotherapeutic strategies achieve results in two directions: the use of targeted cells designed for an antigen on the surface of cancer cells, the so-called CART-T cell therapy and TCR-T cell therapy. The other is to achieve positive regulation by targeting regulatory targets on T cells.

14.2.1 The cancer-immunity cycle

American immunologist Daniel Chen systematically elaborated seven key aspects of tumor cell immunity in a review published in immunity(Figure 14-1).

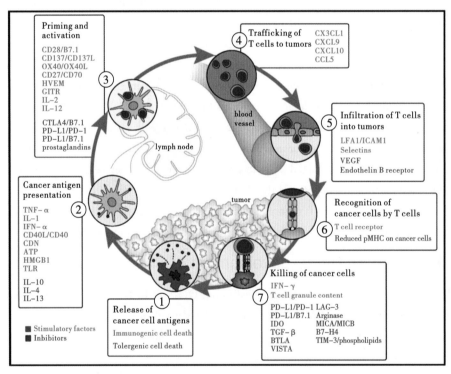

①Tumor cells release tumor-specific antigens (neoantigens). ②Neoantigens are recognized and processed by antigen-presenting cells (APCs) such as DCs in tumors area. ③After APC recognizes the antigen, it migrates to lymphoid tissues such as spleen and lymph nodes, and presents the antigen to CD8+ T cells or CD4+ T cells in the form of MHC I or MHC II peptide complex, then induces its activation, proliferation and differentiation. ④Activated T cells enter the bloodstream from lymphoid tissues such as spleen and lymph nodes. ⑤Lymphocytes in the blood pass through the blood vessels and enter the tumor tissue. ⑥T cells entering tumor tissues (CTLs, Cytotoxic T lymphocytes) recognize tumor cells. ⑦T cells initiate perforin, granzyme and other mechanisms to kill cancer cells.

Figure 14-1　**The cancer-immunity cycle**

The killed tumors further released more tumor-specific antigens, repeating A.

14.2.2 Immunoglobulin superfamily

The immunoglobulin family evolved from intercellular adhesion molecules and later developed into a core molecule in intercellular immune function. In addition to immunoglobulins, MHC, TCR, and BCR on the cell membranes also belong to this family, and they have important functions in intercellular antigen presentation and antigen recognition.

14.2.3 Immunoregulation of T cell function

In addition to the first signal provided by the TCR, the second signal and the third signal are required for APC-induced T cell differentiation. Tumor immunotherapy is the process of increasing the promoting signal and blocking the inhibitory signal.

The second signal (costimulatory molecules), such as, activating pathway: CD28/B7.1, OX40/OX40L, CD40/CD40L, CD137/CD137L, TLRs, etc; inhibiting pathway: CTLA4/B7.1, PD-1/PD-L1, etc (Figure 14-2).

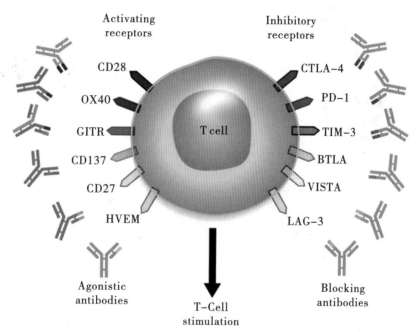

The third signal (cytokines), such as, Activating factor: IL-2, IL-12, TNF-alpha, IFN-gamma, HMGB1, IL-1, etc; Inhibiting factor: IL-10, IL-4, IL-13, etc.

Figure 14-2 Immunoregulation of T cell function

14.2.4 Tumor immune microenvironment

The main feature of the tumor microenvironment is local immunosuppression, which is similar to the immune tolerance mechanism when fertilized eggs are grown. Mechanisms involved in immunosuppression include reduced antigenicity of cancer cells and downregulation of MHC expression, as well as the increase of local immunosuppressive cells, such as Treg, MDSC, M2, and TH2, etc, accompanied by an increase in local immunosuppressive factors.

14.3 Strategies for cancer immunotherapy

Cancer cells use human immune tolerance mechanisms to achieve local microenvironment and systemic immunosuppression, thereby achieving proliferation and metastasis. Cancer lesions in the clinical phase rarely show spontaneous degeneration, and the probability of self-healing is less than one in 60,000. The strategy of immunotherapy stems from an understanding of the mechanisms of immune regulation, and currently proven effective strategies are: antibody therapy, CAR-T cell therapy, and immune checkpoint regulators (Figure 14-3).

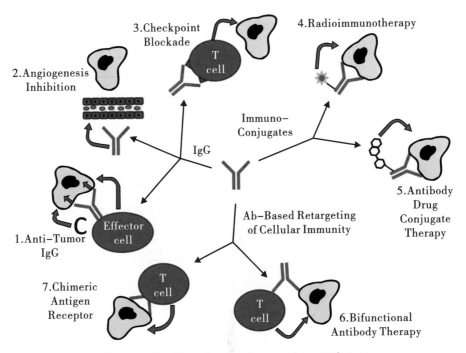

Figure 14-3　The principle of cancer immunotherapy

14.3.1　Antibody therapy against antigens on the surface of cancer cells

There are some special antigens on cancer cells, and targeted therapy based on antibodies can clear cancer cells. For example, Herceptin is a monoclonal antibody against human epidermal growth factor receptor-2 (HER2), a growth stimulator of cancer cells. After the HER2 receptor is blocked, the growth and metastasis of cancer cells are inhibited.

14.3.2　The therapy of targeting interstitial cell in cancer lesions

AVASTIN is an antibody against vascular endothelial growth factor called VEGF, which blocks the VEGF signaling pathway and inhibits the formation of new blood vessels to block the progression of cancer.

14.3.3　Immune checkpoint inhibitors

Immune checkpoints are activated or inhibitory receptor regulatory switches located on effector T cells. Its activation can make T cells in an attack state, and inhibition can leave T cells in a resting state. Blocking inhibitory receptors on T cells such as CTLA-4/B7-1 or B7-2, PD1/PD-L1 pathway, can activate T cell function；PD1/PD-L1 pathway is an important mechanism for cancer cells to inhibit T cell function in tumor microenvironment，and this channel blocker has become an important immunotherapy.

There are many immune checkpoints，other molecules also have potential exploration value，and related drugs are under development now. For example，Anti-4-1BB monoclonal antibodies exert an anti-tumor effect by activating CD8 T cells，promoting IFN secretion and other functions.

13.3.4　Adoptive cellular therapy CART-T cell therapy

Adoptive cellular therapy has undergone a long process of exploration. Early adoptive cellular therapy generally referred to：the first-generation LAK cells，the second-generation CIK cells，the third-generation TIL cells，and the fourth-generation antigen-specific CTL cells.

Most of the early adoptive cellular therapies were inefficient，and the preparation process was difficult to standardize，so it has been eliminated. The fifth generation of adoptive cellular therapy is currently prevalent，which has two main technologies：CART-T cells and TCR-T cells（Figure 14-4）. CART-T cells have developed rapidly，and the fourth-generation therapy has been designed.

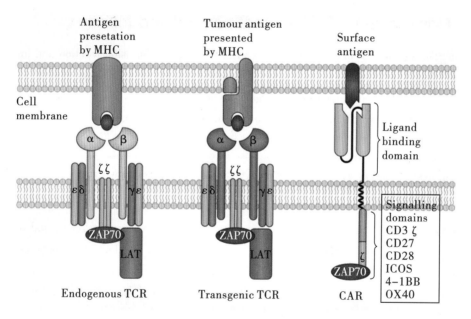

Figure 14-4　The principle of CAR-T cell therapy

14.4　Management of immunotherapy related toxicity

CART cell performs its antitumor function mainly through antigen-specific chimeric single-chain antibody expressed on T cell membrane. And the response rate can reach 80% or more. The response rate of immunological checkpoint inhibitors is between 10% and 40%. Essentially，both of these immunotherapies belong to enhanced immunotherapies，which may result in specific toxicities that are primarily manifested by excessive immune response.

14.4.1 Cytokine release syndrome

It is a common excessive immune response during the CART treatment. Clinical manifestations mainly include : fever, increase of specific cytokines, hypoxia, hypotension, abnormal changes in the nervous system. At least 7 kinds of cytokines have a certain correlation with cytokine release syndrome (CRS) : interferon-γ (IFN-γ), Fracktalkine (fractal chemokine), granulocyte-macrophage colony-stimulating factor (GM-CSF), interleukin-5 (IL-5), interleukin-6 (IL-6), human FMS-like tyrosine kinase 3 ligand (Flt-3L) and interleukin-10 (IL-10).

Effective and powerful medical intervention should be applied to handle the severe CRS, including respirators, vasoactive drugs, antiepileptic drugs and antipyretic analgesic drugs.

High-dose corticosteroids can reverse the clinical symptoms of CRS rapidly. However, corticosteroids can inhibit the proliferation of CAR-T in vivo and reduce the efficacy of CART. The blocking monoclonal antibody for IL-6 receptor (Tocilizumab) can quickly relieve the toxicity related to CRS, without any effect on the proliferation of CART cells.

14.4.2 Management of ICPIs treatment-related toxicity

The toxicity of immune checkpoint inhibitors can be divided into infusion reaction and immune-related adverse events (irAE), or adverse events of special interest (AEoSI). The common clinical manifestation is the inflammation in the skin, colon, endocrine organs, liver and lungs. Although excessive inflammation of some tissues and organs is rare, it may be fatal, such as neurotoxic reactions and myocarditis.

14.5 Comprehensive immune status assessment

No matter what kind of cancer immunotherapy, only part of patients benefit from initial treatment (Figure 14–5). Even if the initial treatment is effective, some patients will develop drug resistance later on. Our understanding for tumor immunity is just beginning, and our ability to predict the effectiveness is very limited for existing therapies. For example, in patients with melanoma treated with anti-CTLA-4 or anti-PD-1, approximately 1/4–1/3 of the patients experienced tumor progression after initial response. Due to our limited ability to understand the therapies and patients, more mechanisms of drug resistance remain unknown (Figure 14–5, Figure 14–6).

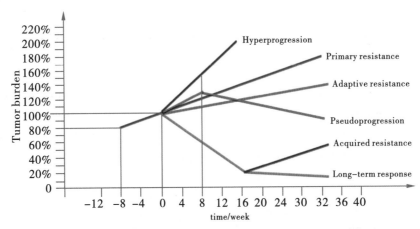

Figure 14-5　The response patterns of cancer immunotherapy

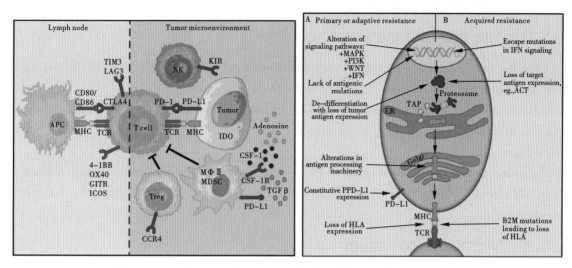

Figure 14-6   Drug resistance mechanism of cancer immunotherapy

Immunological assessment for patients before and after treatment can help us to predict efficacy and toxicity. It also can also help us understand the mechanism of drug resistance in order to design better treatment protocols.

The biological characteristics of cancer cells and the immune system of the host, and even the microecological state of the host, are related to whether the specific immunotherapy achieves the expected therapeutic effect. Immunological assessment requires access to cancer tissue specimens and blood, and even feces. Current progress has suggested that the following should be considered for the immunological assessments.

14.5.1   Genomic instability and immunogenicity of cancer cells

If cancer cells express more neoantigens, cancer cells will have higher immunogenicity. Genomic instability or chromosomal instability of cancer cell is associated with mismatch-repair deficiency (MMR), which can be characterized by microsatellite instability-high (MSI-H) and increased mutation-related neoantigen expression.

Tumor mutation burden (TMB) is a quantitative method for mutation-related neoantigens, which has been confirmed to be related to the efficacy of the immunotherapy.

The expression level of MHC class I molecules on cancer cells is also related to immunogenicity. Some cancer cells obtain immune escape through low expression of MHC class I molecules.

Cancer cells also express PD-L1 with negative feedback that inhibits the killing ability of Teff in TME.

14.5.2   Immunosuppression in tumor microenvironment

The number and function of the TILs in TME determines whether the antitumor response enters the step 6 of the cancer-immunity cycle. The expression of PD-L1 on tumor cells and the number of TILs could probably predict the efficacy of immunotherapy. Therefore, some scholars tailor the cancer immunotherapy based on 4 types of tumor microenvironment on the basis of the PD-L1 status and presence or absence of TILs.

The number of suppressive immune cells or the immune-related cells also reflects the immunosuppressive status of TME, such as Tregs, MDSCs, M2 macrophages.

In addition to the inhibitorymesenchymal cells, tumor cells can also secrete some immunosuppressive cytokines involved in the local immunosuppression of TME.

14.5.3 The immune status of host

There has been a lack of standardized evaluation method, which reflects the status of the hostimmune system. The number of immune cells circulating in the blood, is a alternative tool.

It is not very common that the host immune function has been impeded in the early stage of cancer development. During the treatment or in the advanced stage, the majority of patients have systemic immune function impairment.

The quantity of peripheral blood immune cell can reflect systemic immune function disorder, which can be generally detected through CD3/CD8/CD4/CD19-positive lymphocytes, and CD56-positive NK cells by flow cytometry.

14.5.4 Microbial ecosystem

Microbial ecosystem and human cells are symbiotic relationships, microorganisms in the gastrointestinal tract/skin/mucosa play an important role in a series of human life activities. Studies have shown that the composition of intestinal microbes in cancer patients is related to the effectiveness of ICPIs, and bifidobacterium is beneficial to the anti-tumor effect of PD-L1 inhibitors. Its mechanism may be related to the physiological activity of the metabolites produced by the microorganisms in the body.

14.5.5 Biomarkers that reflect the immunosuppression state in the blood

The increase of blood CRP and IL-6 in cancer patients reflects the chronic inflammatory state of the body, suggesting that there are antigenic foreign bodies in the human body that cannot be removed. LDH in the blood can indirectly reflect the level of aerobic glycolysis in cancer cells. The rise of these three serum markers is associated with systemic immunosuppression state and the efficacy of immunotherapy.

14.5.6 Medical history

Smoking can lead to more neoantigen producing in lung cancer, and the recent history of radiotherapy is also associated with increased immunogenicity of cancer. These two factors are thought to be related to the efficacy of immunotherapy.

14.6 Immunomodulatory effects of traditional anticancer therapy

Before humans made breakthroughs in cancer immunotherapy, the tumors that can be cured are mainly confined to early solid tumors and hematological lymphoid tumors. The therapeutic effects of traditional anti-cancer therapies are mainly manifested as removal, killing or reduction of cancer lesions. From the perspective of immunity, these traditional anti-cancer treatments, such as surgery, physical chemical ablation therapy or vascular embolization therapy (simultaneous local use of chemotherapy agents in most cases), radiation therapy, chemical drugs, molecular targeted drugs (various antibodies or small molecular tyrosine kinase inhibitors) may have certain immunomodulatory effect.

14.6.1   Surgery

Surgical treatment can reduce tumor burden and eliminate immunosuppression; but surgical trauma can inhibit immunity, and inflammation in the wound area can promote tumor development. In some cases, primary tumors release cytokines that inhibit metastases, and removal of primary lesions may also contribute to the growth of metastases.

14.6.2   Ablation therapy

Physical and chemical ablation techniques, such as heat, cold and alcohol can directly kill cancer cells, and their lysates may be immunogenic and even cause residual tumor regression.

14.6.3   Radiation therapy

Radiation therapy not only directly kills tumor cells and induces immunogenic cells death, but also acts as a kind of stress, inducing tumor cells to overexpress heat shock proteins, MHC class I molecules, etc. , improving the immunogenicity of tumors. In addition, radiotherapy can destroy the tumor matrix and induce the expression of ICAM-1, which is beneficial to the infiltration of T cells into tumor lesions.

14.6.4   Chemotherapy

Chemotherapeutic agents usually inhibit bone marrow function and immune function, but some can promote anti-tumor immune response. These drugs promote anti-tumor immunity by inducing immunogenic cells death, increasing immunogenicity of cancer cells, removing immunosuppressive cells, and activating immune effector cells. For example, low-dose cyclophosphamide can selectively remove Treg cells, gemcitabine can activate macrophages, and 5-FU can enhance the immunogenicity of tumor cells.

14.6.5   Molecular targeted therapy

Some studies have shown that Imatinib could initiate DCs to activate NK cells to promote host immune response and thus kill cancer cells.

Systemic therapy is mainly through drug. Chemotherapy is based on the synthesis, stability andmaintenance mechanism of the cancer genome. It is designed to eliminate tumor by interfering with the critical metabolism of cancer cells. Molecular targeted drugs and endocrine therapeutic drugs target some signal pathways or regulatory molecules related to the growth and division of cancer cells. However, the strategy of immunotherapy is different from foregoing methods, of which the target is immune cells in tumor microenvironment. The results have shown that once immunotherapy is effective, it will have "tail effect", which means the patients could obtain long-term remission or even cure. Local treatments such as surgery and radiotherapy are difficult to cure cancer and the remission time of chemotherapy and targeted therapy is relatively short, but these traditional treatments have certain immunomodulatory effect. Therefore, the combination of the immunotherapy and traditional treatments has the potential to enhance the treatment effect.

It has been found that traditional anticancer therapy can promote anti-tumor immune responses by inducing immunogenic cell death, modulating cancer cell immunogenicity, eliminating immunosuppressive cells, and activating immune effector cells. At present, it is believed that the anti-tumor effect of radiotherapy and chemotherapy is partly due to directly killing, and partly due to the immune response induced by this. There are many influencing factors in tumorigenesis. Single-target therapy often has poor efficacy; while based on the tumor microenvironment and the evolution mechanism of cancer cells, the joint strategies is an important way to improve the efficiency of anti-cancer treatment programs. The exploration of anti-cancer therapeutic strategies targeting immune system has just begun. With further understanding of tumor immune escape mechanisms and tumor microenvironment, anti-tumor immunotherapy will continue to progress.

Qin Jianyong, Cui Jiuwei, Zhang Hongmei, Li Yize

Chapter 15

Minimally Invasive Tumor Therapy

15.1　Introduction

Minimally invasive therapy is technically based on the quickly developing modern medical imaging science, which is a newly developed tumor treatment that synthesizes the medical imaging technologies, tumor drug therapy, biogenetics and high-tech medications (such as radio-frequency ablation, microwave ablation, cryoablation, radioactive seeds implantation, laser interstitial therapy, high-intensity focused ultrasound, endoscope, photodynamic therapy, irreversible electroporation ablation, etc.). It has been attested by more and more clinical practice that minimally invasive therapy has its unique advantages including specific targeting, less injury and pain, quicker recovery, affirmative efficacy and repeatability, making it the forth mainstay besides the traditional methods of tumor treatment, i. e. surgery, chemotherapy and radiation therapy.

Early in 1886, Menetrier made the first lung puncture in order to diagnose a mass of malignancy located in the thorax, however, his attempt was with a low success rate but a high rate of complications due to the thick puncture needle and a lack of imaging-guide and assistant cytoscopy technology. Then with the development of X-ray, computed tomography (CT), magnetic resonance imaging (MRI), imaging-guided needle aspiration biopsy achieved an accuracy of 85% –95% in the late 1950s. In 1953, Swedish radiologist Seldinger first invented the manipulation of percutaneous vascular puncture which priorly set a fundamentation for the interventional oncology. In 1971, Ansfield reported the transarterial perfusion of fluorouracil (FU) through the hepatic artery to treat primary hepatic cell carcinoma (HCC). Then the transarterial chemotherapy (with mixture of iodinated oil and chemotheraputic drug) with subsequent embolizing hepatic artery using resorbable gelatin sponge was first employed by Japanese radiologist Nakakuma et al. in 1979 to deal with primary hepatic cell carcinoma, which was considered a breakthrough in the HCC treatment, and is now the first choice for unresectable and/or recurrent disease. Intraluminal stent implantation is another important branch of interventional oncology which was developed in the 1990s. Stenosis and obstruction of the physiological tract caused by tumor mass are commonplaces during the course of the disease, which could be partially or even totally relieved by the stent placement giving rise to the recanalization. Meanwhile, several tumor ablation techniques including cryoablation, radiofrequency ablation, microwave ablation, etc. , also get a take-off with the help of image guide and spread rapidly.

Minimally invasive therapy in China begins in the late 1970s, and nearly 40 years later, remarkable achievement has been made. The very strategy continues to improve patients' outcomes while minimizing toxicities. And this chapter provides us an overview of the concepts and principles commonly used in the clinical procedure. Basically, minimally invasive tumor therapy, according to its interventional approach, is divided into two categories, intravascular minimally invasive tumor therapy and nonvascular minimally invasive tumor therapy. The intravascular way refers to selective or ultraselective intubation of the target vessel (mainly artery) to treat local mass and/or its associated complications, and mainly includes: transcatheter arterial infusion chemotherapy (TAI), transcatheter arterial embolization (TAE), transcatheter arterial chemoembolization (TACE), percutaneous port-catheter system (PPCS), percutaneous transluminal angioplasty, etc. The nonvascular way refers to imaging-guided interventional approach directly targeting the local disease without passing through the vasculature, and mainly includes: tumor ablation, radioactive particles implantation, photodynamic therapy (PDT), percutaneous transcatheter drainage, transluminal stent implantation, endoscope, etc.

Moreover, it is also of great importance for us to know the advantages over the other kinds of treatments and its particular benefits to patients given its prevalent use:

- Minimized injury, small incisions or even no incisions are needed which recover quickly.

- The ability of specific targeting with imaging guide gives the best protection of normal tissue.

- Both eradication and palliative therapy could be achieved-through technology, by which better life quality is improved.

- A comprehensive scheme encompassing minimally invasive therapy could be decided by multidiscipline cooperation and applied to one patient aiming at individualized medical service and better efficacy, which has been a promising trend recently.

15.2　Intravascular minimally invasive tumor therapy

15.2.1　Mechanisms

The growth of neoplasm, whether it is malignant or not, is largely dependent on blood supply which brings nutrients and oxygen and take away the metabolites, also on which metastasis relies. At the same time, the capillaries passing through the parenchyma bring a lot of convenience to the interaction between cancer cell and surrounding microenvironment. It has been proved that tumor growth will be sharply inhibited if the blood supply is cut off. For example, normal liver simultaneously receives double blood supply of the hepatic artery and hepatic portal vein. The former provides 75% –85% of the blood and 50% of the oxygen, while the latter provides a percentage of 20% –25% of the blood and a percentage of 50% of the oxygen. Nevertheless, it is totally different under the circumstance of primary hepatocellular cancinoma, for which almost 95% of blood supply comes from the hepatic artery and barely comes from the hepatic portal vein. This special feature provides the pathophysiological fundamentation for interventional therapy, where chemotheraputic drugs or embolization material or both are delivered through targeted hepatic artery. This usually results in efficient necrosis and subsequent shrinkage of the tumor, leaving the normal tissue less damaged and local therapy achieved.

15.2.2　Techniques

15.2.2.1　Seldinger's technique

Seldinger's technique is a prerequisite for interventional oncologists to carry out the following treatments. First invented by Swedish radiologist Seldinger, this technique actually refers to vascular (usually artery) intubation through percutaneous puncture, which replaced the traditional method of angiography, where direct puncture of the vessel or intubation of exposed vessels through an incision is usually implemented. Due to its obvious advantages including safety, easier operation and less complications, the technique spread promptly and is still in use today.

A brief introduction of the process is as below: puncture needle with a core stylet in it is used to rapidly pierce through the artery in an angle of $30°–40°$, resulting in penetration of anterior and posterior wall of the vessel, then withdraw the stylet smoothly till blood eject from the tail of the needle. Operator now needs to induce the guidewire into the hollow needle, then the needle is supposed to pull out when the guidewire enters into the targeted vessel. After that, a catheter sheath is percutaneously pushed into the lumen of the same vessel following the pathway of the guidewire. Afterwards, guidewire is drawed out with the completion of the sheath placement, and now we have access to the next treatment. However, no technique is perfect, improvement could always be possible to be overlayed throughout the clinical practice, Seldinger's technique is improved by the way that puncture needle only penetrates the anterior wall of the vessel, and less probability of hemorrhage is achieved.

15.2.2.2　Digital subtraction angiography

DSA, an abbreviation for digital subtraction angiography. Clear images of the desired artery are underpinnings to bring the targeted therapy about. DSA is just created to solve the problem. The technology with a digital processing method could eliminate needless background tissue images in the angiograpy, giving only clear images with high resolution of the targeted vessel. The aforementioned traits provide great convenience of observing blood supply of the tumor and of applying the interventional manipulation. Nudelman got the first DSA image in 1977, and nowadays it has been widely used.

15.2.2.3　Selective vascular catheterization

This technique is based on DSA guiding. According to the diameter of the artery catheterized, it has been divided into selective catheterization or ultraselective catheterization. The aim is actually to achieve angiography with contrast media injected into the targeted artery through the catheter, or to deliver theraputic mediator. Selective catheterization aims at medium-sized arteries, whose lumen diameter is usually above 1.0 mm. In most cases, the first-grade branches of the aorta belong to this kind of condition, and commonly there are anatomy names for the vessel, such as arteriae bronchiales, arteria coeliaca, mesenteric artery, renal artery. As for the second, third grade or even smaller branches of the aorta whose diameters are 0.3 – 1.0 mm, catheterization belongs to ultraselective operation which gives more accuracy of the treatment. Catheters are shaped to fit into different forms of targeted arteries.

15.2.2.4　Transcatheter arterial chemoinfusion

Most of chemotheraputic agents exert its anti-cancer effects in aconcentration-dependent way, i. e, the higher concentration of the drug in the local region of the tumor, the better treatment effect. On the contrary, if the concentration is too low to meet the effective threshold, it will never attain any theraputic effects no matter how long the treatment lasts. Transcatheter arterial chemoinfusion(TACI) has substantially elevated the drug concentration in the local region, which partially handles the "hot potato" burning hands of medical oncologists that chemotherapuetic drugs could have had the ability to kill chemo-insensitive cancer cells but failed to achieve it due to a lack of enough local concentration. TACI is a procedure integrated the techniques mentioned above, which perfuses the drug directly into the blood supply artery of the tumor through selective or ultraselective artery catheterization, increasing the concentration dozens of times. Simultaneously, the first-pass effect has also to some extent been circumvented by this, where 90% of the drug will be absorbed by the liver and lose its efficacy. Once the drug enters the blood, it will combine with the plasma albumin, then the drug could no longer get into tumor cells owing to the high molecular weight of the protein. One instance for this is 98% of the cisplatin will be attached to ALB if it is applied in an intravenous way. And the advantage stands out because of a shorter distance the drug travels to the foci.

15.2.2.5 Transarterial embolization

Catheter-directed embolization is one of the fundamental image-guided therapies that has shaped the speciality of interventional oncology. The term embolization refers to the act of delivering an agent or device into a target vessel to produce intentional vascular occlusion. This occlusion may be permanent or temporary depending on the clinical indication and the agent or device utilized. Catheter-directed embolization was first reported in 1972 when autologous blood clot was used to treat a patient with gastrointestinal hemorrhage. The indications for embolization emcompass a wide spectrum of clinical situations including tumor devascularization, tissue ablation, organ protection against nontargeted embolization, blood flow redistribution, control of hemorrhage secondary to malignancy, and delivery of theraputic agents. Embolic agents and devices range from liquid and particulate agents that are flow directed to mechanical devices deployed in a precise position. The agents and devices are chosen for their unique properties, the territory or target site being embolized, and the desired endpoint of the theraputic intervention.

Permanent embolic agents and devices include anhydrous ethanol, stainless steel coils. They mostly aim at a thorough treatment of some malformation of vasculature like devascularization of tumors and hemostasis of bronchial arteriovenous malformation causing hemoptysis. Temporal embolic agents or resorbable agents like the gelatin sponge instead aim at occluding the target vessel which supplies blood for the tumor just for a period of time, by doing that, the rich blood supply could be shut down to a very low level, which enables subsequent surgery resection or ablation.

15.2.2.6 Transcatheter arterial chemoembolization

The difference between transcatheter arterial chemoembolization(TACE) and the two above-mentioned techniques lies in the agents used, a fused emulsifier of chemotherapuetic drugs and embolic agents are perfused and deployed throughout the tumor vasculature generating a combined effect of topical chemotherapy and embolization. In other words, chemotherapuetic drugs, by virtue of embolic agents, could stay longer with a relative high concentration. The pivotal issue of TACE still lies in understanding the basic principles of embolization that include the level or depth of penetration of the planned occlusion so that the appropriate embolic and chemotherapuetic agents can be applied to the appropriate vasculature territory to assure the best chance for both technical and clinical success.

15.2.2.7 Percutaneous transluminal angioplasty

Upon completion of Seldinger's procedure, some other instruments (balloons, stents, laser probe, etc.) are delivered to the pathologic stenosis of the vessel to conduct the angioplasty. Such techniques includes endovascular thrombolytic therapy, transluminal extraction-atherectomy therapy, percutaneous transluminal laser angioplasty, etc. (Figure 15-1).

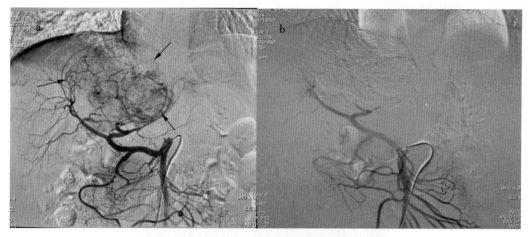

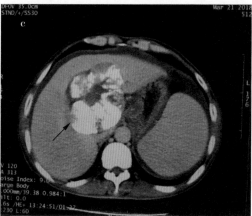

Celiac angiography (a) by DSA demonstrates a diffusion zone (arrow) of contrast agent. (b) shows that the gray zone disappeared after embolization. The computed tomography (c) is one of the follow-up examinations, which shows a high-density area (arrow) in the liver resulting from contrast agent deposition in the tumor vasculature.

Figure 15-1   **TAE in a patient with primary hepatocellular carcinoma**

15.2.3   Complications

Even if properpre-procedureis planned and interventionalists have enough familiarity with the indications, advantages, and shortcomings of each toolavailable in the procedure, complications still happen. So knowing these situations is vital importance to render optimal care to cancer patients.

15.2.3.1   Tissue ischemia

It happens when hemodynamics of the target vessel changes or an inappropriate embolic material is chosen. For instance, portal hypertension in cirrhosis gives rise to a reduced blood supply to the liver, if embolization of the hepatic artery is employed on this occasion, infarction of the liver or even hepatic failure possibly happens due to ischemia.

15.2.3.2   Postembolization syndrome

It is associated with ischemia and resultant necrosis of the tumor among those patients who undergo treatments of embolizaion. Clinical manifestations include fever, nausea, vomiting, paralytic ileus, etc. These syndromes are usually transient, which last for a few hours to a few days or so.

15.2.3.3 Accident embolism

Improper placement of the catheter (not in the target vessel) , inappropriate embolic material and/or releasing at the incorrect time during the procedure will lead to an accident embolism, where vessels of lung, spleen, bile duct, gastrointestinal tract, extremities, nerve system, or even the skin, etc. Accidently embolized as well as infarcted, which could be result in a series of complications of varying severity depending on its location and degree.

15.2.3.4 Chemotheraputic agents associated side effects

In TACI and TACE, chemotheraputic agents associated side effects are commonplaces just as in the standard intravenous chemotherapy, which include digestive tract reaction, myelosuppression, hepatotoxicity, nephrotoxicity, cardiotoxicity, etc.

15.3 Nonvascular minimally invasive tumor therapy

15.3.1 Mechanisms

Nonvascular minimally invasive tumor therapy includes several theraputic modalities that can achieve local and regional diagnosis and/or control of malignancy in addition to providing palliation. With the advent and development of image guidance (X-ray, CT, MRI, ultrasound, endoscope, etc.) , these treatments are bringing into practice through physiological cavities or directly aims at the viscera in a percutaneous way.

15.3.2 Techniques

15.3.2.1 Percutaneous needle biopsy

Pathological or even molecular diagnosis must be acquired before treatment to make optimal treatment scheme for cancer patients. Percutaneous needle biopsy is employed at this time using special puncture needle by aspiration or incision to get some tissues in the local foci, rendering laboratory test. This minimally invasive way has mostly replaced the traditional surgical incision way, which largely extends the application of pathological diagnosis before operation.

15.3.2.2 Percutaneous transhepatic choledochus drainage

Jaundice in cholangiocarcinoma, pancreatic head carcinoma and ampullary carcinoma which is caused by occlusion resulted from local tumor mass does not only impair life quality of cancer patients, but more importantly endanger patients' survival if not handled properly. The jaundice could be relieved by percutaneous transhepatic choledochus drainage(PTCD) bile drainage in an intra bile duct way or an extracorporeal percutaneous way, providing conditions favorable for surgery operation or just for palliation. Percutaneous transhepatic cholangiography is needed before PTCD in order to make sure the exact position of occlusion in bile duct and lesion associated nature (whether it's benign or malignant) , severity, extent of the lesion, etc. The drainage is divided into internal one and external one according to whether finally the bile is drained into the digestive tract (duodenum) or into a drainage bag extracorporeally. The first step of the procedure is to deliver a guidewire into the bile duct by percutaneous transhepatic puncture, then the operator needs to draw back the puncture needle followed by delivering a drainage tube with side holes. At the moment, if the tube is placed at the position upstream to the obstruction, then naturally the bile has to be drained into a bag, which names external drainage; if the tube is placed at the position downstream the obstruction and the opening of the tube reaches distal end of bile duct or duodenum, into which the bile could finally flow, this is called internal drainage.

15.3.2.3   Dilation of nonvascular luminal stenosis

The approach to luminal stenosis depends on the specific type of disease. In term of lumen with an opening to the surface of the body such as digestive tract, airway, urinary tract, routine interventional operation is delivered through the external opening. In contrast, enclosing lumen without an opening to the external environment like bile duct needs a percutaneous puncture way to approach the stenosis. A common flow path is as follows. The first step is to make sure that the catheter is in the right position of the lumen by contrast imaging. After that, a flat dilation balloon is sent to the stenosis where the balloon is inflated for dilation. In case of prolonged lesion hindering one-off balloon dilation, the flat balloon is then placed to the distal end of the stenosis for a gradual retrieving and concomitant dilation. The extent of dilation depends on the nature of the lesion as well as the experience of the interventionalist. After validating treatment effect with reimaging of the stenosis, if satisfying result is confirmed, the balloon could be removed and the therapy is accomplished.

15.3.2.4   Cryoablation

Cryoablation is a thermal therapy choice used to apply freezing temperature to destroy target tissues. The cellular response and energy transformation of ablative therapies that initiate the spectrum of inflammation, repair or death are distinct mechanisms depending on the ablative modality selected. This is especially true concerning cryoablation compared with the heat-based ablative modalities. Frostbite injury, which is essentially devitalized tissue, has long been known to occur secondary to prolonged or extreme-low temperature exposure. Not surprisingly, cryoablation is the oldest of the applicator-based ablative techniques. Oncologic cryotherapy was first performed in England in 1845 by James Arnott. He used a self-designed apparatus to treat cancers of the skin, breast, and uterine cervix, using a salt and crushed ice concoction that reached a tempetature of −20 ℃. Although Arnott's treatment at the time was strictly palliative, he proposed that cryotheraputic techniques had the potential to cure. In 1913, an American neurosurgeon named Iriving S. Cooper developed the first liquid nitrogen surgical probe, which he used with variable success to treat movement disorders such as Parkinson disease and unresectable brain tumors. This spawned further interest in cryotherapy, which led to investigations and applications for the treatments of the liver, prostate, kidneys beginning in the 1960s. The early applicators were of large caliber that required open or laparoscopic access to treat visceral organs. It was not again until the 1990s that cryotherapy experienced a revival as a result of the development of safer and minimally invasive applicator system (endoscopic and percutaneous) and enhanced imaging techniques. Improvements in ultrasonography, which allow for real-time evaluation of cryoablation treatment, and cryoablative equipment with enhanced freezing capacity and smaller diameter of cryoapplicator together have heightened cryotherapy's potential to become a more practical and well-tolerated alternative to oncologic surgery in many clinical settings.

The therapeutic goal of cryoablation is to create a localized area of cell death in targeted tissue which extends approximately 1 cm beyond the tumor margin (for eradication purpose mimicking surgical excision) or to create a cell death area as large as possible within the tumor (for palliation purpose). The treatment is divided into two phases respectively characterized by fast freezing and slow thawing. In the first phase, extracellular matrix freezing creates a hyperosmotic environment outside of the cells which still have intact and thermal-protective membranes. Intracellular fluid is cooled but unfrozen, following its osmotic gradients and diffusing out of the cells. As the temperature goes down, ice accumulates extracellularly and creates a high intracellular solute concentration, and at approximately −10 ℃, proteins are denatured, which allows intracellular ice formation causing mechanical shearing of organelles and irreversible cell death. The thawing process permits ice melting, reversing the osmotic gradient and causing hypotonic extracellular water to diffuse back into the cell, and promoting cell rupture. In theory, this will cause release of the tumor antigen, which to some extent will enhance anti-tumor immune response. At the same time, the repeated freeze-thaw process also causes harms to local microvasculature resulting in thrombosis and ischemia, which is the second mechanism of cell death during cryoablation(Figure 15−2).

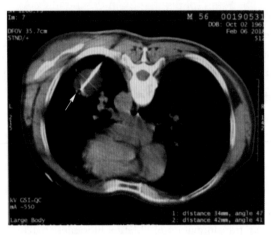

The tumor lesion is of a round shape as shows in the computed tomography (arrow). The white needle-shaped one is the cryoapplicator, which is deployed in the tumor transcutanously.

Figure 15−2　Palliative cryoablation for a 56-years-old male with primary lung cancer

15.3.2.5　Radiofrequency ablation

Radiofrequency (RF) ablation has become an accepted treatment option for focal primary and secondary malignancies in a wide range of organs including the liver, lung, kidney, bone, and adrenal glands. The largest experience has been for hepatic malignancies, where long-term outcomes similar to surgical resection have been reported in some matched patient populations. Benefits of minimally invasive, image-guided RF ablation include reduced cost and morbidity compared to standard surgical resection, and the ability to treat patients who are not surgical candidates. However, limitations in ablative efficacy exist, including persistent growth of residual tumor at the ablation margin, the inability to treat larger tumors, and variability in complete treatment based upon tumor location. Extensive investigations into potential strategies to improve ablation outcomes continue and focus on technological development of ablative systems, improving ablative predictability and combining RF ablation with other kinds of treatments such as chemotherapy and radiation. Given the potential complexity of treatment types and paradigms in oncology and the wider application of thermal ablation techniques, an understanding of their basic principles provides comprehensive clinical perspectives.

One electrode or multiple electrodes are placed within the center of the tumor by percutaneous puncture for high-temperature tissue heating, for which two specific mechanisms account. One is energy-tissue interaction. Electrode delivers radiofrequency current to the local foci causing ion agitation and heat generation. Thermal conduction, the other mechanism, allows for the lethal high-temperature to diffuse to the surrounding tissue inducing irreversible cell injury, which occurs at around 50 ℃. The basic pathologic change is coagulation necrosis encompassing protein coagulation of cytoplasm and mitochondrial enzymes, along with nucleic acid-histone protein complexes, which may give rise to a delayed cell death over a duration of a few days. Meanwhile, incorporation of adjuvant therapies, for instance chemotherapy, are also deployed to increase uniformity of cell death around the sublethal hyperthermic zone.

15.3.2.6 High-intensity focused ultrasound

Ultrasound is most widely known for its imaging capabilities, however, the passage of ultrasound through tissue can lead to biological changes that can be reversible or irreversible. The biological significance of these effects depends to a large extent on the energy in the ultrasound beam and the goal of the exposure. For theraputic high intensity focused ultrasound(HIFU), these effects are divided into two aspects. Tissues will absorb part of the ultrasound energy which leads to localized temperature rising that are required to achieve immediate thermal necrosis. Non-thermal effects or mechanical effects are those arising either from the formation and activity of the micron-sized bubbles in the field(acoustic cavitation) or from the flow of fluids that are induced by ultrasound pressure wave(acoustic streaming).

The principle behind HIFU treatments is very simple. Just as sunlight can be brought into a tight focus using a magnifying glass and used to light a dry leaf or a piece of paper, ultrasonic can be focused, resulting in energy concentration in the focal region which may be sufficient to induce immediate cell death. The focused ultrasound beam is produced by a transducer capable of delivering high power. This may use a lens to shape the beam, a shaped crystal, a phased array, or a combination of these. The transducer parameter determines the shape and position of the focal volume. The HIFU treatment destroys only tissues lying within the focal region, leaving surrounding tissues undamaged, forming a "trackless lesion"-region of coagulative necrosis. It has been demonstrated by histology that the margin between live and dead cells is very sharp. HIFU thus offers the potential to selectively destroy tissue targets at depth without damaging of overlying structures.

15.3.2.7 Microwave ablation

Microwave ablation is one of the several options in the ablation armamentarium for the treatment of malignancy, offering several potential benefits when compared with other ablation, radiation, surgical and medical treatment modalities. The basic microwave system consists of the generator, power distribution system and antennas. Often under image (computed tomography or ultrasound) guidance, a needle-like antenna is inserted percutaneously into the tumor, where local microwave electromagnetic radiation is emitted from the probe's active tip, producing frictional tissue heating, capable of causing cell death by coagulation necrosis. Half of the microwave ablation systems use a 915 MHz generator and the other half use a 2,450 MHz generator.

The mechanism lies in heat generating effect of dipole molecules rotating. Within in biological tissues, charged ions with ion vibration such as potassium ions, sodium ions, chloride ions, and polar molecules with polarization and rotation such as water molecules and protein molecules, will rub against each other in the changing electromagnetic fields, consequently resulting in fast local temperature rise, where at 54 °C for 1min or 60 °C almost at once coagulation of the tumor tissue will be achieved.

15.3.2.8 Irreversible electroporation ablation

Currently, most of the energy sources used in a focal manner utilize a thermal effect to destroy tumor tissue: cryotherapy uses temperatures below −40 °C HIFU therapy uses temperatures above 60 °C. Thermal tissue destruction may have some drawbacks. First, it is non-selective towards the different structures (nerves, stroma, vasculature, glands) and collateral damage could still occur. Second, especially with high temperatures, the heat-sink effect of intra-and extra-tumor vessels (which can dissipate the energy) can lead to under-treatment. Third, the precision required to treat an area of tumor to sometimes within millimeter accuracy may be lacking. New technologies in the field might combine better cancer control outcomes with enhanced tissue preservation.

Irreversible electroporation ablation, also called nanoknife, is a promising new technology. By using high voltage direct electric current, IRE permanently damages the cell membrane with nanopores which give rise to cell death and/or apoptosis with no thermal effect. IRE has been used for the treatment of localized and metastatic tumors in solid organ malignancies such as kidney, liver, pancreas and lung. It has some potential advantages that might lend itself to wider use. First, the tissue outside the electrical field is theoretically not compromised since there is no effect in those areas. Second, the treatment has shown tissue-selectivity in pre-clinical studies, so that collagenous structures such as vessels, nerves and some anatomical tracts like pancreatic duct, bile duct, ureter, urethra, etc. , seem not to be affected.

15.3.2.9   Chemical ablation

Percutaneous chemical ablation is a relatively safe and effective procedure used in the treatment of small confined tumors. It is well tolerated by patients and has very low reported major and minor complication rates (2%). Although the technique requires adequate expertise in placing the needle with imaging guidance, the procedure is simple and does not require any specialized equipment, except multi-side-hole needle if one chooses. Chemical agents for percutaneous ablation include ethanol, acetic acid, and sodium hydroxide. Percutaneous ethanol injection (PEI) is well established and the most commonly used chemical ablation technique. However, due to multiple session numbers, high local tumor progression rate, and variable ablation zone in PEI compared with radiofrequency (RF) ablation, the use of PEI is now limited to situations when RF ablation should not be performed, such as when the tumor is in close proximity to large vessels or critical organs. In one study evaluating the treatment of small HCC, RF ablation demonstrated an approximately 20% higher survival rate at 3–4 years and fewer treatment sessions than PEI in three randomized controlled trials. The basic mechanism of action of ethanol is through cytoplasmic dehydration, denaturation of cellular proteins, and microvascular thrombosis. These changes eventually result in coagulation necrosis of tumor tissue.

15.3.2.10   Radioactive seeds implantation

Radioactive seeds implantation, which is a form of brachytherapy, can be performed repeatedly. It has been successfully applied for treating inoperable solitary tumors for nearly 100 years. In the early days, high-energy radioactive isotopes such as Radium-226 and Cobalt-60, were used in such treatment. These radioactive nuclides release γ-rays with relatively high penetration, bringing radiologists great difficulties in protection, thus severe radioactive injuries should possibly happen. And restricted by experience and technology, whether proper preprocedure scheme or precise image guidance could not be achieved. All of these factors contribute to build a blockade on the way of its wide clinical application. Benefit from development of material science and physics, new low-energy radioactive isotopes like Iodine-125 and Palladium-103 were developed and have been used in therapy with problematic guidance solved by CT and US, radioactive seeds implantation once more gets promising potential.

Clinically, brachytherapy using Iodine-125 seed implantation is capable of delivering a sufficient dose of radiation to the tumor mass. The seeds implanted in the target lesion gradually release γ-rays with low-energy and soft X-rays, the former lead to direct ionization of DNA chains in the tumor cell nucleus, while X-rays cause indirection ionization of the DNA chains by intermediary reactive oxygen radicals. The advantages are obvious: ①the radioactive particles are distributed to the target region in a highly conformal way; ②sustained energy application;③shorter shot-range (about 1.7 cm) with less radiation exposure to surrounding tissues. Given the noticeable benefits to patients, radioactive seeds implantation has been accepted in the treatment of prostate cancer, pancreatic cancer and head and neck cancer. However, in many recurrent and metastatic lung cancers, important organs, large vessels, or bone structures often block the pathway to the lesions, making these tumors inaccessible to needle puncture, and leading to an unsatisfactory distribution of the implanted iodine-125 seeds. In addition, brachytherapy would become very risky when conducting implantation in metastatic lymph nodes located near the mediastinal macrovascular area.

15.3.3 Complications

A brief introduction of common complications.

15.3.3.1 Restenosis and stent-induced perforation

Restenosis is almost inevitable in the luminal stenosis caused by local tumor oppression, which has already been treated with dilation and stent implantation, as this kind of treatment is often used in palliative care, in which systemic anti-cancer therapy has failed and tumor's continuous growth cannot be stopped. Stent-induced perforation in esophagus, bile duct, ureter could lead to serious infection, namely infectious peritonitis, in case of delayed diagnosis as it is not that prevalent and often confused with other complications under the circumstance of advanced stage. Thus, it is not an unnecessary thing for us to be cautious all the time.

15.3.3.2 Pneumothorax

Pneumothorax is a commonplace in the biopsy diagnosis and ablation treatment of lung malignances, techniques which include percutaneous needle biopsy, cryoablation, radiofrequency ablation, microwave ablation and so on. Needle-like probes or electrodes or antennas are employed to pierce into the foci in the lung. When the patient used to be a heavy smoker or at a senior age or have a bad pulmonary function, the odds for pneumothorax increase dominantly. In general, the air could be absorbed without any treatment in the mild case, but closed drainage of pleural cavity is needed for the serious one.

15.3.3.3 Visceral hemorrhage

Visceral hemorrhage happens at times when puncture-associated treatments including various ablations and percutaneous needle biopsy are applied to internal organs. Reasons accounting for this and corresponding clinical presentations vary as the bleeding site changes. Usually, it presents as hemoptysis in the lung, and the severity changes from mild spitting with little blood to fatal asphyxia, which is decided by bleeding volume. Bleeding in the abdominal cavity takes place while liver or kidney is punctured. It's rare but sometimes fatal. Another common situation is upper gastrointestinal tract ulcer and thus bleeding due to stress. Reasonable and timely measures from careful nursing and medicine application to even stopping bleeding by surgery should be taken in case of sudden deterioration.

15.3.3.4 Postablation syndrome

Clinical presentations include fever (under 38.5 ℃), weakness, overall feeling of discomfort, nausea, vomiting, etc. These discomforts usually sustain for 3–5 days. The wider the ablation zone is, the longer the discomforts last. It is noteworthy that if the temperature rises above 38.5 ℃, we should take the hazards of post-surgery infection into consideration.

15.3.3.5 Transcoelomic metastasis

Tumor cells could be implanted along the pathway of puncture, either within the abdominal wall or in the peritoneum cavity. But it's rare to see. Repeated puncture of the tumor, insufficient ablation of puncture pathway (relative low temperature below lethal threshold or retreating the needle too fast), or ablation within pneumoperitoneum all contribute to implantation metastasis.

15.4 Integrated therapy

To date, it is appreciated during the procedure of tumor treatment schedule design that life quality lies at least the same importance to survival. Simply applying one kind method of minimally invasive treatment hardly brings satisfying treatment effects for cancer patients. Integrated therapy that synthesizes several kinds of techniques makes it easier to get prolonged survival on account of less impairment and better effect. So, it is of vital importance to grab the basic principles and clinical ongoing schedules so as toget an illustration of possible development orientation and trend of minimally invasive treatment.

15.4.1 Sequentially combined therapy

Several kinds of minimally invasive therapies are applied to cancer patients in a specially organized spacial-temporal way with the aim both of treating tumors and protecting normal physiological function to the best extend. Taking the interventional treatment of primary hepatocellular carcinoma for example, TACE with subsequent ablation therapy greatly improves the 5-years survival of HCC, which now has been a standard treatment. The advantage lies in the complementarity of the two methods. Firstly, TACE could block the blood supply of the tumor, which reduces the "heat-sink" effect that possibly leads to an inefficient ablation of the tumor margin. Secondly, TACE alone sometimes could not achieve complete necrosis of the whole lesion, but a subsequent ablation can inactivate the residual tumor. Thirdly, embolization material like iodized oil could deposit on the local foci and get the tumor labled, which guides deployment of ablation devices.

15.4.2 Precisely guided therapy

As previously mentioned, minimally invasive therapy is technically based on thequickly developing modern medical imaging sciences. For example, HIFU ablation with real time monitoring necrosis range of the treating region has been brought into reality by MRI guidance. Functional imaging by PET/CT with high spatial resolution is of high diagnostic value for metastatic disease, which is also commonly used for guiding the targeted ablation with an accuracy of nearly 90% –100%. It could not be denied that modern medical imaging technologies including US, CT, MRI, etc. have been the indispensable "eye" guiding precisely targeted treatment of minimally invasive therapy, which build the basis of advantages over tradition methods including surgery and intravenous chemotherapy.

15.4.3 Biology and immune therapy

Biology and immune therapy might be the most promising therapy for cancer treatment in the near future. So it is of vital importance to realize the part it plays among all the treatment instruments. If it is properly used as a complementary medicine during the treating course, better efficacy longer survival and less harm could be anticipated. The main aim of biology and immune therapy is to eliminate micrometastatic foci that is invisible on imaging and those circulating tumor cells. Minimally invasive therapy followed by biology and immune therapy could maximally reduce tumor burden with immune function protected and activated, thus results in a lower rate of local relapse and longer survival without disease progression.

In conclusion, minimally invasive therapy is at a juxtaposition to internal medicine and surgery in clinical oncology and is a promising subject, which is taking its due responsibility and doing its due contribution on the journey of fighting against cancers.

Li Quanwang, Ma Longfei

Chapter 16

Molecular Targeted Therapy For Cancer and Precision Medicine

How to distinguish tumor cells from normal cells in treatment is always the direction of oncology exploration. With the development in the field of molecular biology technology and cytogenetics, the molecular mechanisms of the occurrence, invasion, diffusion and metastasis of cancer have been further recognized, and some protein molecules that play a key role in this process have been discovered. With the protein molecules as the target of attack, some molecular targeted agents have been developed to specifically inhibit cancer cell proliferation, promote cancer cell apoptosis. Within recent 10 years, more and more molecular targeted agents aimed at different target were used in cancer treatment, rapidly expanding the field of drug therapy of cancer, promoting the development of the concept and theory of cancer treatment.

16.1 Molecular targeted therapy for cancer

16.1.1 Definition of molecular targeted therapy

Molecular targeted therapy refers to the treatment modality targeting the cell signal transduction and other biological pathways involved in cancer development. Generalized molecular targets, include the molecule participating in cancer cell differentiation, cell cycle, apoptosis, migration, aggressive behavior, lymphatic metastasis and systemic metastasis process, from DNA to protein and enzyme level.

16.1.2 Characteristics of molecular targeted therapy

16.1.2.1 High selectivity

Completely different from traditional cytotoxic anticancer drugs widely used in more than 50 years, molecular targeted agents are not a role in cancer cell DNA, RNA or protein macromolecules, but specifically targeting tumorigenesis, development, proliferation, diffusion, and transfer related protein micro-molecules, with generally higher selectivity. Molecular targeted drugs against targets including cancer gene, tumor-suppressor genes, growth factor and its receptor, angiogenesis factor, protein kinases and signal transduction pathways, ubiquitin regulatory factors and cell membrane differentiation related antigen.

16.1.2.2　Broad source

Molecular targeted drugs can come from a small molecular compound, artificially modified monoclonal antibodies, the monoclonal antibodies coupled radionuclides and toxins, antisense oligonucleotides, as well as natural products from plants and Marine life, etc. With the further development of molecular biology, it is believed that the new targets and new molecular targeted drugs will appear continuously, and the prospect is very wide.

16.1.2.3　Unique efficacy

According to the existing clinical study, the molecular targeted drugs have good effect for certain types of cancer such as chronic myelogenous leukemia (CML), gastrointestinal stromal tumor, B cell lymphomas, breast cancer, lung cancer; have visible benefits for certain refractory cancer with cytotoxic anticancer drug such as liver cancer, kidney cancer, fully shows that the molecular targeted drugs have strong vitality.

16.1.2.4　Less toxic

Although cytotoxic drugs can effectively kill tumor cells, due to the poor targeting, they can damage the normal metabolic cells of the body, resulting in a series of toxic reactions. Molecular targeted therapy can selectively affect the molecules associated with cancer cells and reduce the degree of toxicity. Most of the molecular targeted drugs do not produce significant bone marrow suppression and gastrointestinal reactions, such as nausea and vomiting, which are common in cytotoxic chemotherapy. Therefore, it can be combined with conventional chemotherapy and radiotherapy. However, special adverse reactions should be noted, such as edema, rashes, interstitial pneumonia, hypertension, gastrointestinal perforation, bleeding, etc.

16.1.2.5　Tumor molecular markers are important

Because of a particular gene or protein may be expressed in different tumor tissues, or the same tumor has different gene or protein expression, applied molecular targeted drugs has certain patients and tumor molecular markers are the key.

16.1.3　Classification of molecular targeted drugs

Molecular targeted drugs are mainly divided into two groups: monoclonal antibodies (mAbs) and small molecular compounds.

16.1.3.1　Monoclonal antibodies

Anti-tumor monoclonal antibodies are usually water-soluble and have large molecules (generally about 150,000), so that cannot penetrate the cell membrane. The antigen binding fragment (Fab) of monoclonal antibody can be specifically identified and combined with antigens, with highly specific targeting. The main role of monoclonal antibodies in treatment is to specifically bind the extracellular components of the membrane receptor (for example, ligand), to block the specific cell proliferation signal of the receptor, such as the vascular endothelial growth factor (VEGF) antibody and the monoclonal antibody of B cell membrane surface antigen CD20.

The birth of monoclonal antibody drugs is the result of comprehensive development of immune technology and genetic engineering technology. Initial monoclonal antibodies were produced by the target antigen in mice, but at that time antibody has strong immunogenicity because of animal origin. When the mouse protein composition is applied to the human body, the human body is at risk of allergic reaction, and also produces human anti-mouse antibody (HAMA). It is easy to be eliminated by the body's immune mechanism, neutralizing the role of therapeutic antibodies. So, it is necessary to "humanize" the antibody to reduce its immunogenicity. Humanization is the process of replacing the molecular structure of non-human antibodies with the molecular structure of human antibodies as much as possible through genetic engineering.

(1) Nomenclature

The current clinical application of monoclonal antibody, retain only monoclonal antibody to specific part in mice, increased the proportion of the amount of human antibody proteins by adopting genetic engineering technology.

Monoclonal antibodies that are derived entirely frommurine gene sequences contain the syllabus "-o" (for example, tositumomab). Chimeric Monoclonal antibodies containing 65% of human elements are named as "-xi" (for example, rituximab). Humanized mAbs containing 95% human composition are named as "-zu" (for example, trastuzumab). Those fully humanize dantibodies containing 100% of human composition are named as "-mu" (for example, panitumumab).

(2) Classification

According to the target molecule of monoclonal antibody, there are currently several kinds as follows.

1) Monoclonal antibodies acting on the human epidermal growth factor receptor (HER/erbB) family

There are four members of HER family, namely HER1 (EGFR/erbB1), HER2 (neu/erbB2), HER3 (erbB3) and HER4(erbB4). They are highly homologous and have similar structures, and the biological effect is cell proliferation and differentiation when the signal transduction is initiated by combining with the corresponding different ligands.

Cetuximab (Erbitus, C225) is a chimeric IgG1 monoclonal antibody anti-EGFR, clinical single-agent or joint with chemotherapy as first-line or second-line treatment of advanced metastatic colorectal cancer, and the joint with radiotherapy or chemotherapy as the treatment of advanced head and neck squamous cell carcinomas.

Panitumumab (Vectibix) is a monoclonal antibody to the whole human sequence and is currently used as a third-line drug to treat advanced metastatic colorectal cancer. Transtuzumab (Herceptin) is a humanized IgG1 monoclonal antibody, which mainly treats HER2 overexpression of breast cancer (including advanced metastatic breast cancer and adjuvant therapy after radical surgery). In addition, another recombinant humanized anti-EGFR monoclonal antibody called nimotuzumab has also been listed in China for the treatment of nasopharyngeal carcinoma, head and neck squamous cell carcinoma and pancreatic cancer.

2) Monoclonal antibody inhibiting tumor angiogenesis

Tumor growth and metastasis must have the formation of new blood vessels. Vascular endothelial growth factor (VEGF) is the key to promote angiogenesis, and plays biology role after combination with its corresponding receptors that vascular endothelial growth factor receptor (VEGFR). VEGF is often excessively expressed in tumor tissues. A synthetic recombinant humanized IgG1 monoclonal antibody bevacizumab (Avastin) can specifically be combined with VEGF, preventing VEGF combined with vascular endothelial cell surface VEGFR, thereby blocking the supply of blood, oxygen and other essential nutrients which are critical to tumor growth, delaying tumor growth and metastasis. Bevacizumab has been approved for first-line treatment in metastatic colorectal cancer and second-line treatment of non-small cell lung cancer (NSCLC). In addition, the world's first endothelial statin anti-tumor agent developed in China, Endostar (human recombinant endostatin, YH-16) prevent the formation of new blood vessels by inhibiting the formation of the migration of vascular endothelial cells. Endostar can be used for the initial or recurrent advanced non-small cell lung cancer.

3) monoclonal antibody targeting the cluster of differentiation

Different tissue cell surface has different cluster of differentiation (CD). With the target of CD20, combined human mouse chimeric monoclonal antibody rituxan (rituximab, MabThera) is used to treat cancers which are expressing CD20, such as B cell non-hodgkin's lymphoma, chronic lymphocytic leukemia, hairy cell leukemia, etc. After combined with CD20 on B lymphocyte, rituxan led to dissolving B cell immune response, including antibody-dependent cell-mediated cytotoxicity (ADCC) and complement dependent cytotoxicity (CDC). Alemtuzumab (Campath), a humanized monoclonal antibody that targets CD52, can be used to develop chronic lymphoma leukemia and non-hodgkin's lymphoma of CD52 positive for alkylation agent and fludarabine resistance.

16.1.3.2　Small molecule compound

Small molecule drugs can penetrate cell membranes and work with the target molecules inside the cells. The research and development process of small molecule drugs and monoclonal antibodies are different. Small molecule drugs research and development process is mainly for large compound screening and optimization, the first thing is to filter one of the most effective compounds interacting with its target molecules in the tens of thousands of compounds, thereafter, chemical modification and re-screening of the selected compounds may finally lead to preclinical studies.

Generally, the structure of small molecule inhibitor is relatively simple, synthesized by chemical method. Small molecule inhibitors are mostly administered by oral administration without intravenous injection. After entering human body, it is mainly metabolized by liver cytochrome P450 enzyme, which can interact with other drugs that interfere with P450 enzyme. The specific targeting of these drugs is weaker than monoclonal antibodies. Currently used small molecule compounds mainly include the following aspects.

(1)Tyrosine kinase inhibitor

Tyrosine kinase (TK) is a set of enzymes phosphorylating amino acid residues, TK activated molecular signaling can result in normal and malignant tissue cell growth, proliferation, migration and angiogenesis, is one of the important ways in cellular signal transduction network. Tyrosine kinase inhibitor(TKI) inhibits the proliferation of tumor cells by blocking intracellular tyrosine kinase signaling pathway.

Imatinib (Gleevec) blocks ATP binding to BCR/ABLPTK and prevents PTK activation. Because CML is associated with BCR/ABL fusion protein encoded by the BCR/ABL fusion gene resulting from the Ph chromosome, imatinib became the first molecular targeted drug to treat cancer, and the treatment of CML was very significant. Later, imatinib was found that also inhibits protocarcinogenic gene product, KIT expressing CD117 or platelet derivation growth factor (PDGF) tyrosine kinase. Treatment of gastrointestinal stromal tumor (GIST) expressing CD117 and PDGF with imatinib also showed obvious curative effect. The newly developed BCR-ABL TKI, nilotinib (enact, AMN107) inhibited the activity of BCR-ABL, which could be used to treat CML patients with imatinib resistance.

Targets to the epidermal growth factor receptor tyrosine kinase inhibitor (EGFR-TKI) include gefitinib and erlotinib (Tarceva), both of which have been allowed for advanced metastatic non-small-cell lung cancer with failure of chemotherapy treatment. Erotinib can also treat advanced pancreatic cancer.

(2)Multiple targets kinase inhibitors

Sorafenib (Nexava) can not only inhibit the RAF-1, B-RAF serine/threonine kinase, but also inhibit a variety of receptor tyrosine kinases, such as VEGFR-2, VEGFR-3, PDFG-β, KIT, FLT-3, with dual antitumor activity of blocking RAF/MER/ERK-mediated signal transduction pathway and inhibiting tumor angiogenesis formation. Sorafenib has significant survival benefit as first-line treatment for advanced metastatic renal carcinoma and primary liver cancer.

Sunitinib (sutent) can block the VEGFR and PDGFR signal transduction pathway, blocking intracellular signal transduction, inhibiting tumor cell proliferation. At the same time, there is a strong anti-tumor angiogenesis effect. This drug has been approved for advanced renal cell carcinoma and gastrointestinal stromal tumors that are not effective for imatinib.

Dasatinib (sprycel) can inhibit the BCR-ABL SRC kinase family, and other kinases such as c-KIT、E-PHA2 and PDGF-R. Dasatinib can be used clinically for various phases CML of imatinib resistance (chronic, accelerated and acute phases), And Ph⁺ ALL adult patients who could not tolerate chemotherapy.

Lapatinib (Tykerb) can inhibit intracellular ATP locus of HER-1 (EHGFR) and HER2, inactivate tyrosine kinase phosphorylation, and block intracellular signal transduction. Lapatinib can be used for the treatment of advanced breast cancer with trastuzumab resistence, which has a preventive effect on breast cancer brain metastasis.

(3) Small molecular compounds of other targets

Bortezomin (Velcade) is an ubiquitin-proteasome inhibitor. Proteasome is responsible for the degradation of most proteins in cells including cell cycle regulation proteins and apoptotic proteins. Proteasome inhibitor has the effect of inducing apoptosis and sensitization of radiotherapy and chemotherapy. This drug is used to treat patients with multiple myeloma and refractory lymphoma.

Mammalian target of rapamycin (mTOR) is a kind of serine/threonine protein kinase, responsible for the transmission of cell proliferation signal and cell cycle, and regulates cell division and growth. Temsirolimus(CCI-779) is a mTOR inhibitor, inhibiting mTOR kinase activity, blocking the progression of cell cycle from G1 to S phase, and has been approved for the treatment of advanced metastatic renal carcinoma, mantle cell lymphoma (MCL) and metastatic breast cancer. Similar drug Everlimus (certican, RAD001) can be taken orally and combined with chemotherapy for non-small cell lung cancer, melanoma, rectal cancer, pancreatic cancer, etc.

Insulin-like growth factor receptor (IGF-IR) combined with its corresponding ligands or IGF-I, mediated by receptor related tyrosine kinase, activateintracellular multiple signal transduction pathways, promote cell growth and enhance cell survival ability to adapt. IGF-IR kinase inhibitors, such as NVP-AEW541, are clinically tested in breast cancer, prostate cancer, multiple myeloma, pancreatic cancer, and colon cancer.

Histonedeacetylase (HDAC) was involved in cell cycle regulation and apoptosis. HDAC inhibitors such as vorinostat (zolinza) inhibit HDACI, HDAC2, HDAC3 and HDAC6, and promote histone acetylation, so as to unscrew the DNA in chromatin, open the chromatin structure, and promote the activation of gene transduction. In vitro studies reveal that HDAC can induce cell cycle suspension and apoptosis. HDAC are approved for treatment of cutaneous T-cell lymphoma with progression and recurrence after two treatment regimens.

Molecular targeted drugs provide a new idea for the treatment of cancer systemic drugs, but the current level is not omnipotent and should not be blindly used. In clinical use, it is necessary to have a strict understanding of the indications, which can be considered in combination with cytotoxic drugs, with special attention to individualized selection, and some drugs may produce serious and even life-threatening toxicity.

16.1.4 Clinical application strategy of molecular targeted drugs

16.1.4.1 Molecular targeted drug single drug application

At present, most of the molecular targeted drugs have limited objective effect when applied alone, but there are new breakthroughs in the treatment of some cancers, which can improve the quality of life and prolong the survival period. Small molecule compounds tyrosine kinase inhibitor treat traditional chemotherapy resistance of cancers, such as Glivec for the treatment of gastrointestinal stromal tumor, sorafenib for the treatment of renal cell carcinoma (TARGET test) and hepatocellular carcinoma (SHARP test), etc.; EGFR tyrosine kinase inhibitors were used for second-line treatment of non-small cell lung cancer such as gefitinib and erlotinib; compared with traditional chemotherapy, the curative effect was similar, and the adverse reactions were decreased, such as gefitinib for the second-line treatment of NSCLC (Interest clinical trial). The IPASS clinical trial of non-small cell lung cancer revealed that EGFR TKI could be used to treat NSCLC patients with EGFR mutations as first-line treatment.

16.1.4.2   Molecular targeted drugs combined with radiotherapy

Experimental results showed that EGFR overexpression decreased tumor susceptibility to radiation therapy, application of EGFR TKI (gefitinib) or EGFR monoclonal antibody (cetuximab) can enhance tumor susceptibility to radiotherapy in animal study. Clinical trials are ongoing; anti-angiogenesis can rebuild disorder of vascular network in tumor, make the structure, function of normalizing, improve local blood circulation, reduce tumor interstitial pressure, and improve the effect of local oxygen partial pressure; other studies have shown that radiotherapy can increase VEGF expression, generate radiation resistance, and support the need for combination of radiotherapy and anti-angiogenesis therapy.

16.1.4.3   Molecular targeted drugs combined with chemotherapy

Currently, this is the main method for the clinical application of anti-EGFR monoclonal antibodies and anti-angiogenesis drugs, which can improve the objective curative effect of cancer therapy and prolong the survival period. In the treatment of colorectal cancer, breast cancer, non-small cell lung cancer and multiple myeloma, it has achieved encouraging effect: herceptin combined with chemotherapy to treat breast cancer; bevacizumab combined with chemotherapy for NSCLC (E4599 and AVAiL trial); Cetuximab combined with chemotherapy for NSCLC (FLEX test); bevacizumab combined with chemotherapy for colorectal cancer and breast cancer (E3200 and E2100); cetuximab combined with chemotherapy for colorectal cancer (CRYSTAL and OPUS test); in addition, small molecule anti-EGFR tyrosine kinase inhibitor and chemotherapy need further study.

16.1.4.4   Molecular targeted drugs combination application

For example, bevacizumab combined with a small molecule EGFR inhibitor (erlotinib) for joint application, showing strong tumor growth inhibition effect, it showed an objective curative effect of 20% for second-line treatment in non-small cell lung cancer. However, the combination of bevacizumab and sunitinib, both of which are anti-VEGF drugs, aggravate the side effects and the clinical trials were stopped.

16.1.4.5   Clinical application of multi-target drugs

Some tyrosine kinase inhibitors have been found to have multiple anti-tumor targets, such as sunitinib and sorafenib. The effect of sorafenib is on EGFR and VEGF and is effective in the treatment of metastatic renal cell carcinoma and hepatocellular carcinoma. Lapatinib is a target for EGFR and HER2, and has achieved good results in the treatment of HER2 positive metastatic breast cancer that resistant to trastuzumab. Sunitinib works on PDGF, VEGF and Kit, with good results for the treatment of metastatic renal cell carcinoma, and GIST that resistant to imatinib.

16.1.4.6   Low dose rhythmic chemotherapy

Folkman, puts forward the concept of low dose rhythmic chemotherapy, namely anti-cancer drugs given in the form of low dose short interval. For mice bearing solid tumor, this anti-angiogenesis scheme inhibited the apoptosis of endothelial cells and tumor growth in tumors. There are two possible mechanisms to explain the anti-angiogenesis of low-dose continuous chemotherapy. The first one is the direct pathway, that is, the activation and differentiation of endothelial cells is essentially sensitive to low-dose chemotherapy, and so may the original endothelial cells in the circulation. The second one is indirect pathway that the concentration of low dose rhythmic chemotherapy drug is too low, cannot cause endothelial cell growth retardation or apoptosis, but induced endogenous angiogenesis inhibiting molecules in these cells. The molecules played in a role, which is inhibiting tumor angiogenesis and shrinking tumor.

16.1.5 The efficacy of molecular targeted drugs

Molecular targeted therapy plays an important role in the treatment of cancer in the past 20 years, and the two most important targeted therapies are antibody drugs and small molecule kinase inhibitors. So far, the FDA has approved 45 antitumor targeted drugs, including 19 monoclonal antibodies and 26 kinase inhibitors. Their names, indications, targets, general side effects and severe side effects were introduced in detail.

Clinicians need to know not only adopting what kind of targeted therapy and its clinical significance, but also need to know about the side effects and impact of these targeted therapies on patients' quality of life, the treatment cost, especially how to give the judgement of the end-of-life care at the right time.

In view of the above issues, Nature Reviews has recently written a summary and guidline for clinicians and other related professionals on the treatment of patients with malignant diseases. Details are as follows.

The efficacy of targeted drugs is closely related to the ability to accurately identify the important target molecules associated with tumor cell proliferation and survival. For example, most chronic myeloid leukemia (CML) occurs ralated with t (9;22) chromosomal abnormalities, which make the partial ABL gene on chromosome 9 fuse with the BCR gene on chromosome 22. ABL gene encoding protein—ABL, is an important signal molecule to regulate cell proliferation. The gene fusion of BCR-ABL enables ABL molecules with tyrosine kinase activity to be continuously active, leading to the continuous proliferation of granulocytes and the occurrence of CML. BCR-ABL is the key molecule of cancerous cells, small molecular targeted drug mesylate imatinib can specifically suppress the tyrosine kinase activity of BCR-ABL, so has significant curative effect on CML, making more than 90% of the patients with CML clinical hematology relief and 60% cytogenetics relief.

The efficacy of targeted drugs is related to whether cancer cells have a suitable target. For example, tyrosine kinase inhibitor of EGFR, gefitinib, has become one of the major treatment options for advanced non-small cell lung cancer. But gefitinib has an effective rate of nearly 80% in patients with EGFR mutations and very low effective rate in patients with no mutation. Similarly, anti-angiogenic drugs are more effective in renal clear cell carcinoma, hepatocellular carcinoma, and thyroid cancer with rich blood supply.

Molecular targeted drugs are therapies aiming at targets, even tumors with different pathological types may be effective as long as there are corresponding targets. For example, anti-EGFR monoclonal antibody, which has been confirmed effective in partial head and neck squamous cell carcinomas, colorectal cancer, and non-small cell lung cancer, because EGFR has expression in most tumors of epithelial origin. For example, BCR-ABL tyrosine kinase inhibitor imatinib, has the specific inhibitory effect of c-Kit kinase activity, therefore, its treatment efficiency can reach more than 80% for gastrointestinal stromal tumor harboring c-Kit kinase mutations, while the traditional cytotoxic drugs for this type of tumor is generally invalid. It can be seen that individualized treatment targeting specific target is the development direction of future medical treatment(Table 16-1, Table 16-2).

Table 16-1   Overview of 19 FDA-approved mAbs for cancer treatment

Drug	Approved indications	Common adverse events	Serious adverse effects	Target
Ado-trastuzumab emtansine (*Kadcyla*)	Metastatic HER2 over-expressing breast cancer	Nausea, vomiting, diarrhoea, constipation, fatigue, cytopenias, hepatotoxicity, hypokalemia, hypertension, headaches, musculo-skeletal pain, epistaxis	Hepatotoxicity, left ventricular cardiac dysfunction, embryo-fetal death or birth defects	Extracellular domain of HER2
Alemtuzumab (*Campath*)	B cell CLL	Myelosuppression, cytopenias, hypotension, respiratory infections, fever, chills, rash, headache	Cardiac arrhythmias, cardiomyopathy, CHF, autoimmune diseases, Grave's disease, CMV-and/or EBV infections, increased risk of secondary malignancies	CD52 on T and B lymphocytes
Bevacizumab (*Avastin*)	Metastatic CRC, RCC and NSCLC. Platinum-resistant, recurrent epithelial ovarian, fallopian tube, or primary peritoneal cancer. Cervical cancer. GBM	Abdominal pain, nausea, vomiting, diarrhoea, constipation, headaches, hypertension, proteinuria, asthenia, upper respiratory infections	Hypertension, thromboembolic events, hemorrhages, bowel perforation, wound dehiscence	VEGF
Blinatumomab (*Blincyto*)	Philadelphia chromosome-negative relapsed/refractory B cell precursor ALL	Fever, cytopenias, nausea, constipation	Cytokine release syndrome, neurologic toxicities, neutropenic fever, sepsis	Bispecific: CD19 on B lymphocytes and CD3 on T lymphocytes
Brentuximab vedotin (*Adcetris*)	Relapsed/refractory Hodgkin and anaplastic large T cell lymphomas	Sensory neuropathy, cytopenias, diarrhoea, nausea, vomiting, rash, cough, fatigue	Supraventricular cardiac arrhythmias, pneumonitis, pneumothorax, pulmonary embolism, PML	CD30. The microtubule disrupting component MMAE binds to tubulin
Cetuximab (*Erbitux*)	Metastatic *KRAS* negative CRC; SCCHN	Acneiform rash, alopecia, pruritis; hypomagnesemia; diarrhoea, nausea, constipation, insomnia; depression (especially in patients receiving irinotecan), sensory neuropathy	Sudden cardiac death, renal failure, interstitial lung disease, pulmonary embolism, infusion reactions	EGFR
Denosumab (*Xgeva*)	Unresectable giant cell tumor of the bone	Arthralgia, headache, diarrhoea, nausea, vomiting, back pain, fatigue, and pain in the extremity	Osteonecrosis of the jaw, osteomyelitis	RANK ligand

Continue to Table 16–1

Drug	Approved indications	Common adverse events	Serious adverse effects	Target
Ibritumomab tiuxetan (*Zevalin*)	Relapsed/refractory non-Hodgkin lymphomas (NHL)	Hypertension, cytopenias; rash, abdominal pain, diarrhoea, nausea	Infusion reactions, severe cytopenia, with haemorrhage, Stevens-Johnson syndrome, toxic epidermal necrolysis, increased risk of myelodysplasia and AML	CD20. Tiuxetan is a chelator and binds to Ytrium-90
Ipilimumab (*Yervoy*)	Unresectable or metastatic malignant melanoma	Rash, pruritus, diarrhoea, fatigue	Pericarditis, adrenal insufficiency, hypopituitarism, hypothyroidism, intestinal perforation, enterocolitis, hepatitis, pneumonitis, Guillain-Barré syndrome	CTLA4
Nivolumab (*Opdivo*)	Unresectable or metastatic malignant melanoma unresponsive to other drugs. Metastatic squamous NSCLC	Rash, pruritus, electrolyte derangements, transaminitis, cough, upper respiratory tract infections, oedema	Immune-mediated colitis, hepatitis, nephritis or pneumonitis	PD1
Obinutuzumab (*Gazyva*)	Previously untreated CLL (in combination with chlorambucil)	Cytopenias, fever, cough, musculoskeletal disorders	Hepatitis B virus reactivation, PML	CD20
Ofatumumab (*Arzerra*)	Refractory CLL. Previously untreated CLL (in combination with chlorambucil)	Rash, diarrhoea, nausea, anaemia, pneumonia, fatigue, fever	Bowel obstruction, viral hepatitis, infectious diseases, PML	CD20
Panitumumab (*Vectibix*)	EGFR-expressing CRC	Acneiform rash, pruritis, exfoliative dermatitis, paronychia; hypomagnesemia, hypocalcaemia; cough, dyspnoea, peripheral oedema, fatigue	Dermatological toxicities, interstitial lung disease, pneumonitis, pulmonary fibrosis	EGFR
Pertuzumab (*Perjeta*)	Metastatic HER2 overexpressing breast cancer, in combination with trastuzumab and docetaxel	Alopecia, diarrhoea, nausea, vomiting, mucous membrane inflammation, rash, peripheral neuropathy, anaemia, fatigue	Neutropenias with or without fever, hypersensitivity reactions, left ventricular cardiac dysfunction	Extracellular dimerization domain of HER2

Continue to Table 16–1

Drug	Approved indications	Common adverse events	Serious adverse effects	Target
Ramucirumab (*Cyramza*)	Advanced/metastatic gastric or GEJ adeno; metastatic NSCLC (disease progression on or after platinum chemotherapy combined with docetaxel） Metastatic CRC （in combination with FOLFIRI）	Hypertension, diarrhoea, neutropenia, stomatitis	Hemorrhage, hypertension, cardiovascular events, liver cirrhosis, bowel obstruction, impaired wound healing, febrile neutropenia	VEGFR2
Rituximab (*Rituxan*)	B cell NHL, CLL	Infusion reactions （fever, hypotension, shivering）; abdominal pain, diarrhoea, nausea, arthralgias, myalgias	Cardiac arrhythmias, cardiogenic shock, cytopenias, renal toxicities, angioedema, tumour lysis syndrome	CD20
Siltuximab (*Sylvant*)	Human immunodeficiency virus-and human herpes virus 8 negative multicentric Castleman's disease	Oedema, arthralgia, upper respiratory infections, fatigue, skin rash	Gastrointestinal perforation, anaphylactic reaction, infectious diseases	Soluble and membrane-bound interleukin6
Tositumomab (*Bexxar*)	CD20 positive NHL lymphoma	Abdominal pain, nausea, vomiting, Hypothyroidism, asthenia, headache, cough, fever	Cytopenia, increased risk of myelodysplasia/AML, pleural effusions, pneumonia, anaphylaxis	CD20 given as "naked" mAb followed by mAb linked to radioisotope I-131.
Trastuzumab (*Herceptin, Herclon*)	HER2/neu overexpressing breast cancer, some gastric adenocarcinomas	Loss of appetite, diarrhoea, nausea, vomiting, stomatitis, cough, dyspnoea, oedema	Cardiac dysfunction （especially with anthracycli-nes）; respiratory failure, hepatotoxicity	Extracellular domain of HER2

Table 16–2 Overview of 26 FDA-approved kinase inhibitors for cancer treatment

Drug	Approved indications	Common adverse events	Serious adverse effects	Target
Afatinib (*Gilotrif*)	Metastatic NSCLC with EGFR exon 19 deletion or exon 21 （L858R） mutations	Acneiform skin rash, paronychia, stomatitis, diarrhoea, decrease of appetite	Left ventricular dysfunction, diarrhoea, hand-foot skin reaction, hepatotoxicity, interstitial lung disease	EGFR, EGFR1/2 HER2 and HER4
Axitinib (*Inlyta*)	RCC	Hypertension, hand-foot skin reaction, diarrhoea, nausea, vomiting, transaminitis	Hemorrhages, arterial/venous thrombosis, pulmonary embolism	VEGFR1, VEGFR2, VEGFR3, PDGFR, cKIT
Bosutinib (*Bosulif*)	Philadelphia chromosome positive CML	Diarrhoea, nausea, vomiting, abdominal pain, skin rash, thrombocytopenia	Prolonged QT interval, pericardial/pleural effusion, hepatotoxicity, acute renal failure	Bcr-Abl kinase and Src-family kinases

Continue to Table 16–2

Drug	Approved indications	Common adverse events	Serious adverse effects	Target
Cabozantinib (*Cometriq*)	Metastatic medullary thyroid cancer	Electrolyte abnormalities (calcium, phosphorus), hypertension, cytopenias, transaminitis, hair colour change, fatigue	Hand-foot skin reaction, arterial and venous thromboembolism, cytopenia, gastrointestinal perforation and fistula formation	cMET, VEGFR2, FLT3, cKIT, and RET
Ceritinib (*Zykadia*)	Metastatic ALK-positive metastatic NSCLC unresponsive or intolerant to crizotinib	Fatigue, transaminitis, anaemia, diarrhoea	Nausea, vomiting, diarrhoea, hepatotoxicity, hyperglycaemia, cardiac bradyarrhythmia, prolonged QT interval, seizures, pulmonary symptoms	ALK, IGF1R, insulin receptor
Crizotinib (*Xalkori*)	Metastatic ALK-positive NSCLC	Vision disorder, diarrhoea, nausea, vomiting, constipation, oedema	Prolonged QT interval, transaminitis and hepatotoxicity, neutropenia, pulmonary embolism, pneumonitis	ALK, cMET
Dabrafenib (*Tafinlar*)	Metastatic or unresectable malignant melanoma with BRAF V600E or V600K mutation	Hyperglycaemia, hypophosphatemia, headache, hyperkeratosis, alopecia, hand-foot skin reaction, arthalgias, fever	New primary skin cancer (malignant melanoma, squamous cell cancer), pancreatitis, interstitial nephritis	BRAF V600E, V600K and V600D kinases, wild-type BRAF and CRAF kinases, MEK
Dasatinib (*Spycel*)	Philadelphia chromosome positive CML, Philadelphia chromosome positive ALL	Body fluid retention, rash, headache, dyspnoea, electrolyte abnormalities	Congestive heart failure, pericardial/pleural effusion, prolonged QT interval, haemorrhagic colitis	Bcr-Abl kinase and Src-family kinases
Erlotinib (*Tarceva*)	Metastatic or locally advanced NSCLC, with EGFR exon 19 deletion or L858R substitution Metastatic or advanced pancreatic cancer in combination with gemcitabine	Oedema, diarrhoea, nausea, vomiting, loss of appetite, abdominal pain, rash, alopecia, cough, depression, fatigue, fever	Rash, Stevens-Johnson syndrome, toxic epidermal necrolysis, cardiac dysrhythmia, myocardial infarction, syncope, bowel obstruction, interstitial lung disease, corneal perforation/ulceration, abnormal eyelash growth	EGFR, PDGFR, cKit
Gefitinib (*Iressa*)	Metastatic NSCLC with EGFR exon 19 deletions or exon 21 (L858R) substitution mutations	Acneiform or pustulous rash, folliculitis; paronychial inflammation, diarrhoea	Respiratory compromise (especially in patients with prior chemotherapy or radiation), interstitial lung disease, tumour haemorrhage	EGFR

Continue to Table 16-2

Drug	Approved indications	Common adverse events	Serious adverse effects	Target
Ibrutinib (*Imbruvica*)	Mantle cell lymphoma, CLL after at least one prior therapy or with 17p chromosome deletion Waldenstroem's macroglobulinaemia	Diarrhoea, nausea, vomiting, thrombocytopenia, increase in serum creatinine and/or uric acid levels, fatigue	Pneumonia, atrial fibrillation, subdural haematoma, gastrointestinal haemorrhage, renal failure, secondary malignancies (for example, skin cancers)	BTK
Idelalisib (*Zydelig*)	Relapsed CLL. Relapsed follicular Bcell NHL. SLL	Hyperglycaemia, hypertriglyceridaemia, fatigue, fever, cough, gastrointestinal upset, neutropenia	Hepatotoxicity, colitis, diarrhoea, intestinal perforation, cytopenias, dermatological toxicities, pneumonitis	PI3K delta
Imatinib (*Gleevec*)	Philadelphia chromosome positive ALL and CLL. MDS, chronic myeloproliferative disorder. Chronic eosinophilic leukaemia. Hypereosinophilic syndrome. Dermatofibrosis protuberans; GIST	Rash, diarrhoea, vomiting, arthralgia, oedema, headache, weight gain	Left ventricular dysfunction, congestive heart failure, cardiac tamponade, cardiogenic shock, gastrointestinal perforation, sensorineural hearing loss, acute respiratory failure, increased intracranial pressure	Bcr-Abl kinase
Lapatinib (*Tykerb*)	HER2 overexpressing breast cancer	Diarrhoea, nausea, vomiting, hand-foot skin reaction, rash, anaemia, transaminitis, hyperbilirubinaemia, fatigue	Prolonged QT interval, left ventricular dysfunction, hepatotoxicity, interstitial lung disease	EGFR, HER1 and HER2
Lenvatinib (*Lenvima*)	Locally-recurrent or metastatic radio-iodine-refractory differentiated thyroid cancer	Hypertension, constitutional symptoms, diarrhoea, nausea, vomiting, stomatitis, proteinuria, hand-foot skin reaction	Heart failure, prolonged QT interval, arterial thromboembolism, hepatotoxicity, gastrointestinal perforation and fistula formation, reversible posterior leukoencephalopathy syndrome	VEGFR1,-2,-3 and other kinases involved in angiogenesis and tumour growth
Nilotinib (*Tasigna*)	Philadelphia chromosome positive CML	Pruritus, night sweats, rash, diarrhoea, nausea, vomiting, arthralgias, myalgias, headache, cough, fatigue, alopecia	Prolonged QT interval, cytopenias, gastrointestinal haemorrhage, intracranial haemorrhage, peripheral arterial occlusive disease	Bcr-Abl, PDGFR, cKIT
Palbociclib (*Ibrance*)	Metastatic HER2 negative, ER positive breast cancer in postmenopausal women in combination with letrozole	Cytopenias, nausea, stomatitis, alopecia, upper respiratory infections, fatigue, peripheral neuropathy	Severe cytopenias, pulmonary embolism	Cyclin-dependent kinases 4 and 6

Continue to Table 16–2

Drug	Approved indications	Common adverse events	Serious adverse effects	Target
Pazopanib (*Votrient*)	Advanced RCC. Advanced soft tissue sarcoma	Hypertension, changes of hair colour, diarrhoea, nausea, vomiting, loss of appetite, arthralgias, myalgias, headache, electrolyte abnormalities, dyspnoea, fatigue	Haemorrhage, hepatotoxicity, congestive heart failure, myocardial infarction, hypothyroidism, reversible posterior leukoencephalopathy-syndrome, pneumothorax	VEGFR1, VEGFR2, VEGFR3, PDGFR, FGFR, cKIT and other kinases
Ponatinib (*Iclusig*)	CML. Philadelphia chromosome positive ALL	Hypertension, abdominal pain, constipation, nausea, headache, fever	Arterial and venous thromboembolism, hepatotoxicity, body fluid retention, congestive heart failure, cardiac arrhythmias, myocardial infarction, cytopenias, pancreatitis	Bcr-Abl kinase
Regorafenib (*Stivarga*)	Metastatic CRC, GIST	Hypertension, electrolyte abnormalities, acral erythema, cytopenias, transaminitis, hyperbilirubinaemia, difficulty speaking, proteinuria, fever	Haemorrhage, hepatotoxicity, hypertension, myocardial infarction, gastrointestinal fistula, gastrointestinal perforation	Multiple kinases including VEGFR2 and TIE2
Ruxolitinib (*Jakafi or Jakavi*)	Myelofibrosis. Polycythaemia vera unresponsive to or intolerant of hydroxyurea	Confusion, dizziness, headache, anaemia, thrombocytopenia	Cytopenias. Herpes zoster or serious infections may occur	JAK1 and JAK2
Sorafenib (*Nexavar*)	Advanced RCC. Unresectable HCC. Locally advanced or metastatic thyroid cancer refractory to radioactive iodine treatment	Diarrhoea, nausea, loss of appetite, abdominal pain, electrolyte abnormalities, fatigue, rash, hand-foot skin reaction, alopecia	Haemorrhage, congestive heart failure, myocardial infarct, prolongation of QT interval, severe skin reactions, cutaneous epithelial tumours	Multiple kinases including VEGFR, PDGFR and Raf kinases
Sunitinib (*Sutent*)	Advanced RCC, GIST. Unresectable or advanced pancreatic neuroendocrine tumour	Diarrhoea, nausea, vomiting, loss of appetite, altered taste sensation, yellow skin discoloration, rash, elevation of uric acid, hypothyroidism, cough, fatigue	Thrombocytopenia, tumour haemorrhage, prolongation of QT interval, left ventricular dysfunction, tissue necrosis, aseptic necrosis of jaw bone, hemoptysis, hepatotoxicity	Multiple kinases including VEGFR, PDGFR and KIT
Trametinib (*Mekinist*)	Unresectable or metastatic malignant melanoma with BRAF V600E or V600K mutation	Rash, diarrhoea, transaminitis, anaemia, lymphoedema, hypoalbuminaemia	Cardiomyopathy, haemorrhage, dermatological toxicities, interstitial lung disease, pneumonitis, visual disturbances	MEK 1 and-2

Continue to Table 16-2

Drug	Approved indications	Common adverse events	Serious adverse effects	Target
Vandetanib (*Caprelsa*)	Medullary thyroid carcinoma	Rash, acne, hypertension, hypocalcaemia, trans-aminitis, headache, fatigue	Prolonged QT interval, ischaemic stroke, interstitial lung disease, respiratory failure/arrest	EGFR, VEGF
Vemurafenib (*Zelboraf*)	Unresectable or metastatic malignant melanoma with BRAF V600E mutation	Nausea, arthralgias, alopecia, photosensitivity, pruritus, rash, skin papillomas	Squamous cell carcinoma, hand-foot skin reaction, prolonged QT interval, ophthalmologic reactions (iritis, photophobia, retinal vein occlusion)	BRAF V600E kinase

16.1.6   Adverse effects of molecular targeted therapy drugs and their treatment

Unlike conventional cytotoxic chemotherapy, molecular targeted therapy drugs block the growth and progression of cancer cells by interfering different pathways which are essential for the development of cancer. Conventional chemotherapy non-selectively interferes the proliferation of all rapidly dividing cells, such as the bone marrow haematopoietic cells, gastrointestinal epithelial cells and hair follicles cells. The rationale of developing molecular targeted therapy agents has been to specifically block one or more molecules which are either upregulated or overexpressed or mutated in cancer cells, therefore minimizing toxicities while improving curative effect.

Since 1997, the first monoclonal antibody Rituximab was approved by the United States Food and Drug Administration (FDA) applied in cancer treatment, the development and use of molecular targeted drugs have grown substantially, more and more molecular targeted therapy drugs have entered the clinic. However, as they gradually change the cancer treatment mode and obtain the remarkable curative effect, they also attracted the attention of the oncology community due to the different adverse reaction spectrum with traditional chemotherapy drugs.

Adverse drug reaction (ADR) refers to in the case of normal doses and methods of use, the drug may have an accidental or adverse reaction that is not related to the therapeutic purpose.

Clinically, the adverse drug reactions are divided into four categories, which are convenient for physicians to record and evaluate:

● Category 1: allergic reactions that occur immediately after administration of the drug, with little relation to the dose. Such adverse reactions are difficult to predict and avoid, requiring more clinical observation and timely treatment.

● Category 2: caused by the enhancement of the pharmacological action of the drug, with more relation to the dose. After drug withdrawal or reduction, the symptoms can reduce or disappear quickly, namely the maximum tolerated dose (MTD) of phase I clinical trial. In the CRF table, it is generally divided into 0, 1, 2, 3 and 4 degrees, which can not only be predicted but also can be used as dose adjustment or withdrawal and corresponding treatment indicators.

● Category 3: adverse reactions caused by the dose or long-term use of dose limited toxicity (DLT).

● Category 4: long-term adverse reactions after long-term administration and treatment.

Molecular targeted drugs directly aim at the targets, which have less damage to surrounding normal tissues and have a significant therapeutic effect, so that the application space is wide, but it does not mean that there is no adverse reaction.

16.1.6.1 Common side effects of mAbs

The most common adverse effects of mAbs are allergic reactions, such as infusion reactions, hives and/or pruritus, flu-like symptoms and skin rashes. The common side effects of mAbs are summarized in Table 16–3. Resistance to mAbs may be the result of the combination of tumor-related and host-related factors, but complement-dependent and antibody-dependent cellular cytotoxicities are considered to participate in the development of drug resistance mechanisms.

Table 16–3 Common side effects of mAbs

Adverse effects	Durgs
Cytopenias and infusion reactions	Alemtuzumab, ibritumomab, rituximab, trastuzumab
Infections	Alemtuzumab
Gastrointestinal perforation, wound dehiscence/healing problems and increased risk of haemorrhage	Bevacizumab, ramucirumab
Neurological toxicities	Blinatumomab
Possibly fatal progressive multifocal leukoencephalopathy due to viral infection	Brentuximab vedotin, rituximab
Cardiac failure	Ado-trastuzumab emtansine, trastuzumab
Severe Tcell activation	Ipilimumab
Dermatological toxicities	Panitumumab
Severe allergic reactions	Tositumomab
Cytokine-release syndrome	Blinatumomab
Embryo/fetal death and birth defects	Ado-trastuzumab emtansine, pertuzumab
Hepatotoxicity	Ado-trastuzumab emtansine
Cardiopulmonary arrest and/or sudden death	Cetuximab

16.1.6.2 Common adverse effects of kinase inhibitors

There are at least 100 signaling pathways in humans. According to the specific targets inhibited, the adverse effects of kinase inhibitors can differ considerably. Moreover, based on the oral administration, plasma concentrations measured in pharmacokinetic studies and the bioavailabilities of the kinase inhibitors can vary considerably between patients.

Generally, most kinase inhibitors cause different degrees of cytopenias, and also affect the digestive system, which include nausea, vomiting, diarrhoea and/or heartburn; some kinase inhibitors cause headaches, muscle cramps, periorbital oedema, and various types of skin rashes. Kinase inhibitors might induce or worsen symptoms of depression. Moreover, female patients of reproductive age should prevent pregnancy and/or stop breast-feeding by taking appropriate measures during treatment due to the teratogenic effect of the durgs. The common side effects of kinase inhibitors are summarized in Table 16–4.

Table 16-4   Common side effects ofkinase inhibitors

Adverse effects	Durgs
Hepatoxicity	Idelalisib, lapatinib, pazopanib, ponatinib, regorafenib, sunitinib
Colitis and gastrointestinal perforation	Idelalisib
Fistula formation	Cabozantinib
Severe arterial thrombotic events	Ponatinib
Myocardial infarction and stroke	Ponatinib
QT interval prolongation with increased risk of torsades de pointes and sudden cardiac deaths	Nilotinib, vandetanib
Pneumonitis	Idelalisib

16.1.6.3   Pretreatment and premedication assessment

Before the administration of kinase inhibitors or mAbs, patients must receive assessments, such as laboratory evaluation (complete blood count, urine analysis, pregnancy test, thyroid function test), and cardiovascular and pulmonary assessments. When the drugs are administrated intravenously, pre-treatment of acetaminophen, antihistamines, steroids and non-steroidal anti-inflammatory drugs (NSAIDs) are usually given to patients. If undesirable symptoms occur, according to the degree and nature of the symptoms, management will be taken and the targeted drugs might be discontinued.

16.1.7   The challenge of molecular targeted therapy

As a new treatment, molecular targeted therapy makes the medical cancer treatment have more choices. More and more patients got benefit from it, and the understanding of cancer has risen to a new height. But the time for targeted therapy to enter the clinic is relatively short, and many problems remain to be solved.

First of all, most of the mechanism of cancer is complex, its regulator control system is a composite, multi-factor complex networks. It is difficult to achieve the goal of eradicating the tumor with only one or two targeted drugs, and the effective rate of most molecular targeted drugs is only about 10%. In addition, the tumor may arise from a single gene mutation in the initial stage of development. With the proliferation of tumor cells, new gene mutations and drug resistance may occur. In the case of imatinib for the treatment of gastrointestinal stromal tumors for 2 years, most patients will develop resistance, and the mechanism may be associated with secondary mutations in c-KIT or PDGFRa genes.

16.1.7.1   How to find the dominant crowd

(1)Select the appropriate population according to the clinicopathological features of the patients

For example, the appropriate population of TKIs in the treatment of NSCLC include: female, Asian, non-smoking, adenocarcinoma. Cetuximab combined with chemotherapy for the treatment of NSCLC, a rash (early rash) occurring in 3 weeks can predict the curative effect (FLEX test). Although clinically some of the so-called "dominant crowd" can be found, but the clinical pathological features need a large sample of clinical test and multiple tests validation, is not conducive to drug research and development, also is not conducive to the treatment of patients; in addition, due to the lack of specificity of these dominant groups, the blindness of treatment guidance is large. Whether these populations can really benefit from targeted drug therapy is lacking in theory. Therefore, it can only be used as a reference when there is no predictive marker of curative effect.

(2) Genetic testing seeking for predictive markers of curative effect

For example, C-kit gene (GIST/MM), HER2 (breast cancer, gastric cancer); EGFR exon 19 mutations and 21 missing detection in TKls treatment of NSCLC; CD20 detection in Rituximab for the treatment of malignant lymphoma; kras mutation detection in cetuximab combined with chemotherapy for colorectal cancer; detection of Kit gene mutation site 9, 11 in imatinib for the treatment of gastrointestinal stromal tumors. The exploration and discovery of curative effect prediction markers may have a significant impact on the clinical application of molecular targeted drugs, i. e. , individualized treatment. There are many clinical researches had joined the potential biomarkers in the design of experiment, we look forward to the results of these studies to change our understanding of the molecular targeted treatment and application.

16.1.7.2 Evaluation criteria for the efficacy of molecular targeted drugs

With the clinical application of molecular targeted drugs, the objective curative effect criteria evaluating the effect of antitumor drug has also been a new challenge. Simply using CT/MRI cannot response the curative effect of the molecular targeted drugs, for example, there is no change in CT/MRI assessment of the primary tumor size after the molecular target drug treatment, but PET-CT shows significantly decreased tumor metabolic (SUV value) or tumor cells had no activity; another example, after anti-angiogenesis therapy, the primary tumor occurs necrosis, appearing low density and low signal. It has always been controversial for us to evaluate the efficacy of drugs for this kind of imaging changes. Released today, there is no evaluation standard, but fortunately PET-CT evaluation to explore the efficacy of targeted drugs have been added to some cancers, with the research going on, PET-CT may have a broader prospect.

16.1.7.3 The cause and treatment of main toxicity of targeted drugs

With the widely application of the molecular targeted drugs, the toxicity reaction of molecular targeted drugs caused the great attention of clinical doctors. The main toxicity of anti-VGFR drugs includes cardiovascular toxicity, hypertension, proteinuria, hypothyroidism, etc. Causes of high blood pressure include VEGF making endothelial cells/platelets secrete less NO/PGI2, vascular density abnormalities (small blood vessels and capillaries), vascular stiffness, endothelin dysfunction; EGFR and VEGF also express in renal distal convoluted tubules and collecting system, VEGF expresse in renal tubular podocyte, anti-VGFR treatment can lead to reducing renin proteins which play an important role in glomerular filtration, thereafter proteinuria ensues. Clinically, it is very important to discuss the causes and treatment of toxicity.

16.1.7.4 Targeted drugs resistance problem

In recent years, with the clinical application of targeted drugs, drug-resistant problem has gradually been known. EGFR TKI, such as gefitinib or erlotinib for treatment of advanced NSCLC show resistance after gaining good curative effect. The study found that the mechanism was related to the activation of the PI3K pathway caused by the re-mutation of EGFR (T790M) or c-met gene amplification. Primary drug resistance is associated with ALK expression in a small number of NSCLC. Therefore, it is very important to find the relevant target inhibitors to overcome the resistance.

For molecular targeted therapy, it has been called the "magic bullet", but reviewing the development of targeted therapy, it is easy to find this is just a portion of the iceberg. As the problems mentioned above, the combination of monoclonal drugs and chemotherapy may improve curative effect, however, TKIs combined with chemotherapy shows a poor performance. More importantly, the combination of blocking multiple signaling pathways drugs designed by signal channels has not seen a significant increase in efficacy.

In view of the above problems, it is one of the hot spots to actively seek new targets of tumor and predictive biomarker of curative effect. With the development of the research, the emergence of new biomarkers for the prediction of clinical results, creative clinical trial design is more important. It is of great significance to understand the toxicity caused by molecular targeted therapy, clinical rational application of molecular targeted drugs and the treatment of toxicity.

16.2   Precision medicine

Precision medicine, also known as personalized medicine, is for the purpose to individualize treatment interventions, according to genomics, proteomics, and metabolomics data, combined with histopathological observation, and the type, stage, and grade of the disease, as well as the potential response of patients to the treatment regimen. With the development of next-generation sequencing technologies, now it is possible to affordably identify all germline mutation of an individual, and therefore paving the way for clinical doctor to provide medical service from an individual perspective. The neologism "Omics" refers to a field of study in biology ending in-omics, such as genomics, proteomics or metabolomics. Omics has become the new mantra in molecular research. Omics technologies include genomics, transcriptomics, proteomicsand metabolomics.

16.2.1   Propose

In 2011, the American academy of sciences, the American academy of engineering, the national institutes of health and the American scientific committee jointly issued the "march toward precision medicine" initiative, a combination of genetic association studies and clinical medicine to achieve accurate treatment and effective early warning of human diseases.

On January 20th, 2015, President Barack Obama put forward "Precision Medicine" program in the State of the Union speech, called on the US to increase the medical research funding, promote individualized genomics research, on the basis of individual genetic information to set individual health care for patients with cancer and other diseases. On January 30th, Obama formally launched the "precise medicine plan", proposing to spend $215 million on the plan in fiscal 2016 to promote the development of personalized medicine.

16.2.2   Application

(1) Diagnosis and treatment intervention

It can give patients more accurate diagnosis and effective treatment. The genomes of different patients can be compared and referenced by detailed understanding of individual gene sequences. For example, the possibility of genetic mutations in existing diseases can be assessed through the human genome project. Now, many companies have developed gene sequencing services for public consumers. At the same time, the different genetic makeup of individual also determines the different response to treatment regimen of patients. Hence, it's very important to understand their different genetic information of patients for effective treatment. In addition, it is also a major step forward in preventing intervention. For instance, many women exist the possibility of breast cancer, ovarian cancer and other diseases due to family heredity. With the help of precision medical, we can for the possibility of individuals suffering from the disease screening, and according to the difference of the individual to take corresponding measures to prevent the happening of the disease. With the help of precision medicine, we can screen individuals for the possibility of the disease, and take appropriate measures to prevent the disease from occurring depending on individual differences.

(2) Drug development and use

Understanding of individual genetic information is vital for the development of drugs. Knowing details of individual genetic makeup is a determining factor of whether the patient can participate in the final phase of drug clinical trials. By knowing what kind of patients the drug is best for and which patients will have adverse reactions in clinical trials, not only can enhance the safety of the drug usage, but also speed up the drug clinical trial and reduce test cost.

(3) Cancer genomics

Measurements of large-scale gene, protein and metabolite have driven the biological resolution to a system-oriented perspective. In the past ten years, With the rapid advancement of high-throughput technologies, such as mass spectrometry and Next Generation Sequencing (NGS) for precise genomics analysis examining biological systems at different levels become possible, such as whole genome, exome sequencing, metabolome and proteome, with high resolution and affordable costs.

In recent decades, with the deepening of cancer research, there has been a growing awareness of the genetic differences between different types of cancer and individuals. Cancer genomics is the use of genomics and precision medicine for cancer research and treatment. In this way, the relationship between cancer and genes can be better described, as well as individual differences and the risk of cancer.

16.2.3　Development

(1) Translational research of bioinformatics and clinical medicine

The integration of precision medicine into large-scale genomics data and clinical medical information. The research of translational medicine is an important part of precision medicine. Although the emergence of big data has important contributions to accurate diagnosis and drug research and development, it is still necessary to have more in-depth precision medicine research for building a new disease knowledge network and classification system. Disease knowledge network will become an integrated information, for searching personal genome, transcriptome and proteome, metabolome, clinical symptoms and signs, laboratory examination, environmental exposure, and socioeconomic factors and related information. The establishment of knowledge network will be an in-depth understanding of disease mechanism, pathogenesis and treatment, and will drive the development of new classification system for disease, thus defining disease subtypes.

(2) New classification system based on molecular phenotype

The development of new classification system based on molecular phenotype plays an important role in precision medicine, which is helpful to explore new therapeutic strategies and new drug development to further improve clinical efficacy. However, the genetic complexity of the disease determines that a single genomics study is difficult to systematically and completely explain the overall biological behavior of the disease for making precise disease segmentation. Therefore, the integrative research of different Omics studies is the key to develop new classification system of diseases. At present, the data standardization of different Omics platforms has not been unified. It is urgent to set up a standardized model of Omics data integration.

(3) Molecular targeted drugs

The large-scale Omics approaches have contributed to the understanding of the molecular pathways of mutations resulting in transformation from normal cells into cancerous cells, and tumor-specific biomarkers identification, which leads to the discovery and development of pathway-related molecular targeted drugs and diagnostics. Several dozens of pathway-related molecular targeted drugs have been approved for breast cancer, hematological malignancies, ovarian cancer and colon cancer in clinical use. These molecular targeted drugs are generally categorized into two groups: therapeutic monoclonal antibodies, targeting overexpressed or specific receptors on tumor cells and subsequently mediating cytotoxicity through antibody dependent cell cytotoxicity (ADCC), complement dependent cytotoxicity (CDC) mechanisms or by carrying toxic factors (i. e. radioisotope, toxin). The second group is small molecule inhibitors, specifically inhibiting intracellular enzymatic activity or receptor signaling pathways, therefore promoting apoptosis of target cancer cells.

Molecular targeted drugs have made great advances in the field of improving clinical curative effect. The choice of therapeutic regimen for specific genetic targets can provide a safer and more effective treatment for patients. Therapeutic targets are usually key molecules of signal transduction or transcriptional activation in signal pathways. Drug toxicity and therapeutic resistance are great challenges in the clinical application of molecular targeted drugs. New molecular targeted drug toxicity can affect the heart, lungs, skin, endocrine and gastrointestinal organs. More specific and effective, but less toxic, targeted drug development is urgently needed. The drug resistance mechanism needs further research to find potential solutions and to develop a new generation of targeted drugs.

16.2.4   Challenges and opportunities

While the precision medicine in cancer is very promising, its full realization faces many challenges and opportunities. Apart from cancer molecular characterization via whole genome and transcriptome sequencing, additional cancer biology complexities need to be considered.

1) Basic research of epigenetic alterations reveals how gene expression is regulated by methylation, which contributes to our perspective of individual cancer.

2) New Omics approaches of proteome and metabolome reveal additional cancer biology information. As the practicability of new Omics approaches increase, new standards for integrating data analysis and transparency in clinical trials should be considered.

3) Additional aspects of cancer biology, such as tumor heterogeneity, drug resistance mechanism, tumor microenvironment, and cancer stem cell properties can influence the treatment response of patients.

16.2.5   Future directions

Integrative analysis via DNA and RNA sequencing has opened new doors to basic and clinical cancer research. Cancer molecular classification based on alterations in genomic and transcriptome may reveal new biomarkers for diagnosis, prognosis, and prediction of therapeutic response. Continuing multi-disciplinary collaboration of oncologists, pathologists, basic scientists, and computational biologists are required. Additional resources and funding are needed to support ongoing basic genomics research, clinical tumor sequencing, and data sharing networks for precision cancer medicine.

Zheng Yanfang

Chapter 17

Traditional Chinese Medicine Anti-tumor Therapy

17.1 Historic evolution of cancer concepts

It had been known for thousands of years in the oncogenesis and treatment by traditional Chinese medicine(TCM) in our country.

1) Malignant tumor is called as "癌病(cancer disease)" in TCM, which is characterized by abnormal hyperplasia of tissue or organ, and its mainly clinical features include mass, uneven surface, hard texture, ache and fever. They are usually accompanied with some symptoms such as inappetence, fatigue and waste away.

2) "癌病(Cancer Disease)" is a kind of ancient diseases and the word "癌" is derived from the ancient word "嵒", which is found to have a tumor of "as high as the top of rock and as deep as a chasm" by the ancients in the breast of a woman. The "疒" was added to "嵒" as "癌(cancer)" in order to highlight the tumor being a kind of diseases.

3) As early as the age of Yin ruins oracle, there had the records about "瘤(tumor)", which was "瘤 (tumor), swelling, stems from disease, and made a sound for pain" and it had been recorded by *Shuowen Jiezi*, which be same as to the meaning of "accumulation" in *the General Records of Shengji*.

4) In ancient literature, the understanding for tumor was mainly came from some diseases, such as "lip cancer" "lingual carcinoma" "cervical malignancy with cachexia" "carcinoma of larynx", "stony goiter", "dysphagia", "pulmonary retention", "breast rock", "abdominal mass", "accumulation", "female abdominal mass", "obstinate sore", "necrosis" and "cauliflower-like sore".

5) "癌(Cancer)", as one of the Yongju Wufa of the diseases, was first seen in the book of *Weiji Baoshu* (1171 AD), which was written by Dongxuan in the Song Dynasty.

17.2   TCM theories of carcinogenesis and pathogenesis

There are some TCM theories of carcinogenesis andpathogenesis.

(1) The carcinogenesis and pathogenesis of tumor is related to the struggle between vital Qi and evil Qi

According to the classic book of *Huangdi Neijing*, it was recorded that the struggle and balance of vital Qi and evil Qi would played an important role in the course of diseases, and the evil Qi wouldn't disturb you if sufficient vital Qi to exist in your body while invasion of pathogen was due to the deficiency of vital Qi. In the later literature of TCM, there were many depictions about the relation between evil Qi and vital Qi. For instance, it was discussed the cancer pathogenesis just for deficiency of vital Qi and organism being attacked meantime by evil Qi in the book of *Yizong Bidu* which written by Zhongzi Li who was an outstanding TCM doctor in the Ming Dynasty.

(2) The tumor occurring is related to the constitution

According to the constitution theory, people differ in their susceptibility or protection against disease, and the tumor constitution mainly includes Qi deficiency, Yang deficiency, Qi depression, phlegm dampness, blood stasis, wet poison and stasis. It was considered that those differences mainly involved in pathogenesis, constitution and the type of disease.

(3) The formation of tumor is related to the inner deficiency

It is pointed out that visceral deficiency is the one of the most important reasons in the process for tumor development in the theory of inner deficiency, and invigorating the spleen and kidney is one of the most important principles in tumor therapy based on this theory.

(4) The formation and metastasis of tumor is related to condensation of pathogenic toxin

In the theory of Chuanshe, it is believed that the tumor formation and metastasis are related to condensation of pathogenic toxin. Whereas, for deficiency of vital Qi not enough to ensure stability and govern retention, these factors result in to the diffusion of pathogenic toxin and tumor metastasis. The evil toxin is the source of malignant tumor metastasis, especially the meridians is an important route of tumor metastasis.

(5) The tumor metastasis is related to the meridians

According to the meridional theory, there will have a tendency of tumor metastasis by some line bias and some difference in the probability and time of metastasis, especially some tumors will have certain organ transfer tendencies instead of occurring randomly.

(6) The tumor metastasis is related to the phlegmatic toxin and deep multiple abscess

In the other hypothesis of metastasis which is called "phlegmatic toxin and deep multiple abscess", it is believed that tumor metastasis is based on the sputum poison injected into the meridian, viscera, Qi and blood. In postoperative tumor, because of the deficiency of vital Qi, much endogenous phlegm damp and residual toxic were been gathered, as a result, the channel of Qi and blood was damaged and then a lump was forming in other parts of our body gradually.

17.3   Etiology and pathogenesis

The TCM etiology and pathogenesis is the theoretical knowledge about diseases. The cause of cancer is not still clear fully. The occurrence of cancer is related to the external six evils and pathogenic toxin, the inner seven kinds of emotions depression, eating disorder, old disease, long illness, and old age in TCM.

1) The etiology and pathogenesis of cancer mainly include imbalance of Yin and Yang, damaged by excess of seven emotions and viscera damage. As a result, Qi stagnation, blood stasis, "pelvic mass" and "accumulation" was occurring gradually.

2) The formation of accumulation and mass is closely related to sputum. It will become an accumulation for phlegm-fluid gathering and coagulating. The mass of the body is often coagulated by phlegm and static blood, and phlegm coagulation is an important pathologic factor of tumor occurence.

3) The characteristics of the phlegm decides that tumor is easy to come into being. The phlegm fluid will become hot with the passing of time and produces evil poison which is called phlegm poison. It can also produce water damp and phlegm fluid, and become more serious disease of phlegm toxin intermingling if evil poison attacked the body.

4) The phlegm fluid will produce blood-stasis, and both have the same homology. It is a summary of the pathological changes of fluid and blood. There will appear syndromes of intermingled phlegm and blood stasis, and the tumor will slowly occur in a long time for phlegm and blood stasis staying in body, Qi movement disordering and the channels being blocked.

5) Phlegm-fluid can carry with blood, stasis, and toxin. The stopping fluid will become phlegm, and blood flowing slowly will become stasis. The phlegm and blood stasis affect each other, with the time goes by, and the poison, phlegm poison and stasis poison will be produced. The phlegm, blood stasis and toxin will coalesce into a lump, which is increasingly large, and form a masse. In summary, stagnation of phlegm, blood-stasis and toxin are the root causes of tumor formation.

6) Although the formation of cancer has many factors mentioned above, the basic pathological changes of the disease are deficiency of vital Qi, Qi stagnation, blood stasis, phlegm junction, wet clustering and heat toxicity. The Pathological properties are asthenia in origin and asthenia in superficiality. It is because of the deficiency, excess resulted from deficiency, and is an asthenia syndrome in whole but deficiency in local.

17.4　Principles and methods of treatment

The rapeutic principles are some rules of TCM including the principles and methods of treatment in the treatment of diseases. TCM has a history of several thousand years in the prevention and treatment of tumors, and the combination of syndrome differentiation and disease treatment is a basic therapeutic principles.

1) The principles and methods of treatment about cancer have been described by doctors in different times. Jingyue Zhang, the writer of *Jingyue Quanshu*, in the chapter of this book *Abdominal Mass*, had said that the treatment of accumulation. . . there had four measures which were named the attacking, dispelling, dispersing and tonifying in Ming dynasty. All the treatment methods of accumulation were highly generalized.

2) In addition, the treatment ways of cancer are different for various stages and the diverse between vital Qi and evil Qi. In the book of *Yizong Bidu*, it was recorded that at the initial stage, the vital Qi was strong, the tumor could been treated by attacking. At the middle stage, evil Qi was stong while the vital Qi was weak, the tumor could been treated by purging and tonifying therapies. At the late stages, tonifying was suggested to widely use for evil Qi having been encroached yet while vital Qi dissolved.

3) People-oriented and holistic view are the major principles of tumor in TCM treatment. These therapy

ways such as operation, radiotherapy, chemotherapy and targeted therapy, all belong to attacking evil but consuming vital Qi leading to the imbalance of Yin Yang and the spread of tumor. So people-oriented and holistic view are been placed in high value on the principles of tumor in TCM treatment.

4) The micro-environment for the growth of tumor will be destroyed, and the symptoms, quality of life, immune function, balance of Yin and Yang will be improved, vital Qi will be stimulated, and reach the purpose of inhibiting tumor, prolonging survival period and reducing tumor recurrence and transfer, regulating Qi, blood, Yin, Yang and physiological function of viscera's channels and collaterals.

5) There has developed a preliminary consensus about TCM treatment of cancer by extensive researches and practices. Firstly, it can reduce the toxic and side effects of chemotherapy or radiotherapy, such as vomit, fatigue, poor appetite and myelosuppression, can enhance sensitivity, resist immunosuppressive effect and improving effectiveness. Secondly, it can improve immunity, mental state, physical strength and the quality of life. Thirdly, it can quickly relieve clinical symptoms in the patients with malignant tumor. Fourthly, it can effectively remove residual cancer cells and small lesions and prevent recurrence and metastasis after surgery, radiotherapy and chemotherapy. Fifthly, we should differentiate syndrome and disease, especially study how to choose the drugs with anti-cancer roles in pharmacology, so the combination of syndrome differentiation and disease treatment is a basic therapeutic principle.

17.5   Treatment of different syndrome

TCM syndrome differentiation is the basic principle to know and treatment disease and a kind of special research and treatment method.

17.5.1   Insufficiency of vital Qi

The occurrence of cancer is mostly vital Qi recession, the internal environment is unstable, the carcinogenic factor accumulates in the body and the viscera is disturbed, so that the combination of phlegm wet and poison stasis becomes cancer diseases gradually. Insufficiency of vital Qi is the basis of the pathogenesis of cancer. After the occurrence of cancer, the toxic factors of cancer will damage vital Qi and it is the most important factor of cancer metastasis while vital Qi is weaker than evil Qi. Rampant advanced cancer cell always begin when vital Qi decays. Therefore, strengthening resistance and tonifying deficiency is a very important principle in the overall treatment ways and the vital Qi will play an active role in anti-cancer and prevention metastasis. The Chinese herbal medicines mainly include ginseng, radix astragali, dendrobium, privet fruit, and glossy Ganoderma, etc.

17.5.2   Deficiency of spleen and kidney

Radiotherapy or chemotherapy is a positive and effective way for the treatment of cancer in modern medicine, but it can damage the spleen and kidney while killing cancer cells, resulting in a deficiency of spleen and kidney. We Can use ginseng, astragalus, ganoderma lucidum, tuckahoe, pinellia, ginger, orange peel, amomum villosum, japonica rice, ginger and other medicines to protect the spleen and stomach, and medlar, dwarf lilyturf, epimedium, rhizoma polygonati, fructus ligustri lucidi, dry grass, mulberry and other to invigorate kidney for consolidating semen.

17.5.3   Viscera disorder

The primary cause of cancer is that the carcinogenic factors disturb the related viscera function in disorder, so it is necessary to adjust the relevant viscera and restore their function as one of the targets. In lung cancer, firstly lung Qi is injured. We can use the radix pseudostellariae, ginseng and straight ladybell to fill the lung Qi and regulate the viscera. In gastric cancer, we can use astragalus, ginseng, atractylodes, pinellia ternata, fructus amomi, fructus aurantii to regulate stomach transport function for functional decrease of stomach accommodating and spleen transporting. In colorectal cancer, it is can not to transporting effectively mainly for the deficiency of spleen Qi. For stasis in the intestine, we can use astragalus, radix, angelica, angelica, fructus aurantii, and wood incense to invigorate, pass, drop and eliminate waste so as to restore the function of the intestinal tract.

17.6　TCM characteristic therapy

TCM characteristic therapy is one of the most important components of the integrative medicine and complementary therapies. In addition to the treatment of TCM decoction, the external treatment is the most important component of these characteristics. External therapy is a kind of technologies such as hydrotherapeutics, plastering therapy, acupoint injection, acupuncture point injection, fumigating and washing therapy, enema therapy, injunction, medicated bath, moxibustion, pressing bean on auricular point, cupping therapy, music therapy, psychological therapy and dietary aftercare by drugs, techniques or instruments in the skin (mucosa).

There had a long history in the treatment of a tumor by external therapy. It was found that the lump which under the armpit, red and hard, treated by stone, the ointment, injunction, not wrapping, six days being cured was Miju in the classical document of *Lingshu, Yongju*. External therapy was relative to the internal medicine treatment method. In Jin dynasty, for the application of paste, treatment of diseases had been developed gradually from external treatment of the skin to the external use of internal medicine. In the document of *Zhouhou Baiyifang*, diseases in ear and nose, were plugged the holes with plasters wrapped by a piece of cloth by mangcao cream. The writer Shiji Wu of *Liyue Pianwen* said that both of external and internal treatment were highly valued for the treatment mechanism and medicine, and then the difference was just methods. It is commonly to treat incurable diseases by roning therapy, fumigation, hot compress, especially in the diseases such as immaculate, gangrene and so on.

The external treatment of TCM is the same as that of internal medicine, and both are guided by the holistic concept and the thought of syndrome differentiation, and some drugs or appliance were used by different methods in skin, bore or acupoints to develop their roles of meridian treatment, harmonizing Qi and blood, detoxification, removing blood stasis, strengthening vital Qi to eliminate pathogens and so on, to readjust and improve lost balance of Yin and Yang in viscera organs, so as to enhance the recovery of body function and have the effect of preventing and curing disease.

17.7　TCM rehabilitation

TCM rehabilitation is a discipline that studies the basic theory, medical method and application based on the guidance of Chinese medical theory.

There have various rehabilitation methods and other useful measures to be adopted to improve the dysfunction of the patient and go back to the society.

17.7.1   Pay attention to the food intake

One can live by his stomach Qi while he will die without it, and keeping his stomach Qi will have an opportunity of living in the theory of TCM. There fore, the food intake is an important sign of the survival of stomach Qi and advance or retreat of disease. Loss of appetite in cancer patients will appear gradually thin in an early stage. Almost all cancer patients don't like food or feel no hunger, meanwhile transport function of spleen and stomach decline in mid-stage. Death is due to not eating in the end of the patients, life in advanced stage cancer. Therefore, the food intake should be promoted to the important status in the treatment of cancer, and to restore the function of the stomach and spleen as much as possible to make the "it would be nice to eat some food".

17.7.2   Emphasis on syndrome and pharmacological

Cancer occurring is always related to phlegm, Qi, poison, and blood stasis. Cancer treatment emphasizes the principles of syndrome differentiation, invigorating vital Qi, regulating the viscera, dissipating mass and anticancer drugs. It is found that a great variety of TCM including clearing heat toxicity, dissipating mass and promoting blood circulation for removing obstruction in collaterals have anti-tumor effect and also have selective organs based on modern pharmacological studies, so it is needed to know the location of disease and tumors' characteristics, and the clinical experience of choosing drugs is important too. For example, sputum coagulation in lung cancer, houttuynia, rabdosia rubesens, thunberg fritillary bulb, taxaceae and so on was suggested. While in bread cancer, those of snake berry, solanum septemlobum bunge, dandelion, cowherb seed, and centipede were suggested to select for the stagnation of Qi and phlegmatic toxin. Especially in Liver cancer or bile pancreatic carcinoma, for wet poison and stasis, herba oldenlandiae, portulacagradifora, Chinese lobelia herb, radix semiaquilegiae, turtle shell, centipede, radix sophorae flavescentis and coix seed are chosen to choose to detoxify, damp elimination, removing the obstruction, and smooth the meridian patency.

17.7.3   Constitution rehabilitation

The constitution refers to the body, nature, and essence, which is the concept of pathophysiology formed during the development of TCM theory. The constitution is the characteristics of physical qualities due to the prosperity and decline of viscera, meridian, Qi blood and Yin Yang. According to the function state and nature of the evil Qi, it can be divided into two categories including the normal and abnormal constitution. The abnormal constitution can be divided into three types, deficiency, excess and intermingling of deficiency and excess. In particular, the constitution mainly includes peace, Qi deficiency, Yang deficiency, Yin deficiency, blood stasis, phlegm dampness, dampness heat, Qi depression. However, in all stages of the disease, the constitution of tumor patients is almost always an intermingling of deficiency and excess, and it is our main objective to achieve peace through the rehabilitation of the patient's rehabilitation therapy.

17.7.4   Maintenance therapy

Traditional Chinese medicine has the principle of removing evil Qi not to destroy vital Qi and keeping vital Qi not to leave evil Qi. After completion of radiation and chemotherapy, maintain treatment with TCM to control tumor, by the local control and the systemic immune regulation of green and safe therapeutic effect, is superior to maintenance therapy with chemotherapy or targeted drugs alone. Therefore, after or in the period of radiation therapy and chemotherapy, it is recommended to use the TCM to maintain the antitumor treatment and it will play an active role in the prevention and treatment of recurrence and metastasis.

17.7.5 Preventive treatment of disease

The preventive treatment of disease is one of the great contributions of *Huangdi Neijing* to the Health medicine and preventive medicine. It was said that there had a sage who did cure preventive treatment of disease instead of the treatment of disease in *Suwen. SiQi Tiaoshen* value... It is a late treatment after illness just like only to start making weapons well if war burst. The preventive treatment of a disease includes three levels of meaning. Firstly, to prevent disease when there is no disease, and to take proactive preventive measures against the tumor to prevent recurrence and metastasis. Secondly, if the disease is still in the light stage, you could see its essence and development trend, and to prevent tumor development by early detection and timely measures through some tiny symptoms signs. Thirdly, the disease was treated as early as possible, and recover in time to prevent further transmission and aggravation.

17.7.6 Concepts of holism and individualization

It was emphasized that the combination of the concepts of holism and individuation in tumor rehabilitation, and human beings is a unified whole in TCM. It had been recorded in *Huangdi Neijing* that where evil Qi invade and where is deficiency, Jingshen guard and there no disease, all of which reflect the whole concept. So we could regard cancer as a whole instead of being isolated from the local, and treatment should be guided by the concept of holism of TCM and the principle of therapy with syndrome differentiation. Considering the patient's constitution, tumor characteristics and different stages, and based on the treatment form of syndrome and disease differentiation, we determine the appropriate treatment plan so as to have a scientific guidance for clinical treatment according to the obtained objective and accurate individual information.

17.8 Progress of TCM research

In recent years, remarkable progress has been made in the study of further improving curative effect to discover the effective components or monomers of TCM with anticancer effect by modern science and technology.

1) The common chemotherapy drug paclitaxel which is obtained from the bark of taxus chinensis, has a good effect on lung cancer and breast cancer. In 1976, Chinese chemist Gao Yisheng obtained the anticancer drug camptothecin from the camptotheca acuminata, which have a good effect in the cancer of gastrointestinal tract or head-neck. What else such as vincristine is an alkaloid extracted from catharanthus roseus, which has a good effect to lymphoma and sarcoma.

2) Kanglaite injection is a drug of antitumor activity which not only could kill cancer cells but also improve immunity function and be extracted from semen coicis, and has a certain synergy and progression combined with chemotherapy or radiation therapy in lung cancer or liver cancer. The tanshinone II A which extracted from salvia miltiorrhiza was found that it has an anticancer role, and it can inhibit the formation of blood vessels and prevent the transfer function, but the biological utilization rate is still very low. Elemene liposome is an effective anticancer component extracted from turmeric, which can induce apoptosis of tumor cells and inhibit the growth of tumor cells. Professor David Adelson, a professor coming from Australia, has found out the mechanism of compound sophora injection to inhibit cancer by system biology method. Brucea emulsion is an antitumor active ingredient made from brucea, which has a good effect on lung cancer, lung

cancer with brain metastasis and digestive tract tumor. It was found that trioxide was a significant therapeutic effect in acute promyelocytic leukemia (APL), and a global gold standard for APL treatment by the research of arsenic.

3) It has been found that astragalus contains a variety of active ingredients of immunoregulation, especially astragalus polysaccharide. It was reported in Science Advances that the molecular mechanism of the production of anticancer by the compounds of scutellaria baicalensis decoction (scutellaria, peony, jujube, licorice) was to enhance the chemotherapy efficacy of colon cancer patients and improve diarrhea or other side effects of being caused by irinotecan. Curcumin is a kind of chemical composition which was extracted from the roots of zingiberaceae (araceae plant) has inhibition to proliferation and metastasis of tumor cells, and it is as a third-generation medicine of tumor treatment in the U. S national cancer institute. Ginsenoside Rg3 is an active ingredient obtained from ginseng and has good anti-infiltration role and antimetastasis effect.

17.9   Prospect of TCM therapy

1) It has a long history and there has accumulated rich experience for thousands of years in treating of tumors by TCM. However, it is still not possible to solve the whole tumor problems alone. The comprehensive treatment model with TCM is becoming popular these years. It can be reduce toxicity and increase curative effect by TCM therapy with radiation and chemotherapy, and promote the functional recovery after surgery by TCM therapy. Maintenance treatment can improve physical fitness, improve the quality of life, enhance immunity, reduce tumor metastasis and recurrence rate after surgery, radiation and chemotherapy by TCM therapy.

2) There are three main aspects to the future outlook. First of all, syndrome differentiation and individualization were emphasized in TCM therapy, but the standardization is not enough. Before and after the operation or chemoradiotherapy, we suggest establishing a standard of TCM therapy to get better, the anti-cancer effect. Secondly, the insufficient understanding to some tumors, and the nature research of tumor needs to be increased, so as to providing a better guide for the treatment. Thirdly, it can enhance the body's immunity, mobilize the human potential, and kill cancer cells with multiple targets by the method of strengthening vital Qi including strengthen spleen, invigorate Qi, nourishing Yin and tonifying kidney, which can achieve the purpose of treating tumor by regulating the state of constitution and viscera function.

We have great confidence in the prospect of cancer by of TCM therapy. In recent years, researching the cytotoxic mechanism of TCM, single drug and compound research, epigenetics, immune regulation, and anti-angiogenesis research has been or is becoming a focus of research with surprise and new achievements.

Yang Zhongming

Chapter 18

Palliative Cancer Care

18.1 Introduction

Each year about 10 million people worldwide are diagnosed with cancer and 6 million will die from it. Up to now, most of the cancer is incurable while diagnosed and most patients will die within years.

The growing incidence and prevalence of cancer makes palliative care a public health issue. Palliative cancer care began as hospice and end-of-life care, but it now has developed into an integral part of comprehensive cancer care. The goals of palliative care are to prevent and reduce suffering and to support the best possible quality of life for patients and their families, regardless of the stage of the disease or the need for other therapies. Palliative care focuses on relief of suffering, psychosocial support, and comfort caring near the end of life.

The World Health Organization defined Palliative Care as an approach which improves the quality of life of patients and their families facing life-threatening disease, through the prevention and relief of suffering by means of early identification, assessment and treatment of pain and other symptoms including physical, psychosocial and spiritual aspects.

In the old model of the cancer treatment, palliative care services would only be involved at the end of life when no further oncological or supportive treatments were available. That was a "terminal care" service for those clearly at the end of life. But, the symptoms that were being controlled occur not only at the end of life but also at different degrees throughout the cancer journey. So now, palliative care is not simply care of the dying patients. The WHO definition refers to "early involvement" in any ultimately life-limiting disease. It is far more than terminal care. The new model attempts to dovetail palliative care with active anti-cancer treatment, gradually increasing its involvement while anti-cancer treatment becomes less appropriate (Figure 18-1).

In west, the oncology team for palliative care include physician, nurse, social worker, chaplain, and volunteer. The principle of palliative care is to neither obstruct nor hasten death.

The standard of care is to treat symptoms proportionately. Palliative care, with its focus on management of symptoms, psychosocial support, and assistance with decision-making, has the potential to improve the quality of care and reduce the use of medical services. Palliative care has traditionally been delivered late in

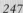

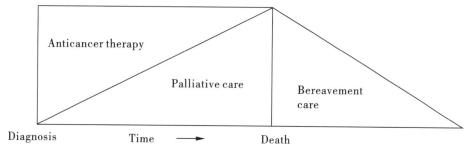

Figure 18-1　Current model of palliative cancer care

the course of disease to patient's. However, late referrals to palliative care are inadequate to alter the quality and delivery of care provided to patients with cancer. To have meaningful effect on patients' quality of life and end-of-life care, palliative care services should be provided earlier in the course of the disease.

The integration of palliative care with standard oncologic care may facilitate the optimal and appropriate administration of anticancer therapy, especially during the final months of life. Patients receiving early palliative care, as compared with those receiving standard care alone, had improved survival. With earlier referral to a hospice program, patients may receive care that results in better management of symptoms, leading to stabilization of their condition and prolonged survival.

Acceptable palliative care should include the following: ①adequate pain and symptom management; ②reduction of patient and family distress; ③acceptable sense of control; ④relief of caregiver burden; ⑤strengthened relationships; ⑥optimized quality of life, personal growth, and enhanced meaning.

18.2　Palliative care screening

The patient with cancer should be screened at every visit for the following: ①unmanaged symptoms; ②moderate to severe distress related to cancer diagnosis and therapy; ③significant comorbidity with serious physical, psychiatric, or psychosocial conditions; ④ potentially life-limiting disease; ⑤ metastatic solid tumors; ⑥patient or family concerns about the course of disease and decision-making; ⑦patient or family requests for palliative care, or patient request for hastened death.

Patients who do not meet the above screening criteria should be re-screened at the next visit. In addition, the oncology team should inform patients and their family members about palliative care services. Anticipation of palliative care needs and prevention of symptoms should also be discussed, and conversations regarding advance care planning should be initiated.

18.3　Palliative care assessment

Patients who meet screening criteria should undergo a comprehensive palliative care assessment by the primary oncology team evaluating the benefits and burdens of anticancer therapy; physical symptoms; psychosocial or spiritual distress; personal goals, values, and expectations; educational and informational needs; and cultural factors affecting care.

Many cancer symptoms can be relieved by control of the cancer with anti-cancer therapy. Special attention should be given to the natural history of the specific tumor; the potential for response to further treatment; the meaning of anticancer therapy to the patient and family; the potential for treatment-related toxicities including impairment of vital organs and performance status; and serious comorbid conditions.

Patients and their families should also be asked about their personal goals, values, and expectations. It is important to share decision-making with patient and the family. The following elements of palliative care are most important for patients and their families: effective communication and shared decision-making; expert care; respectful and compassionate care; and trust and confidence in clinicians.

The patients' priorities for palliative care, including goals, the perceived meanings of both anticancer therapy and quality of life, should be assessed. Goals and expectations that might be better met by the hospice model of palliative care should be identified. When appropriate, it is important to explore the patients' understanding of the incurability of their disease and whether patients wish to know survival statistics.

Assessment of psychosocial distress should focus on illness-related distress and psychosocial, spiritual, or existential needs. The values and preferences of patients and families about information and communication should also be assessed. The oncology team should inquire about cultural factors affecting care and perceptions of the patient and family regarding the patient's disease status.

18.4 Palliative care interventions

18.4.1 Anticancer therapy

Anticancer therapy may be conventional evidence-based treatment or treatment in the context of a clinical trial. In some of the advanced-stage cancers, chemotherapy may be superior to best supportive care and may prolong survival. Palliative radiotherapy also plays an important role in the management of patients with advanced cancer. Furthermore, patients with advanced cancer who are not eligible for systemic chemotherapy may benefit from molecular targeted therapies that may be effective for relieving symptoms, maintaining stable disease, and improving quality of life without the adverse events that may be associated with cytotoxic cancer therapies. Physicians, patients, and their families should discuss prognosis, intent and goals of therapy (palliative or curative), range of choices, benefits and burdens of anticancer therapy, and possible effects on quality of life. In addition, the oncology team should prepare the patient psychologically for possible disease progression.

Anticancer therapy should be in line with stated patient goals and priorities and be accompanied by appropriate prevention/management of side effects as well as palliative care. In patients with progressive metastatic cancer, palliative chemotherapy failed to improve quality of life near death for those with moderate or poor performance status. Patients with months to weeks to live should be provided with guidance regarding the anticipated course of the disease. Physicians should confirm patient's understanding of goals of therapy and preferences regarding prognostic information. These patients are typically tired of therapy and more concerned about the side effects of more treatment. The focus of treatment for these patients shifts from prolonging life towards maintaining quality of life. These patients should consider potential discontinuation of anticancer treatment that is not directly addressing a symptom complex and be offered best supportive care, including referral to palliative care or hospice.

Patients with weeks to days to live (i. e. , dying patients) should discontinue all treatments not directly contributing to patient comfort. Intensive palliative care focusing on symptom management should be provided in addition to preparation for the dying process. Refer the patient to hospice when possible.

18.4.2   Symptom management

The most common symptoms that need to be controlled are pain, dyspnea, anorexia, cachexia, nausea, vomiting, constipation, malignant bowel obstruction, fatigue, weakness, asthenia, insomnia, daytime sedation, and delirium. Palliative interventions for these symptoms are discussed individually below.

18.4.2.1   Pain control

Pain is one of the most common symptoms associated with cancer. Pain is defined by the International Association for the Study of Pain as an unpleasant sensory and emotional experience associated with actual or potential tissue damage, or described in relation to such damage. Pain was reported in 59% of patients undergoing cancer treatment, in 64% of patients with advanced disease, and in 33% of patients after curative treatment. Pain is one of the symptoms patients fear most. Unrelieved pain denies patients comfort and greatly affects their activities, motivation, interactions with family and friends, and overall quality of life.

The importance of relieving pain and the availability of effective therapies make it imperative that health care providers must be adept at cancer pain assessment and treatment. This requires familiarity with the pathogenesis of cancer pain, pain assessment techniques, and common barriers to the delivery of appropriate analgesia. Providers should be familiar with pertinent pharmacologic, anesthetic, neurosurgical, and behavioral interventions for treating cancer pain, as well as complimentary approaches such as physical/occupational therapy.

The most widely accepted algorithm for the treatment of cancer pain was developed by the WHO, which was called as "three ladder principle for cancer paintreatment". It suggests that patients with mild pain be treated with acetaminophen or a nonsteroidal anti-inflammatory drug (NSAID) as the first ladder. If this is not sufficient, the patient should be escalated to a "weak opioid", such as tramadol as second ladder. If that is not satisfactory, the patient should be treated with strong opioid, such as morphine as the third ladder. Although this algorithm has served as an excellent teaching tool, the management of cancer pain is considerably more complex than this three-tiered "cancer pain ladder" suggests.

It is important to note that dying patients in their last weeks of life have several specific requirements. For instance, opioid dose should not be reduced solely for decreased blood pressure, respiration rate, or level of consciousness when opioid is necessary for adequate management of dyspnea and pain. In fact, opioids can be titrated aggressively for moderate, severe acute or chronic pain. In addition, palliative sedation can be considered for refractory pain following consultation with pain management/palliative care specialists. Palliativeradiotherapy may be used to address pain associated with bone metastases.

18.4.2.2   Nausea and Vomiting

Chemotherapy-induced nausea and vomiting has a major impact on a patient's quality of life. Patients can also experience nausea and vomiting unrelated to chemotherapy and radiation, resulting from gastric outlet obstruction, bowel obstruction, constipation, opioid use, or hypercalcemia. These causes should be identified and treated. Consider palliative radiotherapy for nausea and vomiting related to brain metastases. Proton pump inhibitors and histamine-2 (H2) receptor antagonists can be used to manage gastritis or gastroesophageal reflux. Gastric outlet obstruction may benefit from treatment with corticosteroids; alternative treatment options include endoscopic stenting or insertion of a decompressing G-tube. Many medications can also cause nausea and vomiting, and blood levels of possible culprits, such as digoxin, phenytoin, carbamazepine, or tricyclic antidepressants, should be checked.

Non-specific nausea and vomiting are often managed with dopamine or 5-HT3 receptor antagonists. For anxiety-related nausea, the addition of benzodiazepines can be considered. If a vertiginous component to the nausea and vomiting exists, anticholinergic/antihistamine agents may be appropriate.

Titrate dopamine receptor antagonists to maximum benefit and tolerance. In the setting of continued nausea and vomiting, consider additional drug classes with potential antiemetic properties: corticosteroids, 5-HT3 receptor antagonists, anticholinergic agents and/or antihistamines. Alternative therapies (e. g. , acupuncture, hypnosis, cognitive behavioral therapy) can also be considered. Palliative sedation can be considered as a last resort if intensified efforts by specialized palliative care or hospice services fail.

For persistent nausea and vomiting, consider the appropriate route of administration. First, prescribe oral agent and titrate to maximum benefit and consider opioid rotation. If nausea and vomiting is persistent, provide IV administration as needed. For continued persistent symptoms, provide scheduled IV administration or continuous infusion of antiemetics. An around-the-clock dosing schedule may provide the most consistent benefit to the patient. Continuous intravenous or subcutaneous infusions of different antiemetics may be necessary for the management of intractable nausea and vomiting.

18.4.2.3　Constipation

Constipation occurs in approximately 50% of patients with advanced cancer and most patients treated with opioids. Although several drugs including antacids, anticholinergic drugs and antiemetics are known to cause constipation, opioid analgesics are most commonly associated with constipation. Providers should discontinue any nonessential constipating medications. In addition to physical discomfort, constipation in patients with advanced cancer can cause psychological distress and anxiety regarding continued opioid use. Opioid-induced constipation (OIC) should be anticipated and treated prophylactically with a stimulating laxative to increase bowel motility with stool softeners. Increasing intake of fluid and physical activity should also be encouraged, when appropriate. Added dietary fiber may be considered for patients with adequate fluid intake.

If constipation is present, the cause and severity must be assessed. Impaction, obstruction, and other treatable causes, such as hypercalcemia, hypokalemia, hypothyroidism, and diabetes mellitus, should be assessed and treated. Constipation may also be treated by adding bisacodyl 10–15 mg, 2–3 times daily with a goal of 1 non-forced bowel movement every 1–2 days. If impaction is observed, glycerine suppositories (with or without mineral oil retention enema) may be administered or manual disimpaction may be performed. Use suppository and enema with caution in patients receiving chemotherapy due to risk of cytopenia.

If constipation persists, adding other laxatives may be considered, such as rectal bisacodyl once daily or oral polyethylene glycol, lactulose, magnesium hydroxide, or magnesium citrate. If gastroparesis is suspected, the addition of a prokinetic agent, such as metoclopramide, may be considered.

Peripherally acting μ-opioid receptor antagonists may help to relieve OIC while maintaining pain management. methylnaltrexone can provide effective relief of OIC while preserving opioid-mediated analgesia.

Several newer agents have also been examined for treating constipation. Lubiprostone is an orally active prostaglandin analog that activates select chloride channels to enhance intestinal fluid secretion. This agent was shown to be effective for treating OIC in patients with chronic noncancer pain. Lubiprostone could be used in combination with a peripherally acting μ-opioid receptor antagonist such as methylnaltrexone. Linaclotide is a selective agonist of guanylate cyclase-C receptors in the intestines to enhance intestinal secretions, and has been effective in the treatment of constipation associated with irritable bowel syndrome and chronic idiopathic constipation. It can be considered 0. 15 mg per kilogram of body weight of methylnaltrexone every other day (no more than once a day) for patients experiencing constipation that has not responded to standard laxative therapy. Methylnaltrexone should not be used in patients with a postoperative ileus or mechanical bowel obstruction.

18.4.2.4   Diarrhea

In patients with cancer, diarrhea can be caused by a number of potential factors, including anticancer treatment-related side effects, infection, antibiotic use, dietary changes, or fecal impaction. Diarrhea is a common side effect of various chemotherapeutics (e. g. ,fluorouracil and irinotecan), as well tyrosine kinase inhibitors and certain biologic agents (e. g. ,ipilimumab, cetuximab, panitumumab). Abdominal and pelvic radiation therapy (alone or as part of chemoradiation regimens) can also induce gastrointestinal toxicity resulting in diarrhea.

The patients should be screened to determine the grade of diarrhea, and providers should provide immediate intervention for dehydration based on grade and assess for potential causes.

For patients with grade 1 diarrhea, treatment should include hydration and electrolyte replacement, antidiarrheal medications, and a bland or clear liquid diet. If chemotherapy-related, decrease dose or discontinue therapy. For treating grade 2 diarrhea, anticholinergic agents such as hyoscyamine or atropine can be considered. Infection-induced diarrhea should be treated with the appropriate antibiotic. Immunotherapy-related diarrhea can be treated with corticosteroids, infliximab, and/or probiotics. Patients with grade 3 or 4 diarrhea should receive inpatient treatment. In addition to fluid replacement, antidiarrheal therapy, anticholinergics, and octreotide can also be considered.

18.4.2.5   Malignant bowel obstruction

Malignant bowel obstructions are usually diagnosed clinically and confirmed with radiography. For patients with years to months to live, surgery following CT scan is the primary treatment option. While surgery can lead to improvements in quality of life, surgical risks should be discussed with patients and families, including risk of mortality, morbidity, and re-obstruction. Also take into account prognosis and relative invasiveness of the intervention proposed. Although surgery is the primary treatment for malignant obstruction, some patients with advanced disease or patients in generally poor condition are unfit for surgery and require alternative management to relieve distressing symptoms. Risk factors for poor surgical outcome include ascites, carcinomatosis, palpable intra-abdominal masses, multiple bowel obstructions, previous abdominal radiation, advanced disease, and poor overall clinical status. In these patients, medical management can include pharmacologic measures, parenteral fluids, endoscopic management, and enteral tube drainage.

Pharmacologic management of malignant bowel obstruction can be separated into two groups of patients: those for whom the goal is to maintain gut function and those for whom gut function is no longer possible. When the goal is maintaining gut function, patients can be treated with opioids, antiemetics, and corticosteroids, alone or in combination. When gut function is no longer considered possible, pharmacologic options also include somatostatin analogs (e. g. ,octreotide) and/or anticholinergics. If octreotide is helpful and the patient has a life expectancy of at least 1 month, it may be beneficial to consider a depot form of octreotide once an optimal dose is established. Antiemetics that increase gastrointestinal mobility such as metoclopramide should not be used in patients with complete obstruction, but may be beneficial when obstruction is partial. Using of octreotide is recommended early in the diagnosis because of its efficacy and tolerability.

A venting gastrostomy tube or an endoscopically placed stent can also palliate symptoms of malignant bowel obstruction. Total parenteral nutrition can be considered to improve quality of life in patients with a life expectancy of years to months.

18.4.2.6 Dyspnea

Dyspnea is one of the most common symptoms in patients with advanced lung cancer and it is defined as "a subjective experience of breathing discomfort that consists of qualitatively distinct sensations that vary in intensity".

Symptom intensity should first be assessed in all patients. Underlying causes or comorbid conditions should be treated using chemotherapy or radiation therapy; therapeutic procedures for cardiac, pleural, or abdominal fluid; bronchoscopic therapy; or bronchodilators, diuretics, steroids, antibiotics, transfusions, or anticoagulants for pulmonary emboli.

There is evidence for the efficacy and safety of small dose opioids for dyspnea in both the malignant and non-malignant setting. It can be used in severe dyspnea. Morphine has undergone the most extensive investigation for treating dyspnea in patients with cancer.

Scopolamine, atropine, hyoscyamine, and glycopyrrolate are options to reduce excessive secretions associated with dyspnea. Glycopyrrolate does not effectively cross the blood-brain barrier and is less likely than the other drug options to cause delirium, but this agent can produce anticholinergic side effects. Scopolamine can be administered subcutaneously or transdermally. Transdermal scopolamine patches are appropriate for imminently dying patients. A subcutaneous injection of scopolamine can be administered when the patch is not applied or if management of secretions is inadequate.

Palliative radiotherapy can be considered for patients with SVC syndrome or those who have respiratory obstruction by tumor mass.

Non-pharmacologic interventions include the use of handheld fans directed at the face, supplemental oxygen, and time-limited trials of noninvasive mechanical ventilation. High-flow nasal oxygen and noninvasive mechanical ventilation may provide temporary improvements in hypoxemia and dyspnea.

As life expectancy decreases, the role of mechanical ventilation and oxygen diminishes, and the role of opioids, benzodiazepines, glycopyrrolate, and scopolamine increases. If fluid overload is a contributing factor, enteral and parenteral fluids should be decreased or discontinued, and low-dose diuretics can be considered.

18.4.2.7 Anorexia/cachexia

Cachexia is physical wasting with loss of skeletal and visceral muscle mass and is very common among patients with cancer. Many patients with cancer lose the desire to eat (anorexia), which contributes to cachexia. Cachexia can also occur independently from anorexia, as proinflammatory cytokines and tumor-derived factors directly lead to muscle proteolysis. Cachexia leads to asthenia (weakness), hypoalbuminemia, emaciation, immune system impairment, metabolic dysfunction, and autonomic failure. Cancer-related cachexia has also been associated with failure of anti-cancer treatment, increased treatment toxicity, delayed treatment initiation, early treatment termination, shorter survival, and psychosocial distress.

Reversible causes of anorexia, such as oropharyngeal candidiasis and depression, should be addressed. Treatment includes the relief of symptoms that interfere with food intake (eg, pain, constipation, nausea/vomiting), as well as metoclopramide for early satiety.

For patients with months-to-weeks or weeks-to-days life expectancy, consider the use of appetite stimulants (eg, megestrol acetate, dexamethasone, olanzapine) if increased appetite is an important aspect of quality of life. A combination therapy approach included medroxyprogesterone, megestrol acetate, eicosapentaenoic acid and L-carnitine supplementation may yield the best possible outcomes for patients with cancer cachexia.

Nutrition consultation should be considered. Nutritional support, including enteral and parenteral feeding as appropriate, should also be considered when the disease or treatment affects the ability to eat and/or absorb nutrients and the patient's life expectancy is months to years. The goals and intensity of nutritional support change as life expectancy is reduced to weeks to days. Overly aggressive enteral or parenteral nutrition therapies can actually increase the suffering of dying patients. Palliative care in the final weeks of life focuses on treating dry mouth and thirst, and providing education and support to the patient and family regarding the emotional aspects of withdrawal of nutritional support. Family members should be informed of alternate ways to care for dying patients.

18.4.2.8　Fatigue/weakness/asthenia

Fatigue is a common symptom in patients with cancer and is nearly universal in those receiving cytotoxic chemotherapy, radiation therapy, bone marrow transplantation, or treatment with biological response modifiers. The accurate mechanisms involved in the pathophysiology of cancer-related fatigue (CRF) are unknown. Proposed mechanisms include pro-inflammatory cytokines, hypothalamic-pituitary-adrenal (HPA) axis dysregulation, circadian rhythm desynchronization, skeletal muscle wasting, and genetic dysregulation.

In patients with metastatic disease, the prevalence of CRF exceeds 75%. Predictors of severe fatigue include higher disease stage and chemotherapy treatment. The female sex and chronic pain are associated with greater fatigue. Fatigue is a disruptive symptom and persistent CRF affects quality of life.

Fatigue is a subjective experience that should be systematically assessed using patient self-reports and other sources of data. However, because it is a symptom that is perceived by the patient, fatigue can be described most accurately by self-report. Patients should be screened for the presence and severity of fatigue at their initial clinical visit, at regular intervals during and/or following cancer treatment, and as clinically indicated. The history and physical examination, laboratory data, and descriptions of patient behavior by family members, especially regarding children, are important sources of additional information.

Patients and families should be informed that managing fatigue is an integral part of total health care, and all patients should receive symptom management. If patients cannot tolerate their cancer treatment or if they must choose between treatment andquality of life, control of their disease may be diminished. Rehabilitation may include physical therapy, occupational therapy, and physical medicine, and should be considered as indicated from diagnosis to end of life.

Education about fatigue and its natural history should be offered to all patients with cancer, especially for patients beginning potential fatigue-inducing treatments (such as radiation, chemotherapy, or biotherapy) before the onset of fatigue. Patients should be informed that if fatigue does occur, it may be a consequence of the treatment and is not necessarily an indication that the treatment is not working or that the disease is progressing. This reassurance is important, as fear of progression is a main reason for the under-reporting of fatigue.

Energy conservation and distraction are useful in coping with fatigue. Energy conservation is defined as the deliberately planned management of one's personal energy resources to prevent their depletion. It encompasses a common sense approach that helps patients set realistic expectations, prioritize and pace activities, and delegate less essential activities. Patients should be counseled that it is permissible to postpone all non-essential activities if they are experiencing moderate-to-severe fatigue. In a situation of escalating fatigue at the end of life, family members may wish to designate individuals to assume activities relinquished by the cancer patient. Daytime naps can replenish energy, but it is advisable to limit these to less than an hour to avoid disturbing nighttime sleep. Patients may also use labor saving techniques such as wearing a bath robe instead of drying off with a towel or assistive devices such as a walker, grabbing tools, and a bedside commode.

18.4.2.9 Sleep/wake disturbances

Most of patients with cancer suffered from insomnia or daytime sedation. If patients have a history of sleep-disordered breathing such as excessive snoring, gasping for air, polysomnography should be considered. Polysomnography should also be considered for patients with head and neck cancers, because obstructive sleep apnea (OSA) is prevalent in patients with this disease. Primary sleep disorders, such as OSA and periodic limb movement disorder, should be treated with continuous positive airway pressure (CPAP) or Bi-PAP. Restless leg syndrome, if present, can be treated with ropinirole, pramipexole with pregabalin, or carbidopa-levodopa. Fears and anxiety regarding death and disease should be explored, and other contributing factors to sleep/wake disturbances should be treated, including pain, depression, anxiety, delirium, and nausea. Cognitive behavioral therapy may be effective in treating sleep/wake disturbances in patients with cancer.

For refractory insomnia, pharmacologic management includes the short-acting benzodiazepine lorazepam; the non-benzodiazepine zolpidem; antipsychotic medications such as chlorpromazine, quetiapine, and olanzapine; and sedating antidepressants such as trazodone and mirtazapine.

For refractory daytime sedation, the central nervous system stimulants methylphenidate or dextroamphetamine should be given with a starting dose of 2.5–5.0 mg orally with breakfast. If the effect of the drug does not last through lunch, a second dose can be given at lunch, preferably no later than 2:00 PM. Doses can be escalated as needed. Another option for refractory daytime sedation is the psychostimulant modafinil, which has been approved in adults for excessive sleepiness associated with OSA/hypopnea syndrome (OSAHS), shift work sleep disorder, and narcolepsy. Caffeine and dextroamphetamine are additional options for refractory daytime sedation. The last dose of caffeine should be given no later than 4:00 PM.

Dying patients should be assessed for their desire to have their insomnia or sedation treated. The doses of their pharmacologic therapies can be adjusted as appropriate. The addition of an anti-psychotic drug (chlorpromazine or quetiapine) can be considered in patients whose insomnia is refractory.

18.4.2.10 Delirium

Delirium may present as either a hypoactive or a hyperactive subtype. Hypoactive delirium was the most prevalent subtype in palliative care patients and that this condition is often underdiagnosed due to its presentation.

Non-pharmacologic interventions (e.g., reorientation, cognitive stimulation, sleep hygiene) should be maximized before pharmacologic interventions are used. Delirium-inducing medications (i.e., steroids, anticholinergics) should be reduced or eliminated as much as possible. Benzodiazepines should not be used as initial treatment for delirium in patients not already taking them.

The symptoms of moderate delirium can be managed with oral haloperidol, risperidone, olanzapine, or quetiapine fumarate. The symptoms of severe delirium (i.e., agitation) should be managed with antipsychotic, neuroleptic drugs such as haloperidol, olanzapine, or chlorpromazine. Opioid dose reduction or rotation can also be considered for patients with severe delirium. Radiotherapy can be considered for patients with delirium due to brain metastases.

Delirium in patients with advanced cancer may shorten life expectancy. In these patients, iatrogenic causes should be eliminated whenever possible. Opioid rotation can be considered if the delirium is believed be caused by neurotoxicity of the current opioid. If delirium is a result of disease progression, palliative care must be focused on symptom management and family support. Neuroleptic and benzodiazepine medications should have their dose increased and/or their route of administration changed to ensure adequate delirium symptom management. Unnecessary medications and tubes should be removed. For refractory delirium in dying patients, palliative sedation can be considered following consultation with a palliative care specialist and/or psychiatrist.

18.4.2.11　Psychosocial distress-social support/resource management

Psychosocial care should be integrated into routine cancer care across all disease stages and in both the inpatient and outpatient settings. For patients with estimated life expectancy ranging from years to months experiencing psychosocial distress, social support/resource management should be offered. Assess prognostic awareness and discuss on an ongoing basis with patient, family, and caregivers. Patients should be cared for in a safe environment with available caregivers. In addition, it is important to ensure that the patient has adequate financial resources and refers to social services (social worker, psychologist, and/or psychiatrist) as needed. Support and education should be provided to the caregivers and family members. Personal, spiritual, or cultural issues related to the patient's illness and prognosis should be discussed. If language is a barrier, a professional health care interpreter, who is not related to the patient or family, should be available for patients, caregivers, and families as needed.

In a dying patient with an estimated life expectancy of weeks to days, the patient's desires for comfort should be evaluated and supported. The process of dying and the expected events should be explained to the patient, caregivers, and family members. Patients and family members should be provided with emotional support to address any intra-family conflict regarding palliative care interventions. Eligibility and readiness for specialized palliative/hospice care should be determined.

18.5　Palliative care reassessment

All patients should be reassessed regularly, and effective communication and information sharing must exist between the patient, caregivers, and health care providers. Patients and family members benefit most from ongoing discussions about the natural history of the disease and prognosis in clear, consistent language. If the interventions are unacceptable upon reassessment, the oncology or palliative care team should intensify palliative care and reassess the patient and family situation. The oncology team should also consult specialized palliative care services, hospice, or an ethics committee. Referral to a psychiatrist or psychologist to evaluate and treat undiagnosed psychiatric disorders, substance abuse, and inadequate coping mechanisms should be considered.

Patients' treatment goals and expectations may change and evolve as disease progresses. Reassessment should be ongoing, with continuation or modification of life expectancy guided palliative care until the patient's death or survivorship.

18.6　End-of-life care issues

18.6.1　Preparing patients and families for end-of-life and transition to hospice care

For patients with an estimated life expectancy of years or years to months, providers should engage in clear, consistent discussion with the patient and family about prognosis and anticipated care needs on an ongoing basis. The team should facilitate advance care planning and assess decision-making capacity and need for a surrogate decision maker. Elicit values and preferences with respect to quality of life and determine need for specialized palliative care or eligibility and readiness for hospice care.

Patients with an estimated life expectancy of months weeks or weeks to days should be referred to hospice agencies. Assess patient and family understanding of the dying process and provide education as needed. Providers should address potential need for transitions in care while ensuring continued involvement of the primary care physician and primary oncology team. Patients should receive information and additional referrals, as necessary, for psychosocial assessment, legacy work, grief counseling, spiritual support, and funeral/memorial service planning.

18.6.2 Advance care planning

The oncology team should initiate discussions of personal values and preferences for end-of-life care while patients have a life expectancy of years to months.

Advance care planning should include an open discussion about palliative care options, such as hospice; personal values and preferences for end-of-life care; the congruence between the patient's wishes/expectations and those of the family/health care team; and information about advance directives. Patients should be asked if they have completed any advance care planning such as living wills, powers of attorney, or delineation of specific limitations regarding life-sustaining treatments including cardiopulmonary resuscitation, mechanical ventilation, and artificial nutrition/hydration.

When the patient's life expectancy is reduced to months to weeks, the oncology team should actively facilitate completion of appropriate advance directives and ensure their availability in all care settings. The team should also confirm the patient's values and decisions in light of changes in status.

The patient's preferred location for receiving end-of-life care should be determined. Most patients with cancer would prefer to spend one's receive end-of-life care in a skilled nursing facility or an in-patient hospice facility.

In patients with a life expectancy of only weeks to days, the patient's decision regarding cardiopulmonary resuscitation and other life sustaining treatments must be clarified and confirmed. Providers should facilitate continued involvement of the primary care physician and primary oncology team. The desire for organ donation and/or autopsy must also be discussed with the patient.

18.6.3 Care of the imminently dying hospitalized patient

An imminently dying patient is defined as one within hours of death. The physical aspects of care for an imminently dying patient focus on adequate symptom management and comfort, keeping in mind the patient's wishes and values. Approaches may include intensifying ongoing care; adjusting medication doses for optimal comfort; discontinuing unnecessary interventions such as diagnostic tests, transfusions, artificial nutrition, hydration, dialysis, needle sticks and so on; ensuring access to symptom-relief medication through alternate routes if oral administration is difficult; improving physical comfort by providing a pressure-relieving mattress and regular repositioning; eye and mouth care to maintain moisture; treating urinary retention and fecal impaction; managing terminal restlessness and agitation with palliative sedation; reducing death rattle/terminal secretion (e. g. , repositioning patient; reducing parenteral and enteral fluids; adding medications such as scopolamine, hyoscyamine, atropine, or glycopyrrolate) ; and preparing for patient and family requests for autopsy and/or organ donation.

The psychosocial aspects of care for an imminently dying patient should take into account individual and family goals, preferences, cultures, and religious beliefs. Open communication should occur between the patient, family, and care team regarding the physical and psychological aspects of the dying process and the importance of honoring any advance directives. The care plan may also include consultation with social workers or chaplains to meet social and spiritual needs; counseling to promote healthy grieving; support for children/grandchildren and education for parents on age-appropriate grieving processes. Patients who are actively dying in their final hours of life should be allowed to spend uninterrupted time with family, if they wish to do so.

18.6.4　Palliative sedation

Palliative sedation may be considered for imminently dying patients (life expectancy of hours to days) with refractory symptoms that persist despite comprehensive, interdisciplinary palliative care. If palliative sedation is being considered, a prognosis of imminent death should be confirmed. Informed consent must be obtained from the patient and/or a surrogate or family member following discussions of the patient's disease status, treatment goals, prognosis, and expected outcomes. Consent for palliative sedation must be accompanied by consent for discontinuation of life-prolonging therapies (such as artificial hydration/nutrition) and withholding of cardiopulmonary resuscitation, as these therapies would only serve to increase suffering in this case.

18.6.5　After-death care interventions

Comprehensive palliative care for the patient's family and caregivers continues after the patient's death. Immediate issues include informing the family (if not present), offering condolences, and providing family time with the body. Chaplain involvement to assess family's desire for religious ritual or spiritual support may be helpful. Additional concerns include ensuring culturally sensitive and respectful treatment of the body, including removal of tubes, drains, lines, and the Foley catheter (unless an autopsy is planned); addressing concerns about organ donation or autopsy; facilitating funeral arrangements through completion of necessary paperwork; and informing insurance companies and other health care professionals of the patient's death.

18.7　Conclusion

The oncology teams should provide the best and most comprehensive cancer treatment for patients with incurable cancer. Patients with advanced disease may be overly optimistic about their chances of cure and survival, and this can have a negative effect on their quality of life. Physician-led discussion of disease progression and death can improve quality of care and quality of life for both patients and families. Providing information in a collaborative manner protects the autonomy of patients to make informed decisions based on potential treatment outcomes. Palliative care can help patients and families set realistic expectations and meet short-and longer-term goals, such as important life-cycle events. Palliative care is geared toward a different hope than that for cure of the disease itself. Even when cure is no longer possible, hope remains: hope for dignity, comfort, and closure at the end of life. The oncology and palliative care professionals should create a better caring for patients and families, with good quality of life for cancer patients.

Min Daliu

References

[1]JORDAN V C, BARRINGTON J A. Hormone therapy in breast and prostate cancer[M]. New Jersey: Humana Press,2009.

[2]RUSSO M D,FACP,IRMA H. Molecular basis of breast cancer[M]. Berlin Heidelberg: Springer, 2004.

[3]林洪生. 恶性肿瘤中医诊疗指南[M]. 北京:人民卫生出版社,2014.

[4]MELMED,SHLOMO. Williams textbook of endocrinology[M]. Amsterdam:Elsevier saunders,2016.

[5]MURPHY K M,WEAVER C. Janeway's immunobiology[M]. New York:Garland Science,2016.

[6]MUELLER P R,ADAM A. Interventional Oncology[M]. New York:Springer-Verlag New York,2012.

[7]YOU W C. Medical epidemiology,the fourth edition[M]. Beijing:People's Medical Publishing House, 2006.

[8]魏于全,赫捷. 肿瘤学[M]. 2 版. 北京:人民卫生出版社,2015.

[9]ANSELL S M,LESOKHIN A M,BORRELLO I,et al. PD-1 blockade with nivolumab in relapsed or refractory Hodgkin's lymphoma[J]. N Engl J Med,2015,372:311-319.

[10]BURNETT A K,RUSSELL N H,HILLS R K. Supplementary material:Arsenic trioxide and all-trans retinoic acid treatment for acute promyelocytic leukaemia in all risk groups (AML17):results of a randomised,controlled,phase 3 trial[J]. Lancet Oncol,2015,16(13):1295-1305.

[11]CHEN D S,MELLMAN I. Elements of cancer immunity and the cancer-immune set point[J]. Nature, 2017,541(7637):321-330.

[12]CHEN D S,MELLMAN I. Oncology meets immunology:the cancer-immunity cycle[J]. Immunity, 2013,39(1):1-10.

[13]CHEN W,ZHENG R,BAADE P D,et al. Cancer statistics in China,2015[J]. CA Cancer J Clin, 2016,66(2):115-132.

[14]GIULIANOTTI P C,CORATTI A,ANGELINI M,et al. Robotics in general surgery[J]. Arch Surg, 2003,138(7):777-784.

[15]HAMID O,ROBERT C,DAUD A,et al. Safety and tumor responses with lambrolizumab (anti-PD-1) in melanoma[J]. N Engl J Med,2013,369(2):134-144.

[16]HERBST R S,SORIA J C,KOWANETZ M,et al. Predictive correlates of response to the anti-PD-L1 antibody MPDL3280A in cancer patients[J]. Nature,2014,515(7528):563-567.

[17]HERRON D M,MAROHN M. A consensus document on robotic surgery[J]. Surg Endosc,2008, 22(2):313-325.

[18]NELSON P S. Molecular states underlying androgen receptor activation:a framework for therapeutics targeting androgen signaling in prostate cancer[J]. J Clin Oncol,2011,30(6):644-646.

[19]SIEGEL R L,MILLER K D,JEMAL A. Cancer statistics[J]. CA Cancer J Clin,2018,68(1):7-30.

[20]THE CANCER GENOME ATLAS NETWORK. Comprehensive molecular characterization of human colon and rectal cancer[J]. Nature,2012,487(7407):330-337.

[21]WATSON P A,ARORA V K,SAWYERS C L. Emerging mechanisms of resistance to androgen receptor inhibitors in prostate cancer[J]. Nat Rev Cancer,2015,15(12):701.

[22] WAXMAN I,SAITOH Y,RAJU G S,et al. High-frequency probe EUS-assisted endoscopic mucosal re-section:a therapeutic strategy for submucosal tumors of the GI tract[J]. Gastrointest Endosc,2002 (1):44-49.

[23] YU H,BURKE C T. Comparison of percutaneous ablation technologies in the treatment of malignant liver tumors[J]. Semin Intervent Radiol,2014,31(2):129-137.